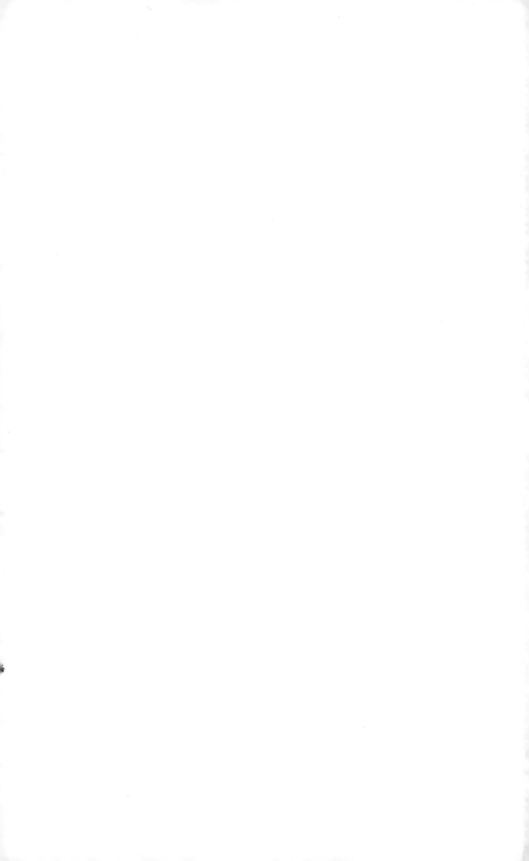

Modern Prometheus

Editing the Human Genome with Crispr-Cas9

Would you change your genes if you could? As we confront the 'industrial revolution of the genome', the recent discoveries of Crispr-Cas9 technologies are offering, for the first time, cheap and effective methods for editing the human genome. This opens up startling new opportunities as well as significant ethical uncertainty. Tracing events across a 50-year period, from the first gene splicing techniques to the present day, this is the story of gene editing: the science, the impact, and the potential. Kozubek weaves together the fascinating stories of many of the scientists involved in the development of gene editing technology. Along the way, he demystifies how the technology really works and provides vivid and thought-provoking reflections on the continuing ethical debate. Ultimately, Kozubek places the debate in its historical and scientific context to consider both what drives scientific discovery and the implications of the "commodification" of life.

JIM KOZUBEK is a computational biologist living in Cambridge, Massachusetts. His science writing has appeared in *The New Hampshire Union Leader*, *The Providence Journal*, *The Boston Globe*, *The Atlantic*, and *Scientific American*.

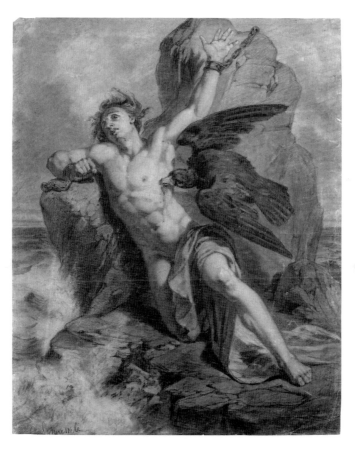

"Prometheus Bound." Christian Schussele, unknown date.

Great gifts to mortal men, am prisoner made
In these fast fetters; yea, in fennel stalk
I snatched the hidden spring of stolen fire,
Which is to men a teacher of all arts,
Their chief resource. And now this penalty
Of that offence I pay, fast riveted
In chains beneath the open firmament.
  Aeschylus (525–456BC), *Prometheus Bound*

Modern Prometheus

Editing the Human Genome with Crispr-Cas9

JIM KOZUBEK

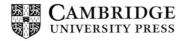

CAMBRIDGE
UNIVERSITY PRESS

CAMBRIDGE
UNIVERSITY PRESS

University Printing House, Cambridge CB2 8BS, United Kingdom

Cambridge University Press is part of the University of Cambridge.

It furthers the University's mission by disseminating knowledge in the pursuit of education, learning and research at the highest international levels of excellence.

www.cambridge.org
Information on this title: www.cambridge.org/9781107172166

© Jim Kozubek 2016

First published 2016

Printed in the United States of America by Sheridan Books, Inc.

A catalogue record for this publication is available from the British Library

Library of Congress Cataloging-in-Publication Data
Names: Kozubek, Jim.
Title: Modern Prometheus : editing the human genome with Crispr-Cas9 / Jim Kozubek, Brigham and Women's Hospital, staff scientist, Department of Neurology Broad Institute of MIT and Harvard.
Description: New York : Cambridge University Press, 2016. | Includes bibliographical references and index.
Identifiers: LCCN 2016034385 | ISBN 9781107172166 (hardback : alk. paper)
Subjects: LCSH: Gene targeting. | Genomes.
Classification: LCC QH442.3 .K69 2016 | DDC 572.8/77–dc23 LC record available at https://lccn.loc.gov/2016034385

ISBN 978-1-107-17216-6 Hardback

Sections of this book previously appeared in *The Atlantic*, *The Boston Globe* and *Scientific American*.

Between 14 October 2013 and 6 May 2016, Jim Kozubek worked as a staff scientist at the Brigham and Women's Hospital which is affiliated to the Broad Institute of MIT and Harvard. Although the Broad Institute is in Crispr genome editing research, development, and sharing, this book was developed independently of the author's Broad affiliation.

Contents

Acknowledgements

Thanks to my editor Katrina Halliday and her colleagues at Cambridge University Press, especially Jo Tyszka, Sarah Payne, and Leigh Mueller, for seeing the value in the story and bringing my manuscript into reality. The project had been in the works more than three years by the time I finally signed it over to the world's oldest publishing house. I first approached Emma Parry to advise my book project in January 2013 just as the Crispr-Cas9 genome editing system was beginning to surface in major science journals. I was aware of the Promethean myth, and it occurred to me that elements of the myth were congruent with the story as it was unfolding. DNA represents a natural power or force that could be expropriated by man, and this expropriation is neither right nor wrong, but comes with a steep learning curve. I was also aware of what Mary Shelley had been doing with her exegesis of the myth in her stunning novel Frankenstein, or The Modern Prometheus. As with most of the Romantic writers, Shelley's writing was primarily concerned with the march of industry and technology, and how the allure of its progress risked a marginalization of the tensions of inner life, existential problems, aptitude for coping with life, its slings and arrows, the kind of hard-won struggle that shapes a soul. Shelley began her novel in a form of epistolary, in other words, delivered as a series of letters. I initially started to build my book based on various scenes of the myth, where I connected scientific research tightly to stages of the myth. I even did try to begin it in a form of epistolary. It was Emma who pointed out that this setup for the book felt like a trap. I was boxing myself in. None of this worked, of course, and I think this is because so much of scientific progress is a gradual grind, based on small technical advances that accrue and build upon each other in stepwise fashion. Rarely do events occur in science that are entirely non-linear, and change the paradigm. Even the application of Crispr-Cas9 depends on a deep edifice of knowledge and applications, for instance, the ability to culture cells, to use viruses and other tools to get the system into cells, and decades of investigation on how genes work. All of these realities came crashing to the surface as I struggled to put the book together. It soon became clear that the only responsible thing was to ditch my artistic impulse to shape the book on the stages of the myth, and to build it upon the more realistic and necessarily chronological events of science. That's when I decided to wrap up a complicated tale spanning more than 50 years into a chronology, and to introduce Crispr-Cas9 right up front in the book. I also made the decision to put myself in the book, as a thread of continuity that tied it up like a string. With these structural adjustments in place, and a deep dive into archive research at MIT, things began to come together. Tim Horvath, Ogi Ogas, Emily Loose, Jennifer Golliday, Lena Yarbrough, Chad Luibl, Erika Goldman, Michael Kozubek, Marcia Kozubek and Melanie Dickerson read excerpts along the way. Many scientists provided feedback on my manuscript, especially David Levine, Erik Sontheimer, George Church, Keith Joung, Janet Mertz, Richard Mulligan, David A. Williams and Emmanuelle Charpentier.

Author's Note

This is a book about Crispr-Cas9. It is animated by many forces. I grew up reading popular science books that could be described as instructive or didactic, but I saw the trade begin to gradually drift into simplistic story-telling which was sold as self-help. To break from this trend, I set out to write in a different style, which is the tragic vein of literature. To this end, the book is injurious throughout, while taking few moral positions. It is not designed to attack or damage anyone, per se, but to describe a more realistic, harder and more complicated situation which we endure. One motivation is my interest in the rise of business elements in science; for example, the Broad Institute draws deeply on public funding, but provides an executive pay structure. In the past few decades, there has been a rise of business elements in science. The federal funding engine is decades old, and biotech-academic partnerships have exploited that to a large degree. Given how robust the biotech industry is, and how competitive academia has become over intellectual property—with substantial partnerships between industry and academia, and elite academic salaries that can exceed $1 million, and which are designed to achieve leverage in an increasingly brutal and competitive climate, I wonder if scientific institutions are maturing to a degree that they may at some point forgo federal funding. If we continue to see scientists in battles for large windfalls and rewards, I think that more taxpayers will just say, OK, then fund and take the risks yourself. Scientists should be allowed to fail, and to be free of public support, if they use the legal system to attract, protect and defend their increasing status and wealth. If anything, science may not be capitalistic *enough*. I am also interested in how scientists develop powerful marketing arms and salesmanship, while most scientists admit that their powers are truly limited, and that the genetic drivers of cancer, autism and schizophrenia will always be with us. The world as Darwin saw it was radically decentralized, deeply unsettling, and a threat to social order. By comparison, the modern scientist has become the social order, seemingly in control of nature through clandestine knowledge and access to the gene, which only a few are said to have the ability to properly interpret. My preferred method for reporting this book is first-person narration, and I made every effort to meet its characters in person. For more than four years, I traveled to Pennsylvania, Illinois, and Washington, buried myself in the archive collection at MIT, and ran up long email correspondence. Jennifer Doudna was also writing a book on Crispr at the time, and I took care to avoid cross-pollination of ideas with her. Thus, she has a minimal presence in the story. My writing also draws on newspaper articles, journal articles, and personal conversations, and references to novels and film. It is written very much how my life is actually like, and evidences my tendency to find truth in a novel or reflection, as much as, or more so than, in primary literature. Indeed, this book arises out of my own conflict over whether to invest more energies into science or the arts and literature, and an interest in which modalities best illuminate reality. In reporting this book, I found the only thing more competitive than Crispr science, was writing about Crispr. I had titled a chapter "Gene Hackers" and written an op-ed for *The Boston Globe* titled "Would You Change Your Genes If You Could?" in 2013, a full two years before *The New Yorker* ran its story "The Gene Hackers" and splashed "Should We Edit Our Genes?" on its cover. Eric Lander wrote a perspectives piece titled "The Heroes of Crispr" after I circulated a draft manuscript of *Modern Prometheus*. Heroism, at least as I use it in my own text, does not emphasize scientific valor as a series of achievements by right-minded people. Rather, to be a hero means to be immersed in a life-world, or lebenswelt, as the philosophers call it, to navigate complicated social, cultural and biological strata where there are no fundamentally right actions. Whereas we once had the archetype of the "Greek hero," who confronted binary decisions of whether to adhere or break with authority, the "Western hero" evolved into a pragmatic model. He knows his own moral character is not higher than his peers, but that does not stop him from enforcing justice or an ethic through a policy of pragmatism. In effect, to be a hero means to pursue one course of action, at the expense of another course. Every "scientific hero" knows he was just following one of many hypotheses and lines of thought. And, just like the valiant hero who steps into traffic to save a child, he denies it was a special act, because he is not entirely confident that he would have done it again. A genuine hero knows full well he could have easily acted otherwise.

1 Crispr, Cas and Capitalists

Genuine tragedies in the world are not conflicts between right and wrong. They are conflicts between two rights.

–Georg Wilhelm Friedrich Hegel

Derrick Rossi is a stem cell biologist at Harvard Medical School. He studies DNA repair mechanisms, the means which cells have to fix themselves when things break down. In the winter of 2013, I worked in his lab on the ground floor in the white marble quadrangle, where I used a computer at a lab space next to a Spanish woman named Paula and a couple of metal chairs with "Rajewsky" written on the back in marker. Rossi has stylish jet black hair, wears a Dr. Seuss watch and sometimes, ironic eye glasses with chunky black frames. His ancestors originated from the tiny island of Malta, near Sicily and off the coast of northern Africa; but he completed his PhD in Helsinki, Finland, and married a Finnish woman who was a former scientist at Genentech, making them a sort of scientific power couple. By now, he and his wife had three smallish children with straight hair who looked like they could appear in an LL Bean catalog, and who scrawled upon the four walls of white board, turning his office into a pop-up art exhibition.

Rossi pointed me to one sharp watercolor which his daughter had painted with shafts of skylight in silvers and blues, a few black snakes slinking along a path. "I had a dream in which my youngest daughter was bitten by a black mamba, and I don't know if you know anything about that, but one bite is lethal. It was frightening, of course, but what was odd was that the snake that bit her was wearing a grey woolen sweater. I recounted the dream to my family over breakfast that morning and a few days later my middle daughter had painted her interpretation of this dream of mine in watercolor – complete with snake sweater."

Ross and his family take adventurous summer trips to Finland, but this year he missed it, too busy with work. But the imagery of his family moved into his office, and at least a little bit of his office into his house. I returned to his office a number of times over the years, and each time I came back there were expanding exhibits of art, so much so, that it began to be almost comical. In his office, the collection of paintings from his children grew. On large cardboard panels. On acid-free paper stuck to the walls with scotch tape. Comingled with his children's drawings were Rossi's own science scribblings. His drawings appeared as schematics of cell lineages or a logical flow of ideas, ordered and analytical. The realm of art deals with deficit and negative space, and a soul that is churning and evolving. It deals with duty and virtue, and questions of option and purpose. The realm of science deals with cause and effect, and predictable outcomes, and focuses on maximizing those outcomes, while the motives are largely assumed. This tension between these realms continued, as Rossi drew experiments, and his children piled back into his office and overwrote his boards with their probing art. The cycle continued, upon any free space, at all, in his office. Rossi drew pathway to deriving a specific blood cell type on the white boards. His children erased that and drew a forest path. The tension replayed, again and again, over what the physician-writer Gerald Weissmann has called the "two cultures" of arts and sciences. That one of these two cultures is more *real* than the other is a question that has a hold on us.

Not that long ago, it became popular for people to send some biological samples away to learn something about ourselves. As the Nobel laureate Jim Watson noted, regarding the push to sequence the human genome, "How could we not do it? We used to think our fate was in our stars. Now we know, in large measure, our fate is in our genes." We want to know if we have Neanderthal genes, which recently have been linked to small tendencies for depression, or genetic variants in there that suggest we are more intelligent or prone to schizophrenia – there are also studies that do this – or that we may have Viking genes. This is the popular idea of genetics which has been sold to the public. In reality, a single gene often has three or four functions. And, a single genetic variant in one of those genes can be pleiotropic, meaning that it causes unrelated effects in different cells, tissues or systems, or that its effects can be enhancing or diminishing, based on genetic background. To complicate things more, most of the genetic variants that explain a complex disease or trait, such as a cancer, height or intelligence, are weak signal variants, meaning they alone are poor predictors of a trait and only exert their effects in the company of other genetic variants, so a lot of the force of a single genetic variant depends on its background. Complex traits are broadly heritable through genetics, but it's improbable that we will ever be able to affect traits through scrupulous genetic editing. The temptation to particularize our character in our genes enormous. We love to put things in boxes. My own father sent away a cheek swab to Family Tree DNA, and learned his Y chromosome, which I also carry, puts us in the haplogroup R-M512 and explains the route some of our ancestors took traipsing through Eastern Europe winding up in the Tatra Mountains in Poland, which we visited. The test reported that I was Austrian, German and mostly Polish, which I knew, but also that there were markers for Ashkenazi descent, which I jumped all over since I tend to think of Ashkenazi people like Noam Chomsky and Albert Einstein as particularly smart. I can still feel the incredulity in my father's email to me after I reported this in an article in *The Atlantic*. ("For your information, we are not Jewish! That is based on hundreds of years of documentation and family history.")

It's not even a safe bet to define our life's trajectory based on immediate family members. My grandfather never graduated past the 6th grade. Surviving the hardscrabble Depression, he was a member of the Army Corp of Engineers, a heavy drinker and amateur boxer who began to lose his memory, probably due to too many punches, a condition called *dementia pugilistica*. My father graduated from Massachusetts Institute of Technology, became a lawyer who helps adjudicated youth and wins contests with his haiku. If I learned anything from this, it is how taxing the 1930s must have been for the immigrant class. One of my instincts is that in our age of neurobiology we rely too much on measured intelligence to decide what our lives should look like and the scope of our horizon. Whenever I talk about intelligence, I am trying to be conscious of what I really mean, which is that I seek to exclude myself as an exception from the drama of life, seeking immunity from social rifts and asylum from nature. In fact, the idea that the street credit of a few outstanding individuals can represent the character of an entire group or that the typecast of a group can define an individual, "Jewish exceptionalism" or "American exceptionalism," is rightly called the exception fallacy. The idea of Jewish identity, or Black identity, for that matter, exists to some extent in our genes and biology, to some extent in our culture and religion, to some extent in our interpretation of our own experience. We all know that identity *emerges* through navigation of layers of substance in these three spheres, the most hardwired of which is our genes. But our genomes are like snowflakes, no two are exactly alike, and which genetic variants – say, a smattering of those on the Y chromosome, or those on 6 chromosome – count as a license to a group, means that ethnicity can often be classified in more than one way. These categories may become all the more flexible, if we were to start slipping snippets of genetic code into our cells, customizing our genomes at will. And this exposes the unsettling existential reality that we are not part and parcel to the categories which are fundamental to existence, but that nature itself changes – we are each just individuals living dangerous lives. The sphere of culture, by comparison, is even more flexible. "Culture" is a crutch, a means to cohesion – science has culture, this book is a piece of culture – and, importantly, entrance into a piece of culture, implies exclusion. It's therefore not surprising that when some people hear the word culture, they reach for their gun.

One of the ideas that animates this book is that science is not higher in its truths, but rather, science is a component of our broader phenomenology. How we assess and use science is deeply subjective, and often dogmatic. Most US taxpayers probably have little appreciation that much of the science they are funding is of dubious value, due to the "replication crisis" which primarily emerges due to scientific studies that reach conclusions based on incomplete information. In 2012, researchers at Amgen reported they could only reproduce results of 6 of the 53 hematology and oncology studies they attempted to replicate.[1] Around the same time, researchers at Bayer uncovered a similar problem in trying to validate published papers to pursue new drug targets, reporting they could not replicate more than 75 percent of the 67 published studies they examined.[2] A study will typically focus on the effect of a genetic variant taken out of context of its genetic background and other types of biological contributions and environmental stressors, which either counter or enhance its effect. Scientists themselves are quite aware that they are probably submitting false positives to the literature. In the words of Paul Thompson and colleagues, "subtle phenomena such as the 'winner's curse' are well known in quantitative genetics, where the effect size of a finding is often not as strong in a replication sample as it is in the initial discovery sample."[3]

Daniel MacArthur and colleagues at Harvard suggested guidelines on reducing false positives in the literature, although those guidelines are merely suggestive, certainly not enforceable.[4,5] To illustrate one of their points, they described a study on autism in which researchers found four *de novo*, or new, mutations in the gene *TNN*. But, it turns out the *TNN* gene is the largest coding gene in the human genome, and just by chance, we might expect to find two mutations. Finding four, then, is not so surprising. The researchers in that study dropped that gene as an autism candidate. But these are only best practices. Within statistics sleeps a demon. Genetic and RNA expression data is expensive – often running into the tens or hundreds of thousands of dollars to generate – and researchers who acquire data *always* find something. In truth, every data set usually includes eight to ten plausible stories for publication, and scientists will typically choose one or two of those stories and ignore the rest. And they often make their picks based on their ability to narrate rather than the strength of the statistics. The temptation to spin a good tale is enormous. Goldstein anticipated the sheer wealth of candidate mutations in the human genome and the allure to tell their story on the impact to traits as the "narrative potential of human genomes."[6]

The emergence of one compelling story often ignores competing interpretations, or downplays the reality that a finding is context dependent. The replication crisis in social sciences is even more severe and controversial.[7,8,9] But, while the data-driven culture of science involves evaluation of cause and effect and results-based assessments, it excludes deontic or virtue ethics, characteristics we pursue for the sake of duty or honor or beauty. But I am not the first person to feel that science and technology has the potential to erode our capacity for introspection, and weaken our sense of reality. At the turn of the century, William James complained that "scientific absolutists pretend to regulate our lives," and explained in his dissenting opinion that "science has organized this nervousness into a *regular* technique, her so-called method of verification; and she has fallen so deeply in love with this method that one may even say she has ceased to care for truth by itself at all. It is only truth as technically verified that interests her. The truth of truths might come in merely affirmative form, and she would decline to touch it."[10]

Institutions, these days, strive to avoid the "merely affirmative," and strive to be data driven in their decisions under the guise that they're being scientific, and thus more authentic. The repression of emotional content which they try out in their writing, is nudging forth today, as the subconscious is not only thought of as primitive, but tainted. At my workplace, talks are given on "unconscious bias," suggestive that intuitive pull not only has little value but jeopardizes our lives and demoralizes our heads. The subconscious is said to lead us astray through preference and bias, but seldom is discussed how it protects and signals against dangers and the wrong choices. But we seek to eliminate it. We evaluate decisions in terms of data science and we extol those who are data-driven. The Yale psychologist Paul Bloom has called empathy a "parochial emotion" and the organizational guru Adam Grant has suggested we find ways to remove "soft" intuition-based influence over our decisions, telling *The Washington Post* "I think we are leaving the age of experience and moving into the age of evidence," he says. "One of my big goals professionally is to get more leaders to stop acting on intuition and experience –and instead be data-driven."[11,12] The allure is obvious: we simultaneously remove our bias and let the data decide for us, removing any tension over how to make a decision on who to hire, or fund, or to bring into our lives, a problem I have written about before.[13]

Erroneously, the "modern impulse," which seeks to particularize and monetize, based on data-driven decision science, is often placed in dichotomy with the "romantic impulse," which values soft intuition and experience, although intuition and experience play a large role in science itself. A dream of a snake is not something to ignore. The German chemist August Kekulé solved the structure of Benzene after dreaming of a coiled black snake with its tail in its mouth. The neuroscientist Eric Kandel, among others, has called this "night science," a visitation that seems to be a strange remnant from the Romantic Period; as Edgar Allen Poe once professed, "they who dream by day are cognizant of many things which escape those who dream only by night."

The way I read it, the irrational or "romantic impulse," does not refer to unconfirmed beliefs, but finds its more authentic definition in its premise that nature is agnostic to its classification, and that it's ultimately accidental at its core – there is no logic at the basis of reality. "Darwin displaced humanity from the pinnacle of the organic world," Nathaniel Comfort, a historian of science at John Hopkins, astutely wrote recently in *The Atlantic*, while "Cheerleaders for Crispr" and their gene-centric history suggest "when we control the gene, its champions promise, we will be the masters of our own destiny."[14] The "subtler gene," as Comfort calls the "rise of genomics," disabuses us of the inclination that we can use Crispr to treat modern maladies such as schizophrenia or autism, and control fate and time. Indeed, such a naïve view on the insistence on genetic science as a wellspring of meaning and an illuminated reality is at odds with the existentialists' observation that personality often finds itself foreign – this foreignness is deeply problematic for science. We think if we only had better data, we'd have complete control. Comfort notes the seductive illusion that we might control our genes with "Crispr, the new, revolutionarily simple method of editing genes, foretells designer babies, the end of disease, and perhaps even the transformation of humanity into a new and better species."

Science emerges, as Noam Chomsky noted, through our "science forming faculties," as phenomenologists called it "bracketing," setting aside questions of real existence to focus on the analysis of the phenomenon of experience, but the brackets are exposed to us through encounters with nature, and through the other, and the alterity of "otherness," elucidated by such writers as Kafka and Kundera, and by Ralph Waldo Emerson, who wrote, "Other men are lenses through which we read our own minds." That nature is not cohesive, and that it's agnostic to its classification, and that it's ultimately accidental, implies that the irrational is unlikely to be eliminated by scientific inquiry, and the danger in repressing the act of framing or bracketing – a tendency that philosophers call "eliminativism" – almost certainly obscures our sense of reality.

The modern science view is that intelligence and personality dynamics are particularized in our genes. We can test it and what we see is what we get. The folk science view is that our character is built as experience seeps into our being. "It takes a while for our experiences to sift through our consciousness," the writer Nathalie Goldberg once observed. "Our senses are themselves dumb. They take in experience, but they need the richness of sifting for a while through our consciousness and through our whole bodies. I call this 'composting.' Our bodies are garbage heaps: we collect experience, and from the decomposition of the thrown-out eggshells, spinach leaves, coffee grinds, and old steak bones of our minds come nitrogen, head, and very fertile soil. Out of this fertile soil bloom our poems and stories. But this does not come at once. It takes time. Continue to turn over and over the organic details of our life until some of them fall through the garbage of discursive thoughts to the solid ground of black soil."[15] Watson is right, but he is only partly right – our fate is in our genes, but at least as much of the human condition we enter into is a blooming, buzzing confusion.

Genetics contains pieces of who we are. It had only begun to percolate. Who was I? Was my identity to be found in science or was it to be found in the space of literature? I had been a journalist for a number of years, when entering the grips of a quarter-life crisis, I went back to school to study genetics – "Be a mensch" my father said. "I think it's funny that you should say that," I said, since that word sounds Yiddish to me. After graduation I was camping on the shore of New Hampshire for six months, which incidentally, was just at the beginning of the "Occupy" movement. I finally got a job. One of the first people I met in the world of working scientists was Derrick Rossi.

Rossi was still a young scientist at age 45 when he landed on *Time Magazine*'s list of 100 Most Influential People in 2011, after just months before demonstrating how to reprogram adult cells into stem cells. That same year, a good year for him, he launched a company, Moderna Therapeutics, which quickly drew more than a billion dollars in investment. Rossi developed the company's core technology, which involves introducing customized RNA molecules into cells to effect a therapeutic outcome. This counts as a "biologic," a means to use biological spare parts to alter or repair a cell signal. Consider that a gene is built from a sticky macromolecule of sugary bases, or nucleotides, which are adenine, guanine, cytosine and thymine, and are themselves composed of carbon, hydrogen, nitrogen and phosphoric acid, which assemble into rings to make those four nucleotides. This is deoxyribonucleic acid, or DNA, and it is in turn copied into ribonucleic acid or RNA. In fact, the "central dogma" in biology is that DNA is transcribed into RNA, which is translated into protein, and modern drugs, for the most part, target the proteins in our cells, that molecular menagerie of enzymes, antibodies, receptors and cell signaling molecules. What Rossi was doing was to move the drug industry a step deeper to the level of the RNA. In effect, by inserting his own engineered RNA molecule he could instruct the cell to produce any type of protein he wanted from scratch. I wrote to him asking for work. Rossi said Moderna didn't hire many computational people, but he could use help on a separate project in his lab at Harvard to characterize the nature of mutations in stem cells, which concerns his other interest, how cells break down and the machinery that repairs them. That's how I got to work at a bench next to Paula.

I work on the computer. Paula sacrifices mice, which Rossi constantly refers to as "sacking mice" as if we are taking a castle. After Paula sacks the mice and harvests a cluster of stem cells, we dose the cells with a treatment to induce mutations, or DNA damage, and Rossi wants me to look at the data and tell him which genes have the mutations, and whether general purpose stem cells are more or less prone to mutations than differentiated adult cells, which build our blood, bones and immune system. "That's a question I've wanted to know the answer to for a long time," he tells me, later acknowledging that it was one of many questions his lab has posed since its inception. The established dogma in the field is that stem cells are more protected, or "uniquely cytoprotected,"[16] against mutations, and Rossi wants to test his theory that the opposite may be true, that stem cells may be *more* at risk to accruing mutations than differentiated adult cells. This all plays into an emerging concept that mutations arising in stem cells give rise to many different types of cancer.

To me, it looks like the "control" cells are littered with mutations. That might be expected because "we dosed the (expletive) out of those cells," Rossi tells me. But, after a few months, it turns out our data was not sequenced adequately at the core lab, which provides a service for next-generation sequencing, and is not of high enough quality to draw any conclusions from our experiments. The core lab at Tufts says they will do it again, for free. We're going to have to start over from scratch, and I can tell that Rossi is annoyed and sometimes he walks by without saying anything. "That's just how he is," Paula says. "He's thinking in his head, 'I've got to get things done, I've got to get things done.'" What was going on in his head was more complicated than I knew. That month, a couple of papers had appeared in the journal *Science* on Crispr-Cas9, a powerful new tool which worked like tiny molecular scissors, and could be programmed to edit a specific genetic sequence in a human cell. This system was discovered as an immune system that a microbe has to fight against phages, which are viruses that can invade a microbe.[17] It was only later repurposed as a technology. In fact, 50 years ago microbiologists first discovered that microbes have *innate* immune systems to fight viruses by using "restriction enzymes," proteins which can chop up phage genomes at specific short sequences, thereby restricting their growth. Scientists then repurposed these enzymes to cut and paste DNA, in effect, giving rise to the biotech industry.[18] A decade ago microbiologists discovered that bacteria also have *adaptive* immune systems, meaning they are equipped with a kind of programmable system that will allow them to acquire intelligence on a phage by capturing a bit of code from it. Once the microbe has a record of the phage on file, it can hack to pieces any invading virus that matches the description. This was the Crispr system. A few small molecular tricks later, scientists had learned to reprogram it as a tool to make precise edits to the genes in human cells, rekindling a debate on what it meant to engineer mankind.

In fact, Crispr stands for "clustered regularly interspaced short palindromic repeat" and it is repetitive genetic code that has nested within it more code, called a "spacer," which records telltale signs of a past invading phage, keeping a record of the phage like a fingerprint or a mugshot. In effect, the spacer captures the code of an invading phage as a genetic download in the genome of the microbe. If a phage that matches the description enters the microbe in the future, an expressed molecule senses and detects the phage and guides a special enzyme called a Cas nuclease to chop up the virus like molecular scissors. In 1987, Japanese researchers first reported these strange repeat sequences in the common bacteria *Escherichia coli*, not knowing what to make of them.[19] But a molecular gumshoe was on the case. In 1989, Francisco Mojica began his doctoral studies at the University of Alicante just up the coast of the "Mediterranean port of Santa Pola on Spain's Costa Blanca, where the beautiful coast and vast salt marshes have for centuries attracted vacationers, flamingoes, and commercial salt producers."[20] Mojica joined a laboratory working on *Haloferax mediterranei*, a single-cell organism which is part of the archaea domain, a vast section of microbial life that includes no nucleus and is thus classified as a card-carrying member of the prokaryote domain, but unique enough in its biochemistry and genetic components to be distinguished from bacteria. Many archaea are "extremophiles," meaning they thrive in extreme niches and include such intriguing bugs as "psychrophiles," which inhabit extremely cold temperatures. In fact, *there are no superior genes*, only genes that provide advantages in specific niches at the expense of weaknesses in other niches. In fact, Mojica was studying a "halophile," which was known for its extreme salt tolerance and isolated from Santa Pola's marshes. He was toying with restriction enzymes to chop up the genetic code of this microbe. In such an experiment, he could delete or add bits of genetic code to a microbe and study the resulting effect on the cell to gain insight into the function of a given genetic element. But "in the first DNA fragment he examined, Mojica found a curious structure – multiple copies of a near-perfect, roughly palindromic, repeated sequence of 30 bases, separated by spacers of roughly 36 bases – that did not resemble any family of repeats known in microbes."[21,22]

Eric Lander is director of the Broad Institute, a non-profit research institute which partners with MIT and Harvard and its affiliated hospitals. He is also a MacArthur Fellow and was a leader in the Human Genome Project, the effort to sequence a consensus human genome. He wrote a sweeping and controversial essay covering decades of research on Crispr which was titled "The Heroes of Crispr," and received much of the territory. "The 28-year-old graduate student was captivated and devoted the next decade of his career to unraveling the mystery. He soon discovered similar repeats in the closely related *H.volcanii*, as well as in more distant halophilic archaea."[23] Mojica scanned the literature and saw a similar repeat sequence had been mentioned by the Japanese group in 1987 in a bacteria separated by a space of random genetic sequence, although the spelling of the sequence was different. "Mojica realized that the presence of such similar structures in such distant microbes must signal an important function in prokaryotes," and that these strange repeats were not an anomaly.[24] By 2000, Mojica had taken a faculty position at Alicante, but his interest persisted, and searching through databases, he had identified similar repeats in 20 different microbes.[25,26]

In 2002, the biologist Ruud Jansen published a paper showing that these repeats are usually neighbored by sets of genes that build "Cas" enzymes. He further showed that 40 to 50 percent of bacteria have Crispr-Cas systems, and 90 percent of archaea have Crispr-Cas systems.[27,28] Mojica had started putting the pieces together declaring Crispr was "not junk DNA." It was becoming increasingly clear this was a conserved and essential mechanism. In correspondence with Jansen, Mojica suggested the name "Crispr," which Jansen liked and adopted.[29]

"During the August holiday in 2003, Mojica escaped the scorching heat of Santa Pola's beaches and took refuge in his air-conditioned office in Alicante. By now the clear leader in the nascent Crispr field, he had turned his focus from the repeats themselves to the spacers that separated them. Using his word processor, Mojica painstakingly extracted each spacer and inserted it into the BLAST program to search for similarity with any other known DNA sequence. He had tried this exercise before without success, but the DNA sequence databases were continually expanding and this time he struck gold."[30]

Mojica had performed a sort of computer background check on Crispr repeats using a simple and widely used computer algorithm. It was only because he could not get funding to do his work that he opened up his laptop to try a test he could do for free. It was then that he found that sections of the "spacer" sequence in between two repetitive Crispr sequences matched the description of a phage named P1; in other words, bacteria were capturing a genetic record of an invading phage.[31] Mojica had stumbled upon a record-keeping system and he was the first to suggest that the microbes were actively learning about the phage that invaded them, trapping pieces of their code. "Mojica opened up the floodgates," genome engineer and Broad Institute scientist Feng Zhang told me. "And the reason he was doing it, was that he was having trouble getting funding to do his research." As Lander wrote, Mojica instantly recognized the importance of his finding, and "went out to celebrate with colleagues over cognac and returned the next morning to draft a paper."[32] But skepticism abounded. Few editors at the top journals believed his findings were important enough to publish. "So began an 18-month odyssey of frustration. Recognizing the importance of the discovery, Mojica sent the paper to *Nature*. In November 2003, the journal rejected the paper without seeking external review; inexplicably, the editor claimed the key idea was already known. In January 2004, the *Proceedings of the National Academy of Sciences* decided that the paper lacked sufficient "novelty and importance" to justify sending it out to review. *Molecular Microbiology* and *Nucleic Acid Research* rejected the paper in turn. By now desperate and afraid of being scooped, Mojica sent the paper to the *Journal of Molecular Evolution*. After 12 more months of review and revision, the paper reporting Crispr's likely function finally appeared."[33,34]

Mojica was right to be nervous about being scooped. Studies began to elucidate a system in bacteria that directs enzymes known as nucleases to clip nucleic acids. In 2005, a Russian émigré working in France, Alexander Bolotin, had been studying the microbe *Streptococcus thermophilus*, which had just had its genome sequenced, when he discovered a Crispr sequence which was neighbored by a gene that coded a large protein, Csn1, soon to be renamed Cas9, which he predicted could snip nucleotides such as RNA or DNA.[35] Separately, the human geneticist Gilles Vergnaud was working south of Paris with the French Ministry of Defense on using methods to trace pathogens, which he had been researching since intelligence reports in the late 1990s raised the prospect that Saddam Hussein had biological weapons. Vergnaud was focused on studying genetic repeats as a means to track pathogenic strains of bacteria responsible for anthrax and plague as it swept through a human population. In case a microbe was weaponized, it might allow forensic departments to trace its origin. Vergnaud and colleague Christine Pourcel found a Crispr repeat including a record of a phage permanently logged in the genome of *Yersinia pestis*, based on a study of 61 samples which had been archived since a plague outbreak in Vietnam in 1964–1966, suggesting the microbe had absorbed the code of the phage to represent a memory of "past genetic aggressions."[36,37] Phage code began to be discovered in the genome of microbes from all corners of the Earth. Jill Banfield, a microbiologist at UC Berkeley, discovered Crispr sequences in "microbes she collected from acidic, 110-degree water from the defunct Iron Mountain Mine in Shasta County, California."[38] Definitive evidence would soon show that Crispr-Cas systems were capturing phage code as a component of a primordial immune system.

Rodolphe Barrangou and Philippe Horvath, scientists with Wisconsin-based Danisco USA, along with assistance from Sylvain Moineau of Université Laval in Québec City, were trying to improve production at a yogurt plant. *Streptococcus thermophilus*, the same microbe that Bolotin had been studying, is a probiotic used in milk culture and is prone to becoming infected with phages that lower production rates. Rhodia Food in Dangé-Saint-Romain in western France, a company later acquired by Danisco USA (itself acquired by DuPont in 2011) had tapped Barrangou and Horvath to study how its cultures protect themselves from phage, which was of scientific interest and economic importance to the dairy fermentation process. If the agricultural scientists could improve the growth of such probiotics and protect those microbes from being attacked by phages, it would make dairy production more profitable. Horvath identified a connection between the incorporation of phage code into microbes' genomes, and a microbes' resistance to those phages. In, 2005, the three scientists reported "resistant strains had acquired phage-derived sequences," and the more phage incorporated "correlated with increased resistance."[39] They provided the first conclusive evidence that Crispr-Cas was an acquired immune system in action. The scientists also had studied the role of a string of "*cas* genes" and it appeared that the microbes required the *cas7* gene in order to gain resistance and download the phage code, but that the *cas9* gene was required to go on the attack and chop up an invading phage.[40,41]

Insights into the mechanisms of the system came fast and furiously. John van der Oost is a scientist at Wageningen University in the Netherlands who had been working on biofuels and studying extremophile microbes such as *Sulfolobus solfataricus*, which thrives in the hot springs of Yellowstone National Park. In 2005, Eugene Koonin, an expert in microbial evolution at the National Center for Biotechnology Information and the National Institutes of Health, introduced van der Oost to current writings on Crispr, shifting his attention to its emerging study. The two scientists and their lab mates began tinkering with the Crispr system, introducing each of its separate parts into an *E. coli* strain that lacked the system, in order to deduce the minimal requirements which would enable the system to function. By doing this, the scientists unraveled a complex of five Cas proteins, which were termed the "cascade," and which is, in more general terms, an "operon," a set of genes in a microbe which are all turned on at the same time and go to work together. The study had elucidated what would be termed a type I Crispr system, which required a cascade of *cas* genes and which was distinct from the type II system in which a single *cas9* gene does the work of the cascade, so easy to engineer it would soon be embraced by biotech as Crispr-Cas 9.

It appeared that two Crispr repeats were "spaced" apart, and code for a phage had integrated into the midst of those two Crispr elements. Neighboring this "Crispr loci" was a set of *cas* genes, which are enzymes or action molecules of the system.[42] In a paper with stunning explanatory force, van der Oost loaded code of four genes from a phage into a type I Crispr locus including a cascade of *cas* genes, and installed the construct into a microbe. The microbe then displayed resistance to a phage that was used to infect it.[43] Eric Lander commented "it was the first case of directly programming Crispr-based immunity – a flu shot for bacteria."[44]

But it was not yet clear whether the cutting action of Crispr systems targeted the DNA of an invading phage at its genetic level, or the RNA molecules produced by the phage genes. Mojica, and also Kira Makarova,[45] in the early days of its study predicted that Crispr would be the "RNAi of bacteria." As it turns out, RNA interference, or RNAi, was a very popular technology that provided the possibility of gene "knock-downs" by inserting custom double-stranded RNA molecules into a cell to stop a gene from being expressed into a product. The technology was based on insights into a natural molecular pathway. In 2006, its elucidation won Andrew Fire and Craig Mello the Nobel Prize. In fact, mammalian cells use this pathway to fine tune its own gene expression, by producing small species of RNA which clasp onto "messenger RNA" to form a double-stranded molecule which gets chewed up by enzymes. Indeed, it is probable that mammalian cells developed this system to attack invading viruses and then reengineered it to fine-tune its own gene expression. Fire and Mello figured out that they could introduce a custom double-stranded RNA into a cell and this would engage the pathway, and, in effect, reduce the expression of messenger RNA with a complementary sequence. Crispr was thought to work as a similar interference system in bacteria. But it turns out that the predominant mechanism Crispr is not an interference system that targets RNA. Instead, it goes right to the heart of the matter to target and cut DNA.

Luciano Marraffini and Erik Sontheimer at Northwestern University designed an elegant experiment using a "self-splicing intron" to show that Crispr systems targeted DNA, articulating the "considerable functional utility" of using Crispr as a technology for gene engineering. Let me back up a step! In 1977, Phil Sharp discovered introns as pieces of code which are clipped out of RNA, resulting in a processed molecule called a "messenger RNA." In fact, a single gene can generate dozens of these messenger RNA species; it's the reason we have about 20000 genes and 100000 proteins. Thomas Cech and Sidney Altman discovered that introns are catalytic or self-splicing, meaning they clip out of RNA on their own, and therefore constitute a class of molecules called "ribozymes" which can *do* things without the help of proteins. In fact, Jennifer Doudna, whose name would later become synonymous with Crispr-Cas9, completed her PhD in biochemistry at Harvard University while working on these self-splicing introns in the lab of future Nobel laureate Jack Szostak, before moving on to do her postdoctorate with Cech at the University of Colorado. Doudna then moved to Yale University, where she would work on solving the three-dimensional structure of self-splicing introns and also a species called the hammerhead ribozyme, which is in viruses that infect plants and gains its name from its resemblance to a hammerhead shark.[46] A decade after graduating Harvard, Doudna had an endowed chair at Yale University and was a Howard Hughes Medical Institute investigator, a force in the world of biochemistry long before Crispr was on the radar.

Marraffini and Sontheimer created an experiment in which they inserted one of these self-splicing introns directly into the midst of a DNA target sequence, such that it would clip itself out of the sequence once it turned into RNA. This snippet of intron was installed smack in the middle of a target sequence and would block Crispr-Cas from recognizing the target in the DNA code, but once it turned into RNA, the snippet would clip itself out, allowing two flanking arms of the target sequence to converge into a single recognizable target, so that Crispr-Cas could snip it. If Crispr-Cas targeted RNA, then it should have shredded it to pieces, but it did not do that. This experiment provided logic and a bit of evidence that the Crispr system targeted DNA. "At that time we didn't have the means to actually observe DNA cleavage," Sonthemier told me. "But we did make it *impossible* to explain our genetic observations by an RNA targeting mechanism." Marraffini and Sontheimer are therefore often credited as the first scientists to provide evidence that Crispr may be repurposed for genome editing.[47]

On September 23, 2008, the scientists used that idea to file the first of what would become a barrage of patents on Crispr-mediated DNA targeting and genome editing. But Sontheimer's patent was denied in 2010. "We didn't know enough in 2008–2010 about how the system worked to engineer it," Sontheimer told me at lunch in Cambridge one afternoon. In truth, Marraffini and Sontheimer were working with yet another "type III" Crispr system that could not be readily used as a tool for biotech. Marraffini told me by email that their seminal work did, however, initiate a landslide of new experiments. Our "findings that DNA, instead of RNA, was the molecule targeted by Crispr, represents a turning point in the field... it opened the possibility of unique applications derived from the RNA-programmed destruction of DNA molecules." More insights soon came rushing to the surface.

Sylvian Moineau had been working to decipher the mechanism of just how the Crispr system clips DNA, reconfirming earlier findings that the Cas9 nuclease is necessary to do it.[48] Importantly, he identified a single, precise break in the DNA which neighbored a three nucleotide code, NGG, whereby N can be any genetic letter, which was termed the *proto-spacer adjacent motif* (PAM) sequence.[49] It is sort of like a shoehorn where the Cas9 nuclease begins to clasp down to make a "blunt-end" cut, meaning the double-strand DNA is cleanly broken without leaving any overhangs. By 2010, the group had demonstrated that Crispr-Cas9

Cas9 creates double-stranded breaks at precise 20 letter sequences in DNA neighboring the PAM sequence. Jennifer Doudna and colleagues showed that the PAM sequence was required for cleavage of target double-stranded DNA.[50]

In 2011, a cast of characters including Sontheimer and Doudna were at an American Society for Microbiology meeting in San Juan, Puerto Rico. Doudna was accosted when "an intense, dark-haired French scientist asked her if she wouldn't mind stepping outside the conference hall for a chat."[51] Charpentier had been studying rare sequences which coded for RNA molecules. "I was obsessed with how bacteria cause disease and working with the right models," Charpentier told me, when we later sat down to talk. In 2006, Charpentier used bioinformatics tricks on her laptop to find novel RNA molecules in *Streptococcus pyogenes* and identified an RNA – now known as tracrRNA – located in the vicinity of the *csn1* gene in an operon or cluster of four *cas* genes. This tracrRNA molecule, as she called it, was forming a nice base-pairing with a gene encoding a microbial protein called CAMP factor, which in *pyogenes* has a role in lysing or destroying red blood cells in a host organism such as a sheep. If scientists could learn more about that, then they could tweak systems within the microbe and perhaps prevent it from destroying red blood cells in the host organism or causing other pathogenic effects. "We had demonstrated that the small RNA, this tracrRNA, targeted the virulent gene but we could not show that it was regulating its expression; it was just a nice interaction," Charpentier told me.[52] But Charpentier soon stumbled on another function of this obscure RNA she was studying. At the time, it was predicted that the protein, Cas9, which has gone by aliases including COG3513, Csx12, Cas5 and Csn1, was an RNA-guided nuclease, meaning that it latched onto RNA molecules that guided it to its destination like a GPS system. But no one knew how it mobilized and went into action. Since tracrRNA was encoded right upstream of the *csn1* gene, she asked if it might be required for the expression or activity of the Crispr-Cas system. Charpentier and colleague Jörg Vogel showed that after tracrRNA and Crispr RNA clasp together, this duplex is stabilized by the protein Cas9 (*csn1*). They then described co-evolution of tracrRNA, Crispr RNA and Cas9.[53]

"I had been studying tracrRNA and was interested in that, and they just happened to be encoded in the vicinity of these Crispr," Charpentier told me. "I think I was the first person to start putting things together" that tracrRNA and crRNA (once Crispr is expressed as RNA it is named crRNA) were two independent components of RNA that needed to clasp together and form a double-stranded RNA complex.[54] Only once this ladder formed, could the Cas9 nuclease latch onto that ladder, while an overhanging spacer sequence that extended from the repetitive Crispr sequence contained the complement code that would merge, through "Watson-Crick base-pairing," to a DNA target that was to be cut by Cas9 after it shoehorned down on PAM. The Crispr system that Charpentier was studying was much simpler than the type I Crispr system that van der Oost had described with its "cascade" of five Cas nucleases or the type III system Sontheimer was studying. As it would soon be shown, the Crispr system in S. pyogenes was a type II Crispr system and made use of a complex of tracrRNA and crRNA, and required only a single Cas9 nuclease rather than a cascade of multiple nucleases to target DNA and cleave it. In fact, it was so simple it might be repurposed as a tool.

Charpentier first demonstrated an interaction between tracrRNA and crRNA, suggesting it was a step that might be required in order for the Crispr system to work, and presented her findings at a large meeting of Crispr scientists in the Netherlands. At the time, Crispr was not yet a name that had entered the public vernacular and was unknown to most scientists. Except for Moineau, whom she met at a conference on phages a couple of years before, Charpentier did not know anyone else studying Crispr. She met Marraffini at the conference. The first experiments by her students showed that tracrRNA and Crispr RNA were processed together into mature forms. Further investigation showed that an "anti-repeat" sequence in tracrRNA allows it to base-pair, or clasp, together with each of the repeats in the Crispr RNA. (The interaction between these two molecules leads to the creation of a hairpin structure that was later presented and engineered into the "extended single guide RNA" that clasps to Cas9 and would soon become the paradigm biotech tool we today refer to as Crispr-Cas 9. When she reported how the mechanism worked in October 2010, scientists in the audience came up to her after her talk, shaking her hand. "To have everyone come up and congratulate you, people who did not know you, that does not happen often," Charpentier told me, remarking on how special that day was, for her. Her lab had been under intense pressure, and she had argued for pushing research in the direction of Crispr while others had claimed it was a dead-end. That day in the Netherlands, Charpentier was vindicated.

Now in San Juan, just months after the Netherlands conference, Charpentier hoped to convince Doudna, the head of a powerful lab at UC Berkeley who had contributed to clarifying the three-dimensional structure of molecules such as ribozymes, to help to deduce the molecular structure of Crispr-Cas. In the words of the journalist Jennifer Kahn, "Among scientists, Doudna is known for her painstaking attention to detail, which she often harnesses to solve problems that other researchers have dismissed as intractable. Charpentier, who is French but works in Sweden and Germany, is livelier and more excitable. But as the pair began discussing the details of the experiment, they quickly hit it off." Amy Maxmen explained what happened next in her article in the magazine *Wired*. "As they wandered through the alleyways of old San Juan, Charpentier explained that one of Crispr's associated proteins... appeared to be extraordinary. It seemed to search for specific DNA sequences in viruses and cut them apart like a microscopic multi-tool." Structural data emerged only later in 2014 to show that "when the Crispr-Cas9 complex arrives at its destination, Cas9 does something almost magical: it changes shape, grasping the DNA and slicing it with a precise molecular scalpel."[55,56,57,58]

In the summer of 2012, Charpentier and Doudna published findings in the now classic Jinek paper, while demonstrating tracrRNA, Crispr RNA and Cas9 were necessary and sufficient for cleavage of a corresponding DNA sequence. The necessary and sufficient components of the Cas9/crRNA/tracrRNA complex for programmable DNA cleavage of what became the widely applied "type II" Crispr systems was not definitive and fully elucidated until the publication of the now historic Jinek 2012 *Science* paper, a result of a collaboration between the Doudna and Charpentier labs, and included important intellectual contributions from colleagues Martin Jinek, a Czech scientist, and the scientist Krzysztof Chylinski from the Charpentier lab, who was able to communicate with Jinek, since, just by chance, they happened to speak the same dialect of Polish.

In parallel, Barrangou, Horvath, and the Lithuanian scientist Viginijus Siksnys, contributed to further elucidate the mechanisms of the system. Siksnys grew up in Soviet-era Lithuania and completed his doctorate at Moscow State University before returning to Vilnius University. His group found that they could transfer the Crispr system from *S. thermophilus* to an *E. coli* bacteria which lacked the system, and that the system would still work; in other words, it was portable.[59] Furthermore, he went on to show that Crispr and Cas9 nuclease, which made a double-stranded break, three nucleotides from the PAM sequence in the target DNA, were at least two components needed to make the system work. Siksnys was not yet convinced of the requirement for tracrRNA, writing in a paper that "the role of tracrRNA in DNA silencing ... remains to be established." Dramatically, he showed that the "spacer" sequence, which separated two Crispr repeats and which typically included a record of an invading phage to target, could be trimmed down to 20 bases and that it was "programmable" to virtually any target.[60] The essential components had been isolated and elements of the sequence could be reprogrammed to order. "This paper was the first to show that Cas9 could be manually reprogrammed – that is, Crispr spacers could be engineered against a Cas9 target chosen in advance," Sontheimer told me. In their definitive review article, Doudna and Charpentier wrote that by that time it was also learned that the Cas9 endonuclease uses two separate "domains," technically, HNH and RuvC-like domains, to cleave each arm of a genetic ladder to create a double-strand break, such that "Cas9 uses its HNH domain to cleave the DNA strand that is complementary to the 20-nucleotide sequence of the crRNA; the RuvC-like domain of Cas9 cleaves the DNA strand opposite the complementary strand."[61,62] Charpentier and Doudna had identified the minimal components of the Crispr-Cas9 system and shown how the parts came together to mobilize it in action in *S. pyogenes* and these essential findings, in effect, were reiterated by Siksnys' work in *S. thermophilus*.

"The field had reached a critical milestone: the necessary and sufficient components of the Crispr-Cas9 interference system – the Cas9 nuclease, crRNA, and tracrRNA – were now known. The system had been completely dissected based on elegant bioinformatics, genetics, and molecular biology. It was now time to turn to precise biochemical experiments to try to confirm and extend the results in a test tube," Lander wrote. Both groups clearly recognized the potential for biotechnology with Siksnys declaring that "these findings pave the way for engineering of universal programmable RNA-guided DNA endonucleases," and Charpentier and Doudna noting "the potential to exploit the system for RNA-programmable genome editing." Charpentier early on predicted the potential of the Crispr-Cas9 system for genome recombination and silencing in eukaryotes, and the treatment of human genetic disorders. She began by working on reducing the system to minimal components, first by looking for the smallest Cas9 proteins in nature and combining domains of that protein with sequences of RNAs. Martin Jinek, a Czech scientist collaborating with Doudna, was able to combine the Crispr (crRNA) and tracrRNA into a "single-guide RNA," or sgRNA, molecule with an extending 20-base spacer sequence that could be reprogrammed to target virtually any site in a genome, simplifying the system as a genome editing technology.[63] If there was an initial engineering feat which transformed Crispr into a "technology," it was the development of the guide RNA, which was published in the Jinek 2012 *Science* paper. The precise design of the guide RNA was later independently being tinkered and worked out in multiple labs. Combining the components of the Crispr system into a single guide RNA, as it became known, was a sensible step to streamline lab work, but it later turned out that longer forms of those guide RNA were more efficient in eukaryotic cells. In the words of Doudna and Charpentier, "Although the Crispr acronym has attracted media attention and is widely used in the scientific and popular literature, nearly all genome editing applications are based on the use of the protein Cas9 together with suitable sgRNAs... Crispr refers to the repetitive nature of the repeats in the Crispr arrays that encode crRNAs, and the term does not relate directly to genome engineering. Nonetheless we prefer to use 'Crispr-Cas9' in a way that is less restrictive than other nomenclatures that have been used in the field."[64]

Doudna's patents were filed under the regents of the University of California, the University of Vienna, and Emmanuelle Charpentier as a provisional application on May 25, 2012, shortly before the Jinek paper was published online in *Science* on June 28, 2012, describing the biochemistry and showing the guide RNA technology could be deployed to cut DNA in a test tube, suggesting it could be a genome editing tool (see Figure 1). In that moment, it was impossible to ignore that Crispr-Cas9 was a paradigm new technology. Amy Maxmen declared "it was elegant and cheap. A grad student could do it."[65,66]

In February 2011, Feng Zhang "heard a talk about Crispr from Michael Gilmore, a Harvard microbiologist, and was instantly captivated. He flew the next day to a scientific meeting in Miami, but remained holed up in his hotel room digesting the entire Crispr literature. When he returned, he set out to create a version of *S. thermophilus* Cas9 for use in human cells."[67] Zhang started reaching out to experts in the field for support and collaboration, including Luciano Marraffini,

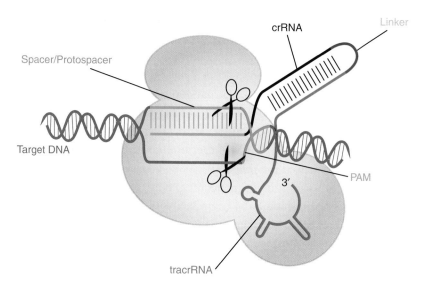

FIGURE I   The blue shape is the Cas9 enzyme, or endonuclease, that does the cutting.
In fact, there are no tiny scissors, but that's what the enzyme does. The tracrRNA and
crRNA are for technology purposes fused into a single gRNA, or "guide RNA." The
gRNA forms a hairpin which binds to Cas9. The spacer includes a 20-nucleotide
programmable sequence (originally a sequence of a phage, but which can be
programmed to be virtually any 20-base sequence) and guides the entire mechanism to
a matching site in the double-stranded DNA, by Watson–Crick base pairing, in our
genomes to make an edit. There is one caveat, and that is that the 20-base target
sequence must end with three more bases that are NGG (where N can be any base) and
this is the "PAM" sequence for the Cas9 from *Streptococcus pyogenes* (Cas9s from
other bacteria have different PAMs). In fact, Cas9 first binds to the PAM sequence and
then "finds" the 20-nucleotide match and cuts it. Imagine the possibilities. If you
make cuts at two sites, you can excise larger swatches of genomic sequence, or if you
also introduce a new gene along with the cut, often the cell's own DNA repair
mechanisms will patch up the break with any genetic material you give it.
(Reprint of Figure 5a from Jinek *et al.*, *Science* **337**:816 (2012) obtained with
permission from Science with issued License OP-00073788.)

who confirmed to me in an email that Zhang "was inspired and sought
my help to carry on these experiments." Over the next year, Zhang was
able to select various versions of tracrRNA and Cas9 endonucleases
from the microbes *S. pyogenes* and *S. thermophilus*, which worked the
best in mammalian cells, and improved upon their fusion into a single
guide RNA by restoring a small, but critical, bit of hairpin code in the
tracrRNA that enabled it to function much more efficiently. The hairpin
is a structure that looks exactly like it sounds, a small buckle in the

RNA that turned out to be important to retain in the fused RNA to enable the system to work in mammalian cells. Around the same time, Prashant Mali and Luhan Yang were postdoc students in George Church's lab and also set out to test crRNA-tracrRNA fusions in mammalian cells as a single guide RNA, unaware of Zhang's efforts to do so, and independently found that short fusions were inefficient in vivo (in a living cellular environment), but that the full-length fusions including the hairpin did work well."[68,69] In fact, Mali and Yang working out of the Church lab at Harvard were the first to show this small molecular tweak made the system high-functioning, doing it before Zhang did it. Restoring this hairpin to the single guide RNA was not necessary for successful gene editing in mammalian or, specifically, human cells. It did make the technique more efficient. Consider that DNA is read in a direction from 5' to 3' which refers to the orientation of the ring of five carbon elements in a nucleotide. By extending the sequence of the tracrRNA component of the "guide RNA" in the 3' direction, scientists had created a range of guide RNA molecules at various lengths, so called "extended guide RNA," some of which turned out to be more efficient. This was accomplished by a number of labs – for example, independently, by Keith Joung's lab – and was by no means a brilliant stroke of insight. "The Jinek 2012 *Science* paper had already demonstrated several months earlier that a guide RNA could successfully use tracrRNAs with a wide range of 3' tail lengths (including full length, which naturally includes the 'additional' hairpins), so using a single guide RNA with a tracrRNA that had a long 3' tail compared to a short 3' tail was not necessarily a 'critical feat'," Doudna wrote me in an email.[70] Zhang and Marraffini submitted a paper reporting mammalian genome editing and Mali, Yang and Church independently submitted a paper on genome editing in human cells, which simultaneously appeared in *Science* on January 3, 2013.[71] On January 29, 2013, Keith Joung, along with colleagues Joanna Veh and Randall Peterson, was the first to show the system could be used to modify a single cell embryo, putting the technology on stunning display in an act of genesis to create a new colony of zebrafish which was genetically engineered to his liking.[72] In the same journal and on the same day, Jin-Soo Kim in Seoul, South Korea reported that Crispr-Cas9 could edit the genomes of human cells.[73] On the same day Doudna published a paper describing Crispr cutting a single genomic site in human cells.[74] "Jennifer and I exchanged drafts, and I certainly felt very collaborative (not competitive, since she was doing biochemistry and I was focused on human genome HDR)," Church told me. All told, five major papers hit publication in January 2013. Two of them, from Zhang and Church, described "homologous directed repair," or HDR, which is a very precise repair, while the other three papers described "non-homologous end-joining," or NHEJ, which is a sort of makeshift fix that cobbles together a jury-rigged repair and often leaves behind a patchwork of small insertions and deletions, like an improvised patch.

In the words of Lander, "In early 2013, Google searches for "Crispr" began to skyrocket – a trend that has continued unabated. Within a year, investigators had reported the use of Crispr-based genome editing in many organisms – including yeast, nematode, fruit fly, zebrafish, mouse, and monkey. Scientific and commercial interest in potential applications in human therapeutics and commercial agriculture began to heat up – as did social concerns about the prospect that the technology could be used to produce designer babies."[75] Crispr-Cas9 was a general-purpose tool for editing genes in living human cells.

In January 2016, the journal *Cell* published Lander's essay "The Heroes of Crispr," which went to print just as a patent battle for the rights to certain Crispr applications was escalating between Doudna's camp at UC Berkeley and Zhang's camp at the Broad Institute. The moment was charged. Jennifer Kahn, a writer who teaches journalism at UC Berkeley, also wrote a profile on Doudna for *The New York Times Magazine* in which she failed to disclose her connections to the UC Berkeley journalism school (I have been employed by Harvard affiliated hospitals, and while writing this book held affiliation to the Broad Institute, meaning I used their office space and computing resources). By comparison, Lander's essay, while promoting Zhang, minimized the work of Doudna and Charpentier. Importantly, many said, the article failed to mention that his institution had a vested stake in the patent battle, as well as close ties to venture capitalists, who stood to gain a king's fortune from research that had primarily been paid for by taxpayers. The right to commercialize Crispr technology was a matter of intense dispute.

Since the 1970s, academic science has been in part driven by corporate elements and has increasingly found its purpose in finance. Lander, who advises President Barack Obama on science, also has started private companies such as Foundation Medicine for personal cancer genomics, and exemplifies the contradictions in advocating for public funding and crystallizing its insights in venture-backed, private entrepreneurship. The blowback against his article as a controlling narrative was harsh and swift. Doudna and Charpentier disputed the accuracy of Lander's *Cell* paper in *The Scientist*, Church logged a dispute, as did a strange mix of new bedfellows, a range of commenters, scientists from all corners of the Earth, sympathizers of the feminist cause, even one justified historian, Nathaniel Comfort.

"I never saw the entire (Lander) piece until publication, and have the email correspondence to prove it. Dr. Lander should name the other scientists he received input from," Doudna reprimanded in a comments section. In STAT News, Sharon Begley tried to explain Doudna's fury. "That is because Doudna is a cofounder of three Crispr companies and the coauthor of several patent applications and has already won a $3 million prize (the Breakthrough Prize) for her work. Meanwhile, Broad, along with MIT and Harvard, owns several patents as well as a multi-million stake in Editas Medicine, a company that is hoping to go public in a $100 million IPO (initial public offering). Lander also has deep financial and personal ties to Third Rock Ventures, one of the venture capital firms that started Editas."[76] Doudna and Charpentier were attracting a circle of supporters in the blogosphere, who noted Lander was writing outside his immediate field of expertise, something rare for a scientist to do, suggesting it was inspired as grist for a looming patent battle. "No conflict of interest declared? Broad can potentially gain billions from patent," wrote the Toronto biochemist Elton Zeqiraj. *The Scientist* weighed in on the controversy in an article suggesting that Zhang's patents were currently being "investigated by the US Patent and Trademark Office (USPTO). And Lander's *Cell* paper does not disclose the potential conflict of interest."[77] Michael Eisen, a UC Berkeley and Howard Hughes Medical Institute biologist "went ballistic" in a "tweet blast of righteous indignation."[78] Eisen noted "The whole thing is about trying to establish Zhang paper as pinnacle of Crispr work," continuing, "it's a deliberate effort to undermine Doudna and Charpentier patent claims and prizeworthiness."

The MIT computational biologist Manolis Kellis, who had been the target of a staccato of fire on Twitter and a blog from Lior Pachter at UC Berkeley a couple of years prior for some nebulous statistical dealings, told me the situation was overinflated. "Eric Lander wrote a perspectives piece for a journal. He was offering his perspective." In fact, Lander did disclose his institute's interest in the patent dispute on a conflict of interest form, but *Cell* didn't include it in print. Antonio Regalado, a journalist for MIT's own *Technology Review*, obtained the original forms. *Cell* released a statement confirming that Lander filed a conflict of interest form, but stating that it only actually prints personal conflicts of interest.

Regalado characterized the Lander essay as "a little Machiavellian" and expanded that "Lander's Crispr tale is clearly an attempt to back up Broad's patents, granted based on the surprise claim that Zhang hit on the technology in 2011 on his own, unbeknownst to anyone outside the institute, and before Doudna's work was ever published. Zhang's discoveries weren't published at the time and so they are not part of the official scientific record. But they're very important if Broad wants to hold onto its patents and score a victory" in patent proceedings. "No wonder, then, that Lander might like to see them described for the first time in an important journal such as *Cell*."[79] The deluge did not stop for days.

Comfort chastened Lander in a blog post for writing a "Whig history," a reference to a political party, which colloquially, has come to represent "a way to use history as a political tool" that "justifies the dominance of those in power." As Comfort describes the characterization: "The term comes from the Europeanist Herbert Butterfield. In a classic 1931 essay, Butterfield wrote that Whig history was "the tendency in many historians to write [English history] on the side of Protestants and Whigs, to praise revolutions provided they have been successful, to emphasize certain principles of progress in the past and to produce a story which is the ratification if not the glorification of the present. The term – now often lower-cased to distance itself from the particularities of British politics – has become historical shorthand for one way to use history as a political tool. It rationalizes the status quo, wins the allegiance of the establishment, justifies the dominance of those in power. One immediate tip-off to a Whiggish historical account is the use of melodramatic terms such as 'heroes' in the title..."

Comfort's position seems to stem from his distrust of scientific authority, and the appropriation of biology and genetics into the full authority of a few high-profile scientists who sense an almost exclusive right to describe its history and define its narrative. He explained "the whig interpretation of history," as the epitome of the ninteenth-century English gentleman: "Protestant, progressive, and whig," a tactic now and increasingly applied to science. In Butterfield's words, the Whig historian "very quickly busies himself with dividing the world into the friends and enemies of progress." The danger of Whig history is that it justifies the dominance of the ruling class as the outcome of inexorable natural forces. It is especially seductive when writing about science, for scientific knowledge does indeed progress."[80]

Comfort went after Lander in the blogs, and Siddhartha Mukherjee's book *The Gene: An Intimate History*, in *The Atlantic*, each of them, for promulgating a "Whig history of the gene," in effect, for transitioning evolution from a theory that was powerful, but inherently unsettling, destabilizing and democratic, into the hands of a small number of scientific whigs, who sought to use it to expropriate a narrative of nature, turning evolution into something a few authorities could comfortably describe and control. "(Charles) Darwin's great insight was that while species do change, they do not progress toward a predetermined goal: Organisms adapt to local conditions, using the tools available at the time. So too with science. What counts as an interesting or soluble scientific problem varies with time and place; today's truth is tomorrow's null hypothesis – and next year's error... If Copernicus displaced the Earth from the center of the universe and Darwin displaced humanity from the pinnacle of the organic world. A Whig history of the gene puts a kind of god back into our explanation of nature. It turns the gene into an eternal, essential thing awaiting elucidation by humans, instead of a living idea with ancestors, a development and maturation."

Mukherjee's explanation that early 20th century researchers dismissed DNA as "comically plain" or a "stupid molecule" are not correct, nor is it accurate to call it the "underdog of all molecules," which was right-sided by valiant researchers who appear on white horses and explain to the forerunning scientists what they were overlooking the entire time, Comfort explains: "Before Watson and Crick described the gene as a sequence of DNA, visualized as a succession of letters – like a line of computer code – terms such as *information* would have been nonsensical. Genes had been imagined as beads strung along the chromosomes. They didn't "encode" anything; they simply carried traits. The term *gene* wasn't coined until 1909. Before the turn of the 20th century, (the monk Gregor) Mendel's *elemente* were not thought of as physical things. They were mere abstractions."[81]

Comfort extends his critique on the history of the gene and its modern heroism to Lander and Crispr-Cas9 scientists, and wider public perceptions that we can edit and alter our genes to affect complex traits, and to control our fate and destiny. In fact, Mukherjee concedes that it is unlikely we will be developing a "forward catalog" of genetic variants which are either diagnostic or actionable for complex disorders such as schizophrenia or autism. Comfort emphasizes the complexity of the genome now puts the early explorers of the gene in the mid to late 20th century into a new perspective. "Ironically, the more we study the genome, the more 'the gene' recedes," he tells us. But indeed, there will be applications of genetic technology to control. And the quest to control the narrative of evolution through the elucidation of gene, and to control its function through Crispr-Cas9 has implications for cancer therapeutics and many diseases that emerge through single genes. And, that's something worth fighting for, and who exactly controls these powers depends in part on who controls the narrative. The Crispr squabble reached a head in Lander's article.

Comfort noted that a Nobel Prize and perhaps hundreds of millions of dollars in revenue are at stake through the patents. "Who claims them will be decided in part by what version of history becomes accepted as "the truth..." He goes on, "Good writers know how rhetoric can be used to persuade. Does Lander use writing techniques to advance a self-interested version of history? On first read, Lander's piece seems eminently fair, even generous. It "aims to fill in [the] backstory" of Crispr, Lander writes; "the history of ideas and the stories of pioneers – and draw lessons about the remarkable ecosystem underlying scientific discovery... By turning his lens on such unsung heroes, laboring away at universities well beyond the anointed labs of Harvard, MIT, UCSF, Johns Hopkins, and the like, Lander creates the impression of inclusiveness, of the sharing of credit among all the "heroes" of Crispr. But when he reaches Doudna and Charpentier's chapter in the story, the generosity becomes curiously muted. Though Lander maintains his warm, avuncular tone, Doudna and Charpentier enter the story as brave soldiers, working shoulder to shoulder with others... Charpentier reported in a note on Pubmed: "I regret that the description of my and collaborators' contributions is incomplete and inaccurate. The author did not ask me to check statements regarding me or my lab. I did not see any part of this paper prior to its submission by the author. And the journal did not involve me in the review process." Lander narrates Charpentier's story alongside that of the Lithuanian scientist Virginijus Siksnys. But Siksnys receives top billing... Now, enter Feng Zhang and George Church of the Broad Institute. They receive the longest treatment of any actor in the story – a solid page out of nine pages of text."

Comfort's deconstruction of the Lander essay would make Jacques Derrida shudder with unexpected relevance. He notes that the first reference to Jennifer Doudna in the essay "is buried in the middle of a paragraph, in the second half of a long sentence, the direct object rather than the subject of the sentence" and that her key accomplishments are couched as occurring "with assistance from Church" while submitting this and three other "short [ie., minor] papers."[82] But, Church also called out Lander in a comments section, attesting that his conversations with Doudna about his work in mammalian genome editing did not, in fact, provide Doudna with "significant assistance." In fact, Doudna and Charpentier had written a sweeping and authoritative review of the history of Crispr-Cas9 a year before in *Science* that covered much of the same ground (but with no mention of Zhang)[83] and in the same issue of *Cell* as Lander's article appeared Doudna dropped a technical review paper demonstrating impressive mastery over Crispr systems.[84]

By now, the feminist impulse was roiling. "How One Man Tried to Write Women Out of Crispr, the Biggest Biotech Innovation in Decades," excoriated Joanna Rothkopf in a January 20, 2016 blog post to Jezebel, suggesting that women scientists were being turned into handmaidens. "It rationalizes the status quo, wins the allegiance of the establishment, justifies the dominance of those in power... The crediting issue evokes that of Rosalind Franklin, the chemist and x-ray crystallographer whose work was largely excluded, despite her crucial findings, from the story of the discovery of the structure of DNA at the hands of her colleagues... Watson and Crick won the Nobel Prize, and remain the names universally associated with the double helix."[85]

Janet E. Mertz, a scientist who holds a chair at the University of Wisconsin Madison School of Medicine and Public Health, was a graduate student in the laboratory of Nobel Laureate Paul Berg from 1970 to 1975. Mertz and other members of Berg's laboratory spliced together molecules to create the first "recombinant DNA." "This is about science politics, not science," Mertz wrote me in an email. "Having previously worked in the Harvard Business School, Eric Lander is a terrific administrator, statesman, and fund raiser for his own and his colleagues' causes as well as a terrific scientist and public speaker." She also noted that "outstanding women scientists" typically don't feel entitled or allowed to "behave in this highly assertive, self-aggrandizing way."

Scientific fields in academia have been hidebound by gender inequities, raising questions of whether these inequities have to do with ability or motivation. The journal *Science* noted that "just 27% of math Ph.D.s go to women. Exactly the same percentage – 27% – of people with careers in science, technology, mathematics, and engineering (STEM) fields are women. Women constitute a very similar number – 30% – of STEM college professors."[86] In 2005, the issue exploded when Larry Summers, then president at Harvard, suggested the prospect of innate differences in gender; as summarized in *The Economist*, he "infuriated the feminist establishment by wondering out loud whether the prejudice alone could explain the shortage of women at the top of science." Mertz then conducted her own cross-cultural analysis to "rule out several causal candidates, including coeducational schools, low standards of living, and innate variability among boys," telling a reporter at *Science* "We have pretty clear data debunking the greater male variability hypothesis" and suggesting "one thing the U.S. might do to improve math performance would be to pass the Paycheck Fairness Act and the Equal Rights Amendment to the U.S. Constitution."[87]

In the spring of 1972, Mertz was a young student at Stanford in Berg's lab when she demonstrated an easy method for splicing together DNA molecules with high efficiency, using her protocol to generate "recombinant DNAs." Stanford University, together with UCSF, filed the first of their patent applications relating to cloning of recombinant DNAs in November of 1974, listing Herbert Boyer and Stanley Cohen as the only co-inventors, despite the ideas behind this invention having already been published in the literature by Mertz, and others, in 1972, striking a rollicking disagreement over who had first demonstrated the "reduction to practice" of the first easy-to-use tools for recombinant DNA. The dispute is highly contentious and evokes deep differences to this day. "Cohen denied the validity and importance of the clearly prior work from the Berg laboratory, claiming to have had a 'eureka moment' in November of 1972, instead, to justify his patents and claim to fame. The Broad Institute folks seem to be doing likewise as best I can tell," Mertz said.

Nancy Hopkins, a Professor Emerita in the Biology Department at MIT and vocal leader on women's rights in science, told me that a long-standing issue is an "unconscious bias" whereby a female scientist voices an idea, leading colleagues to shrug their shoulders, only to have a male colleague reiterate the idea, which then sparks an engaged conversation. The mid-twentieth-century powerhouse biologist, Nobel Laureate Barbara McClintock, once told her that "men would take her data and leave her sitting outside the room while they went inside to discuss her data." Over the decades, Hopkins said, "I saw the situation change dramatically, and I saw women much more fairly credited... Even so, when Crispr came along... I wondered once again... if two women would actually be allowed to get credit... When Doudna and Charpentier won the Breakthrough Prize, I was thrilled. To me it was a measure of just how far women scientists have come – that they were recognized so quickly for this work." But after that "I wondered whether they would be allowed to make money from this discovery or whether all the money would go to men. While the issue of scientific credit has gotten so much better for women during my life time, it has been replaced to some extent by the astonishing exclusion of women faculty scientists from the Biotech companies their male colleagues found – exclusion as co-founders, scientific advisory board members, etc., of startup companies. So I was thrilled when I read that Doudna was part of Editas – and then later, disappointed and curious as to why she had dropped out. Anyway – when the Lander 'history' appeared, I did not read it. Because of the patent fight, and because it is not his field. However, when the criticisms of how he had treated the two women scientists began to fly, I read those and was astonished to learn that women were once again – and publicly – being treated the way women scientists were treated so long ago... On the other hand, that men came to their defense shows how much things have changed in a good way for women."

In the *Harvard Crimson* on January 29, Law School Professor Jennie C. Suk and longtime Lander advisee Pardis C. Sabeti said the attacks were baseless: "The kind of dedication that I saw firsthand, that Eric Lander had, to supporting and furthering the career of his mentees who were women – that is utterly inconsistent with some idea that he is erasing women's role in science," Suk said. Sabeti characterized Lander as an "extraordinary mentor" who pushed many women to have a strong voice at the Broad Institute, and said that the Crispr narrative was not an issue of gender. I think the relevant question in play is not whether men think women have a right to succeed, but whether they are more likely to gamble, put their reputation on the line and go for broke when something valuable is at stake. Lander declined my request to be interviewed.

In 2007, at a meeting of the American Psychological Association in San Francisco, the Florida State University psychologist Roy F. Baumeister gave an address titled "Is there Anything Good About Men?" He noted the "war of the sexes" was somewhat of a misnomer since any biological tactic comes with tradeoffs, hence none is superior. In the 1960s psychology espoused the dogma of male superiority, while for a brief moment in the 1970s there were no real differences. In the contemporary moment, female superiority has become popular in titles such as "Men are Not Cost Effective," or Maureen Dowd's book "Are Men Necessary?" Or Louann Brizendine's book, "The Female Brain," which introduces itself by saying, "Men, get ready to experience brain envy." Nowadays, Baumeister quipped, "Both men and women hold much more favorable views of women than of men. Almost everybody likes women better than men. I certainly do."

Baumeister went on to support the "male variability hypothesis," confiding that "actually, there is some evidence that men on average are a little better at math, but let's assume Summers was talking about general intelligence. People can point to plenty of data that the average IQ of adult men is about the same as the average for women. So to suggest that men are smarter than women is wrong... But that's not what he said. He said there were more men at the top levels of ability. That could still be true despite the average being the same – if there are also more men at the bottom of the distribution, more really stupid men than women. During the controversy about his remarks, I didn't see anybody raise this question, but the data are there, indeed abundant, and they are indisputable. There are more males than females with really low IQs... Almost certainly, it is something biological and genetic."

Baumeister went on to concede that "research by Jacquelynne Eccles has repeatedly concluded that the shortage of females in math and science reflects motivations more than ability." Interestingly, Baumeister's answer to the lack of female motivation for STEM fields was due to an "underappreciated fact." "The first big, basic difference has to do with what I consider to be the most underappreciated fact about gender. Consider this question: What percent of our ancestors were women? It's not a trick question, and it's not 50%. True, about half the people who ever lived were women, but that's not the question. We're asking about all the people who ever lived who have a descendant living today. Or, put another way, yes, every baby has both a mother and a father, but some of those parents had multiple children. Recent research using DNA analysis answered this question about two years ago. Today's human population is descended from twice as many women as men. I think this difference is the single most underappreciated fact about gender. To get that kind of difference, you had to have something like, throughout the entire history of the human race, maybe 80% of women but only 40% of men reproduced."

"If evolution explains anything at all, it explains things related to reproduction, because reproduction is at the heart of natural selection. Basically, the traits that were most effective for reproduction would be at the center of evolutionary psychology. It would be shocking if these vastly different reproductive odds for men and women failed to produce some personality differences," Baumeister said. "We know from the classical music scene that women can play instruments beautifully, superbly, proficiently – essentially just as well as men. They can and many do. Yet in jazz, where the performer has to be creative while playing, there is a stunning imbalance: hardly any women improvise. Why? The ability is there but perhaps the motivation is less. They don't feel driven to do it." In evolutionary terms, "For women, the optimal thing to do is go along with the crowd, be nice, play it safe... For men, the outlook was radically different. If you go along with the crowd and play it safe, the odds are you won't have children. Most men who ever lived did not have descendants who are alive today. In terms of the biological competition to produce offspring, then, men outnumbered woman both among the losers and among the biggest winners."

Baumeister, who also coined the term "ego-depletion," extends these gender dynamics into a "two-spheres" theory that suggests the rise of institutions emerged around the expendability of men, while small-group dynamics have been driven by the individuation of women. "It turns out that in close relationships, women are plenty aggressive." This is not a purely male trait. "Instead, the difference is found in the broader social sphere. Women don't hit strangers. The chances that a woman will, say, go to the mall and end up in a knife fight with another woman are vanishingly small, but there is more such risk for men. The gender difference in aggression is mainly found there, in the broader network of relationships. Now consider helping. Most research finds that men help more than women. Most research looks at helping between strangers, in the larger social sphere, and so it finds men helping more. Inside the family, though, women are plenty helpful, if anything more than men." The "two-spheres" conclusion is "supported in plenty of other places. Playground observation studies find that girls pair off and play one-on-one with the same playmate for the full hour. Boys will either play one-on-one with a series of different playmates or with a larger group. Girls want the one-to-one relationship, whereas boys are drawn to bigger groups or networks. When two girls are playing together and the researchers bring in a third one, the two girls resist letting her join. But two boys will let a third boy join their game. My point is that girls want the one-on-one connection, so adding a third person spoils the time for them, but it doesn't spoil it for the boys."

"Thus, men create the kind of social networks where individuals are replaceable and expendable. All-male groups tend to be marked by put-downs and other practices that remind everybody that there is not enough respect to go around, because this awareness motivates each man to try harder to earn respect. Some sociological writings about the male role have emphasized that to be a man, you have to produce more than you consume. The phrase 'Be a man' is not as common as it once was, but there is still some sense that manhood must be earned. Every adult female is a woman and is entitled to respect as such, but many cultures withhold respect from the males until and unless the lads prove themselves. This is of course tremendously useful for the culture, because it can set the terms by which males earn respect as men, and in that way it can motivate the men to do things that the culture finds productive. Risky jobs extend beyond the battlefield. Many lines of endeavor require some lives to be wasted. Exploration, for example: a culture may send out dozens of parties, and some will get lost or be killed, while others bring back riches and opportunities. Research is somewhat the same way: There may be a dozen possible theories about some problem, only one of which is correct, so the people test the eleven wrong theories end up wasting their time and ruining their careers, in contrast to the lucky one who gets the Nobel prize." Thus, Baumeister argues, "culture exploits men" and uses "individual men for symbolic purposes more than women. This can be in a positive way, such as the fact that cultures give elaborate funerals and other memorials to men who seem to embody its favorite values. It can also be negative, such as when cultures ruin a man's career, shame him publically. The essence of how culture uses men depends on a basic social insecurity. This insecurity is in fact social, existential, and biological. Built into the male role is the danger of not being good enough to be accepted and respected and even the danger of not being able to do well enough to create offspring. The basic social insecurity of manhood is stressful for the men, and it is hardly surprising that so many men crack up or do evil or heroic things or die younger than women. But that insecurity is useful and productive for the culture, the system."

Lander describes his article as seeking to elevate the "unsung heroes" in the molecular story of Crispr. I think it is a complex and interesting set of motives, which at least partly owes something to Friedrich Nietzsche, who codified the concept of "transvaluation," a native drive to reassign value to those with least credit. Consciously, at least, the article emerges due to some admission that the Broad has been overly credited for Crispr-Cas9 by journalists and the public, and the article appears to provide a proper recognition to its pioneering scientists. Lander draws an intellectual line to Mojica, and to Marraffini, in a move of transvaluation to reassign credit, but in doing so, unconsciously draws upon their authority as early pioneers to stabilize his position, and set Zhang as a rightful intellectual heir. And it is also clearly tangled up with a competitive impulse to devalue the work of more direct competitors in Doudna and Charpentier. "Eric Lander tries to downplay the specific discovery and invention of Charpentier and Doudna by describing in his review article how it was simply building upon much prior work of others," Mertz told me, pointing me to a 2010 review article she co-authored with Berg which describes the history behind the invention of recombinant DNA cloning as one example of how "almost all major scientific discoveries come from building upon prior work of others."[88] Lander's "heroes" article articulates a version of history in which Berkeley folks merely made a few small steps in a long scientific progression which culminated in Zhang's molecular tweaks of Crispr and deployment in human cells. By contrast, the Berkeley people and allies in Boston, including Rossi and Sontheimer, argue that early work by Crispr gumshoes like Charpentier made Zhang's deployment of Crispr in human cells nearly inevitable.

In April 2016, Lander addressed the blowback at an Aspen Institute event. Joel Achenbach of *The Washington Post* reported the talk in his column. "'My intention is not to diminish anybody,' Lander said this week. He specifically mentioned Jennifer Doudna, of the University of California at Berkeley, whom he described as 'a spectacular scientist.' Doudna was among the Crispr heroes who didn't care for his essay. Also apparently rankled were some hard-working graduate students, laboring anonymously in the labs of tenured scientists."

Also that month in an article in *Nature* titled "Crispr: pursuit of profit poisons collaboration," Sherkow wrote of the looming patent battle: "One conspicuous aspect of this case, in my opinion, is the degree to which UC Berkeley and the Broad Institute have weighed in on what is essentially a dispute over scientific priority . . . The Broad Institute has produced press releases, videos and a slick feature on its website that stress the importance of Zhang's contributions to the development of the Crispr-Cas9 technology . . . The financial stakes are high. The Crispr-Cas9 patents are widely viewed to be worth hundreds of millions, if not billions, of dollars."

Crispr was a piece of theatre. In play were *ad hominem* attacks and suggestions that special interpretations in policy, and venture capital-ists had an indirect influence on the content of *Cell*. I asked Joe Caputo, a spokesperson for *Cell*, whether or not the journal had a policy in place which allowed scientists to write outside their field of expertise. "*Cell* encourages multidisciplinary thinking and cross pol-lination of ideas at all levels," Caputo told me. Fair enough. One of the ideas that I hope to show in this book is how, since the late 1970s when the first biotech patents emerged, science has progressively come to be dominated by business elements. Caputo's response to me in my email inquiry regarding Lander's "heroes" article was that it was a peer-reviewed article. In effect, this is a strawman that shifts the conversation from a question of motive to the reliability of the content. In our modern times of science, we assess decisions only in terms of results and outcomes, but we need to be asking these types of questions, not only about the replication crisis and value of science, but about motive. We are also at the mercy of scientists, to some extent. As the Harvard science historian Steven Shapin quipped, "if you don't find scientists trustworthy, if you think of them as mere servants of power and profit, then the ultimate price to be paid is that you'll have to do the science yourself – and good luck to you in making your findings credible."[89]

Science is not driven by aesthetics. That is a hard lesson for me. I could never work in finance, for instance, because I would wake up every morning wondering what my life was even about. I had stints with Buddhism. I had once thought of MIT as a kind of cathedral, and it represents itself as this sort of thing, with its dome structure, and names chiseled up high on the substrate of its architecture: Archimedes, Copernicus, Darwin, Faraday, Newton – as Francis Bacon called it, the "scientific priesthood." Bacon wrote that: "If these scientific priests can reach the center of the maze, they will find the 'summary laws of nature' and can use them to grasp immense power for the benefit of humankind." One could add, "as well as immense wealth and personal fortune."

I had thought of MIT as a more perfect place of pure mathematics and ideas that elevated beyond the low-lying violence that permeates through life. But it is not that. I was now alive to the idea that modern science is motivated by business elements as territory in conflict. Life does not aim for pure abstraction as Plato knew it; it is rather organic in its representation as Schopenhauer, Heidegger and Nietzsche saw it. Chomsky showed us that our institutions function to disburse risk and resources, and are not simply power structures, since order is inscribed in the springs and bolts of the brain, broadly distributed and coextensive.[90] Competency is not defined by the institution, it's in us. But, as Steven Pinker mentioned to me, the capacity for intelligence and creativity, this everywhere-ness of it, does not necessitate cooperation, and any evolutionary explanation of altruistic cooperation by means of "group selection" or evolution through broad society goals is "hopelessly incoherent." Crispr-Cas9 is in part a trust for the betterment of man, but its applications would almost certainly convey a differential advantage to a minority, its benefit more tribal than inclusive; striving to attain it as a sort of chalice of life was coming at considerable personal risk. George Church simultaneously grasped the title of my book, with its numerous examples of self-injury, the blowback against Lander's piece and the spectacle the Crispr scientists and science was becoming by "noting that many classic Greek heroes were invulnerable, except to self-inflicted wounds."

On the first sunny day in 2013, Derrick Rossi rode his bike to work and was descending a hill when a car door opened in his path. He broke his collarbone, seven ribs, and splintered bones which nearly nicked major arteries that certainly would have killed him through the auspices of internal bleeding. Boston is marked with "ghost bikes," bicycles that are spray-painted white and chained to the sites of bicyclists' deaths as a token reminder to all commuters what is at risk. Rossi's bike was parked in his office. It had never been painted.[91]

Rossi was bouncing back, just getting off the phone from a conference call, when I strolled into his office. His left arm was in a sling and he was a bit roughish looking. He had just completed a second arthroscopic surgery after the bicycle accident. He had been out of work for just a matter of weeks. I had been stumbling back into his lab every few weeks over the winter and early spring for a short meeting. I was starting to make some notes on Crispr-Cas9, and collecting my thoughts, and poring over his data. The story was grabbing me and I wanted to write about it.

"The gene therapy field is undergoing a renaissance," Rossi told me in his matter-of-fact way of talking. He typically sounds like he's recognized a power in naivety, or near naivety, of living life as if he's only scratched the surface; and when Rossi tells you something, there's never a trace of a hedge. It sounds like facts knocking on the door. Church, who worked across the street in the New Research Building, has been among the chief architects of the system, and I asked if he could introduce me. Not likely, Rossi said. Church was too busy. By that time, Doudna's work had instantly elevated her status to among the most sought-after gene engineers in the field. And by now, calls were shooting back and forth between Harvard and Berkeley. Rossi had just gotten off a conference call with Church and Doudna when I stumbled in. Lander also wanted to get in on the ground floor of the new company, which would be named Editas Medicine. Among the first things I mentioned to him when I entered his office was that I had just emailed Doudna with some questions about the applications of Crispr-Cas9, the microbial trick that scientists were now feverishly pursuing as a new mechanism for editing genes in humans. "That's who the whole conference call was about, Jennifer Doudna." Rossi said. "To see if she would be interested in launching a company with us."

Rossi wanted to get involved for a couple of reasons. The first, as I mentioned, is that he studies repair mechanisms in cells. Cas9 is an endonuclease, which hacks into the DNA ladder and creates what is called a double-strand break. When this happens, the cell automatically patches itself back up with a repair. In fact, a cell must do this hundreds or thousands of times a day as it takes on injuries, patching itself up with spare parts of DNA molecules that are available in each cell. If a double-strand break occurs which leaves overhang, which is called a cohesive or "sticky" end, then it has a template available for a neat and professional repair using machinery in a pathway called "homology-directed repair;" but if the double strand break is "blunt," meaning there is no overhang, then it is more likely to make the repair in an unguided way, patching it up with bits of code, which results in insertions, deletions and ad hoc patches, based on a pathway called "non-homologous end joining." In fact, Cas9 makes blunt cuts, and non-homologous end joining is the favored strategy. But here is the cool trick: if you use Crispr-Cas9 in nearby locations, you can end up removing, or "excising," a number of bases, and if you include some new bit of genetic code with the shuttle, you can get the cell to add your new snippet of code. Rossi was already an expert in these pieces of repair machinery. The second reason he wanted to be involved is that he studies hematopoietic stem cells, the type of stem cells that give rise to blood and immune system cells. It turns out that these cells were among the first type of cells targeted in human genetic engineering. Hematopoietic cells are circulating cells that can be removed from bone marrow or blood. Gene editing is highly applicable to immune disorders, or rare blood disorders, since these can easily be removed and returned to a body. I had been collaborating with Rossi for about six months, as the summer approached. He began digging into the complicated matters of setting up a company, and I left his lab and took a deep dive into writing about the major shift that was happening.

Not long after, I got into Church's office and talked to him for an hour on what was happening with Crispr-Cas9. At the time, Church had just made some colorful comments to the German magazine *Der*

Spiegel and his phone was ringing off the hook with reporters asking for comments on how and whether he was going to use gene engineering to raise Neanderthal to life. He took one of the calls, but it was not what he expected, and I'm sure he wished he hadn't picked it up. "Any question but that one," he told a British reporter before hanging up. Church is a level-headed scientist in person, and he commands a deep knowledge of molecular biology. I think what makes him provocative to the public and mildly subversive to his peers is that he has the wicked imagination of an inventor, while the orthodox tone in science is one of staid understatement. As one scientist told me, speaking of Church, "there are people in this town who take up way too much attention coming up with ideas that can never work in reality." But Keith Joung, a collaborator, told me Church is good for science because he injects the field with a charisma that inspires young people to the moon-shots of science. What I would come to understand after seeing Church talk over the course of the next few years, is how much aptitude he has for prosaic details about drug development, and how wonkish he can be about the Food and Drug Administration. For whatever few charismatic remarks Church can make to a reporter, he can also talk for hours on end about the most boring items on how to bring a drug to market. Church got his name not by doing fantastic things, but by returning to molecular biology and its problems, again and again, in short, through his own persistence. Writing this story over the course of years, it became clear how easy it is as a journalist to distill a scientist's personality into a few sentences, when in actuality, each of them, Doudna, Zhang, Church, Joung, is routinely questioning their own strategies, uncertain about their own plans, ruminating, reconsidering, and obsessed about a wide range of extremely prosaic details that turn out to matter a lot. And when you're writing journalism, there is the constant temptation to distill them into adjectives, and the impulse to expose their vulnerabilities and weaknesses to make them seem more real on the pages. I could not possibility begin to explain the life or complexity of any given character, there is an ocean of subconscious under each of them. If you read interviews and articles on Lander throughout his career, it's clear that his curiosity is ultimately what has driven the trajectory of his life. If you follow Doudna, it's clear not only that she is one of the dominant biochemists of her generation, but that she continues to question her own motives.

It wasn't too long after that, I met up with another big ideas person, Richard C. Mulligan, a MacArthur Fellow whose office is a couple floors removed from Church at Harvard. I had a hard time catching up with Mulligan because he's usually in New York these days. I eventually met him for a couple hours in his office, and the first thing he said was "guess what I'm doing, you'll never guess." In truth, I could not guess. It turned out what he doing was "trying to fix poorly managed companies" with the activist investor Carl Icahn. Mulligan is a fascinating person because he set the field of gene therapy in motion. In fact, he is a one-time student of the Nobel laureate Paul Berg. But the arc of his story goes back a couple of decades. In the late 1960s, the first "restriction enzymes" were discovered as a component of an innate immune system that microbes could use to chop up invading phages. Herbert Boyer's lab members had isolated one of the first such restriction enzymes, which worked as tiny molecular scissors to cut DNA at a specific sequence. Boyer had passed out his molecular scissors to Janet Mertz, a member of Paul Berg's lab. In 1971 and 1972, scientists in Berg's lab performed the first gene splicing experiments, mending together pieces of genetic code from a cancer-inducing virus and a bacterium, touching off a firestorm of a debate. We could engineer life. And this tempest over genetic engineering had only just begun. Berg and his people were the first to cross the threshold, launching a wave of deep debate within the scientific community. No one knew what to make of this at the time. Some people were concerned that a rogue, genetically engineered microbe might run on the loose and spread a blood-clotting infection, or trigger cancer throughout the human population. Michael Crichton wrote *The Andromeda Strain* and Stephen King wrote *The Stand,* each of those novels being about tweaked genes in virulent microbes that decimated the human population. A moratorium was placed on the cloning of such recombinant DNAs, something that had been unheard of except in the case of the construction of nuclear fission power plants, just a few years before. In 1975, a major conference was held at a California resort named Asilomar to take up the matter. Scientists, for the most part, did not want Congress involved, and some of the public was alarmed at playing God with DNA. "You have to remember, it was the 1970s," MIT biology professor and Nobel laureate Phil Sharp later told me in his office. "People were deeply skeptical of scientific authority."

Sharp and David Baltimore were among the 140 attendees at Asilomar. As tensions eased, the technology led to the emergence of the first major biotech patent, the "Boyer–Cohen patent" and major companies such as Biogen (which Sharp co-founded) and Genentech (which Boyer co-founded). Among its first applications was to add genes for insulin to microbes and then scale up the drug, which was protein synthesized from "recombinant DNA." Baltimore was instrumental for so many reasons, but one of them was his development of the eponymous Baltimore Classification System, which was a means to classify all the many types of viruses and clarify how they enter and replicate in cells. In short, there are RNA viruses and DNA viruses and some have one strand of genetic material and some have two strands, and they can be put into categories based on these properties for how they enter cells and replicate. Of course, different viruses enter into unique cell types. Take your pick: retrovirus and lentivirus can enter blood and immune cells, adenovirus can enter cells in tissue, rabies and herpes simplex virus can enter neurons. Baltimore also co-discovered reverse transcriptase, which is an enzyme that enables a kind of RNA virus called a retrovirus to transform itself back into DNA and burrow its way into our genomes like a pest. It was heretical at the time because no one (other than Howard Temin, the originator of this idea) thought that RNA could turn back into DNA code, hence the "retro" in the name. But, what it also meant is that a virus could be gutted and used as a kind of vehicle to deliver any kind of genetic material into our cells. By this point, Berg and others had developed a means to splice pieces of genetic material together, and growing insight into the nature of viruses meant that scientists could cobble together any sort of genetic sequence and use a virus to package and deliver it into human cells. Mulligan graduatedout of Berg's lab at Stanford, and emerged on the scene like a fireball around 1980. Baltimore and Sharp recruited him to MIT and he was one of the key people who was able to splice together human genes and viruses, and get these recombinant products into human cells. But there was only one catch: the virus would end up installing at any random site in any of our chromosomes. If a virus landed next to a gene that regulated the cell cycle, it could cause a cancer. "What we later learned was that, indeed, complications can occur for a great number of genes," Mulligan told me. "It was a surprise that inserting new genes could cause so many difficulties." Baltimore and Sharp both mentioned to me they thought Mulligan was one of the brightest scientists of his generation. Ironically, when I went to see Mulligan, he told me how he had recently been involved in a proxy fight aimed at gaining board seats in Sharp's company Biogen, but by then Sharp had been ready to move onto other things, and the two had remained on excellent terms. In his office, Mulligan told me how he built upon Baltimore's work with retrovirus to develop it into the first system for efficient "gene transfer" in human cells. He spun a story, taking me back to the 1980s, when scientists finally had a set of tools they could use to try in living humans.

Mulligan was sitting on a council called the Recombinant DNA Committee or RAC, a federal advisory committee in the US set up in 1974 at the National Institutes of Health at the time of Asilomar, set to review a proposal by another scientist named W. French Anderson, to conduct what would become the first successful gene therapy treatment.

And at the time, Mulligan was mentoring two young students, one was named Jim Wilson, who was studying liver cells, and one was David A. Williams, who was studying blood stem cells. Scientists were in a scramble to see who would be the first to put this technology to work. As the first trials surged ahead, a patient treated for an immune disease called X-linked severe combined immune deficiency or X-SCID died in France when the retrovirus integrated near a gene in his own cell that controls cell division, throwing it into overdrive, causing a "leukemia-like condition." Near the same time, Wilson decided on adenovirus for a trial on a rare disorder at the University of Pennsylvania called ornithine transcarbamylase (OTC) deficiency syndrome. In 1999, 18-year-old Jesse Gelsinger was enrolled in his trial and died when a feature of the virus triggered an immune reaction, which quickly threw his immune system into a runaway signaling cascade called a cytokine storm. The gene therapy field was thrown to a screeching halt. Months before the Gelsinger trial, a scientist from the Naval Medical research Institute named Bruce Levine had just taken a job at Penn. Levine had been working with Carl June since 1992 when he joined his lab as a postdoctoral fellow. June had a plan to develop a new gene therapy system, called Chimeric Antigen Receptor T-cells (CAR T-cells), whereby he would add new bits of code to our own T-cells, and create a new receptor on those T-cells that did not previously exist in nature. That receptor could be designed to guide the T-cells to a marker on the surface of cancer cells. This was exciting, because it could move gene therapy from fringe orphan diseases into mainstream cancer therapeutics. "The plan was Carl's and was set in motion with a collaboration with Cell Genesys," Levine told me. "We believe this was the first use of CARs in humans."

But June and other vanguards of the field had to retreat. The FDA suspended Penn's gene therapy program, among the largest in the country, on January 21, 2000. Levine continued to collaborate with Carl June at Penn and persisted with his work, but it would be years before June was able to bring CAR T-cells into trial and get the program at Penn back into some state of coherence. Wilson continued to deal with massive grief, but persevered in his dedication to making the technology safer. In the meantime, Williams, now chief of hematology at Boston Children's Hospital, and colleagues transformed the virus technology into much safer forms, stripping viruses of features that can cause immune reactions, and swapping out the promoter and enhancer features with weaker versions so that they will be less likely to trigger strong gene expression, and hopefully, thus, not a cancer. Gene therapy was poised for a rebound. In 2013, by the time I was in Mulligan's office, investment was roaring back into the field and gene therapy companies were filing IPOs. Those included Bluebird Bio, which involved, at the time, one of Mulligan's former understudies, Mitch Finer, as its scientific officer, REGENXBIO, which employed Jim Wilson as its scientific officer, and Intrexon Corp., which had been spearheaded by the billionaire RJ Kirk. Crispr-Cas9 has been introduced as a potent new means for "genome editing," meaning the techniques that allow us to make very specific changes to bases in a sea of our 3-billion-nucleotide genomes.

At this point, I am still interested in the story of using retrovirus to insert genes into random locations in cells, which is a technology that was much farther along in trials than Crispr-Cas9. The use of retrovirus to randomly insert a gene into a human chromosome was known as "gene trapping" and it was of great use for inserting a supplemental gene which could suffice to ameliorate a great number of disorders that could be rescued by simply restoring one copy of a broken gene. These were, in large part, the recessive genetic diseases or enzyme deficiency disorders. Crispr-Cas9 would emerge to allow us to make any mechanical change at a very precise location, providing hope to also treat dominant genetic disorders in which a broken copy of a gene had a deleterious effect on a cell, or tissue. Crispr-Cas9 would allow us to do so much more than just throw an extra copy of a gene into a cell like a monkey wrench. It would allow us to make genetic alterations with high precision. But, as of early 2016, it was not yet in human trials. Retroviral therapy, and "gene trapping," was much farther along, a story I wanted to follow.

David A. Williams and colleagues led a new round of X-SCID, or "Bubble Boy," trials, and so far their patients were recovering, although in the original trials a "leukemia-like condition" did not show up for a couple of years after the treatment. It had been just a year since the patients in William's new trial were treated. No one knew if it was safe or if they would get cancer, but most of the problems seemed to be solved. I wanted to know more. At this point I had to know more. There are not many Bubble Boys in the world. There is one in Illinois. I hit the road, heading west by highway. I arrived in Bloomington, Illinois and met Jennifer and Rob Golliday, who have a two-year-old son named Jamey who was born with X-SCID. Jennifer showed me pictures of how she built an improvised "bubble stroller" and the set of events that led her to learn her baby boy was a Bubble Boy. In short, if you have a Bubble Boy, your whole family becomes "bubbled." You don't have friends. No one can come to your house. When you go to the grocery store you take off your clothes as soon as you come inside, you wash your hands furiously because you don't want to give a cold to your son, because even with a small cold, he could die. She told me the story about how her son was treated with gene therapy months before by using retrovirus to install a gene for the IL2-gamma receptor, which is required for immune system T-cells to mature and function. Jamey's immune system was now on the rebound. He was walking with his mother in the yard and then he came up to me, and asked to hold my hand; I was the first person out of his immediate family that he interacted with since his treatment. I wrote some articles on the trip for *The Atlantic* and *The Boston Globe* that summer. Driving out of Illinois I felt a shiver in my bones for the first time, a sense that this was more than pop science. It was the first time I felt science as something concrete, visceral, non-trivial. Driving out of Illinois I started to well up because I knew that all these things were real.

It is superficial to speak of a moment that changed one's life, as a singular axis upon which everything turns. It is more realistic to speak in terms of micro-moments, pieces of experience that slowly weight and rock a polyhedron of perspective onto a new face. I recall a series of such moments, as I was approaching the age of 30, while reading Stephen Jay Gould's tome *The Structure of Evolutionary Theory* over a winter on the seashore in Maine. I have always taken to winter, when life appears as a photographic negative, stark, its figure more visible where its color and personality recede. When the moon is visible in the morning, when the sea recedes to reveal timeworn rock, its salt and ancient decay, when the staccato of fist-sized rocks roll up and then recede back into the sea with each advancing wave, most of all, the pale, gentle light. When these things happen, I am in love with the winter. But in all of us there lies a negative form, a soul of retreat. I fell into concentration, reading. Over that winter, I had a sense of "deep time," of living on a nameless planet. An ordinary sense of space and temporality is eclipsed by a greater expanse. Its facility to eclipse is what the poet Keats once called "negative capability," which he described as "when a man is capable of being in uncertainties, mysteries and doubts, without any irritable reaching after fact and reason."[92] Almost everyone has experience with déjà vu, an odd familiarity with a foreign place, but few people use the compatible term, jamais vu, which means an eerie sense of seeing a familiar place for the first time, as if it is brand new. So much beauty exists in being able to forget, and also lies in our willingness to be forgotten. I was also aware that raw particulate matter, the "noumenon" as the phenomenologists called it, doesn't know or care a thing about science. Science is something we made up to classify and order life and physical things. Particulate matter is just accidentally related stuff crashing into each other.

"Of all the sciences, biology is the most lawless," wrote Mukherjee in *The Gene*, but lawlessness may transfer even to physics. In *Time Reborn*, one of the most unappreciated books in recent years, Lee Smolin suggested that time is primordial, and even the laws of physics may undergo evolution: "What is needed is relationalism, according to which the future is restricted by, but not determined by, the present." Smolin wrote, "Physics can no longer be understood as the search for a precisely identical mathematical double of the universe. That dream must be seen now as a metaphysical fantasy that may have inspired generations of theorists, but is now blocking the path to future progress." I could be wrong, but my instinct is that life is an accident; to the question of whether laws or matter is primordial, I side with matter. The idea, that, at the basis of the universe lies a single, elegant mathematical equation, or so forth, I don't think it's true. This view entails the moral directive that we can get closer to reality and truths by moving through science and mathematics. Science makes us better people. Not so for Nietzsche. He argued instead that raw nature is utterly without order, at its basis is particular substance and accident. Science is vocation. Math is merely an emergent property. Nietzsche wrote "that my life has no purpose is clear from the accidentalness of my origin: that I can set a purpose for my life is another matter."

I had been writing for *The New Hampshire Union Leader*, that diatribe of news and polemics written by publisher Joe McQuaid, known for his front-page editorials written in boldface or all caps. But that winter, I began reading books. I was awakened to a sense of scientific heritage. For me, the basis of science, and its quest, is not defined by its establishment, but by an awakening to the absence of any requirement, the chaos of the sea, oblivion and violence that permeates life. A structural tension in modern life is presented as a rift between science and religion, but its fissure goes deeper than that, to one between science and the absence of fundamental order in nature. Facts have a strength to them – they are subject to catalytic turnover. This is a subtle but critical point. I don't see the universe as a gestalt, a whole entity with parts, and fundamental laws, but rather I see it as particulate matter that does not assemble into a whole. I don't even think of time as a singular or inclusive term, I only see disparate models in competition. I felt this at a visceral level in my bones while reading *Structure*, with its numerous examples of models of life that have been tried since the Cambrian explosion.

Books have a stabilizing function. It was the cynosure of the book that led me into graduate school and into science. What can be powerfully attractive about science, as with the humanities, is it provides an entry-point into a deep legacy and heritage. After graduate school, I did an internship with Rossi, and then, a few years later, I was working at the Broad Institute, a non-profit research institute based on computation aspects of research, which was founded in 2003 by Eli Broad and his wife, Edythe, after he became a billionaire in post-war America by inventing a model for a cheap basement-less house that could sell for less than $15,000. The Broad Institute is a steel and glass-encased building that rises up 12 floors and includes an elevated bridge that merges two buildings. The windows are virtually sound proof, and up on its top floor, in the winter, steam rises over the pipes and HVAC on the tops of smaller buildings below; all of Boston including the Charles River can be seen below and makes the world seem all that more quiet and frozen and picture-perfect still. I'm still writing. In my day job I am working on a project on how hepatitis C virus disposes us to liver cancer. Viruses can cause cancer for many reasons and most of this happens by natural selection that is purely random and selected for over generations of virus. In short, viruses tweak and alter cellular machinery in a variety of ways to maximize their growth and that can lead to cell stress and damage, and in some cases, viruses even carry bits of code that can drive cells to divide. A virus cannot replicate on its own, but only through the hijacking of machinery in a host cell that it infects. The hepatitis C virus enters hepatocytes, or liver cells, and takes up residency, and it turns out that even if you cure a patient with a hepatitis C drug, which for a three-month treatment course can run to $80000, the patient still has a significantly elevated risk for liver cancer. And all of this is caused by random molecules. The liver is interesting because it is one of the most resilient of organs, and can often regenerate. In the Greek myth, the titan Prometheus is chained to a rock while Zeus takes the form of an eagle and pecks out his liver each day, only for the liver to grow back at night. Interestingly, the ability of the liver to regrow may be one key to understanding how cycles of chronic injury and regeneration may initiate cancer. By comparison, the cells that build heart tissue are "terminally differentiated" and heart tissue does not regenerate, and intriguingly, there is no heart cancer. I had been working on this liver cancer project for about a year with a French scientist named Thomas, and I showed him our data, that we'd found some possible changes in expression of genes in a liver cell after it is infected with a hepatitis virus. The first thing Thomas said is that we're going to Crispr-Cas9 the regulatory molecules which regulate, or turn on, those genes. Presumably, the virus may alter a transcription factor or a regulatory molecule, which in turn activates a number of other genes, which by happenstance, dispose a cell to a heighted risk for cancer. Cancer can start in a single cell. And so if we can use Crispr to activate or deactivate the same regulatory molecules, which the virus also does, and artificially create the same effects that the virus does, then we can learn how to intervene at the precise molecular points that the virus intervenes, and reverse the changes it causes in the cell that contribute to a risk for cancer. I am coming to realize how profound an effect the Crispr-Cas9 system has on basic research. It has transformed the way we do experiments and test hypotheses.

Crispr-Cas9 is used by thousands of labs around the world. Consider that any experiment you do nowadays requires a "functional validation," which means that journals don't care if you disprove something statistically, they want you to knock out a gene in a cell culture or mouse model and show that you're dealing with reality, not just information. Before we got to this point, all we had was RNA interference, which was a way to down-regulate a gene's expression in a cell, meaning the quantity of RNA that is transcribed by a gene. But now we can use Crispr-Cas9 to cut, delete or re-engineer any gene and watch its effect on a cell. If we package Crispr-Cas9 into a virus to deliver it into a cell it allows us to edit or amend a gene at a very specific site. We can test virtually any hypothesis with incredible precision. This is having sweeping effects on science throughout every corner of the world. The capitalists have seen the writing on the wall. Doudna, Church, Joung, Zhang and David Liu started Editas, a company to use Crispr-Cas9 to edit human cells as disease treatment. Rossi, Barrangou, Marraffini, Sontheimer, and now again, Doudna started a second Cas9 therapeutics company called Intellia Therapeutics, following her departure from Editas, a company which had endured deep internal rifts since its inception. Doudna's other company, Caribou Biosciences, began collaborating with DuPont to grow Crispr-edited agricultural crops, which were expected to reach supermarkets within a few years. And by this point, UC Berkeley and the Broad Institute were in an epic patent fight over the claims to Crispr-Cas9. The battle over the patent rights was coming to a head in January 2017.

Marraffini and Sontheimer's initial 2008 patent application on Crispr had been disallowed on lack of description to enable and deploy it. Doudna's patents filed under the Regents of the University of California, the University of Vienna and Emmanuelle Charpentier were registered as a provisional patent which was filed seven months ahead of Zhang's provisional patent (his non-provisional patent was eventually granted) filed under the Broad Institute, Inc., Massachusetts Institute of Technology, and President and Fellows of Harvard College. In fact, the Regents et al. indeed followed up with a non-provisional patent (Patent Application No. 13/842,859), which is still pending and in condition for allowance, pending a proceeding which was filed that suggests that Zhang's patent interfered on the prior patent, a case which is expected to be resolved in early 2017. But Doudna and Charpentier's patent application had become the basis of an interference proceeding, which suggested the prospect of invalidating some of the issued patents. As Sontheimer remarked to me, one thing that any Crispr company must have on staff these days is lawyers. As Jacob S. Sherkow declared in the Stanford Center for Law and the Biosciences Blog, "Without question, this year's – and potentially, this century's – biggest biotech story is the rise of Crispr, arguably the most precise and flexible gene editing technology yet to be created. As others have reported at length, two research teams – Jennifer Doudna's lab at UC Berkeley, and others, and Feng Zhang's lab at the Broad Institute and MIT – are engaged in a patent dispute over fundamental aspects of the Crispr technology. (And to be clear – it's Doudna's and Zhang's attorneys running this show – not the scientists.)"[93]

In practical terms, Zhang's modifications to Crispr-Cas9, which can be ordered in a circular vector called a plasmid from a repository called Addgene, turned out to have the most utility and became the dominant versions ordered by academics. At talks and conferences, Crispr scientists were commiserating and downplaying tensions, but privately there were rifts and small animosities, not surprising when hundreds of millions of dollars in licensing fees, legacies and almost certainly a few Nobel Prize awards were at stake. I met with Charpentier in person at the Broad Institute, and she is largely credited as the first person to put the pieces of the Crispr-Cas9 system together in 2011, and shortly afterward elucidating the mechanism and then the details of the biochemistry leading to the guidelines of how to design the system as a genome editing tool, tracing the footsteps of the 2007 work from Horvath and Barrangou. Charpentier had started a third company together with co-founders Shaun Foy and Rodger Novak, Crispr Therapeutics, and landed $90 million in pocket money to begin working on using genome editing to treat sickle cell disease and cystic fibrosis, and while talking to her I was awestruck by this one thing: the NIH recently suggested it would phase out one of its funding branches and was instituting a new funding schema based on "translational research," which means they want you to do science that results in medicines and impacts lives. Microbiologists have complained for years how their journals have been demoted in impact score, and how scientists who work on eukaryotic or "higher" cells have all of the prestige. In the modern era, no one takes microbiologists that seriously, but with the reemergence of the "microbiome" and the discovery of Crispr in the machinery of microbes in seas and mineshafts, it was irrefutable that the microbiologists were on par if not dominant to the eukaryote medics in changing the landscape of human medicine.

I was talking to Charpentier, with this in the back of my mind, and she was telling me how she was studying these rare RNA repeats in a microbe, which is obscure research. And what amazed me, was how her work on basic science enabled the emergence of the hottest research field in therapeutic research. And even now, no one knows how deep this will go. Charpentier and I met in a small conference room with an oval table, and she told me the story of her discoveries, and how things began to unfold. At the time, she brushed off issues of competition, arguing that there was enough elbow room for so much research to blossom, but was also sensitive to patent battles that were emerging over Crispr-Cas9 technology. When I pushed her about the status of patent fights, her voice lowered and her gaze sharpened, and she started pressing me: "Who do you work for?"

Charpentier suggested that Zhang is supported by the Broad's tremendous platforms and high-throughput sequencing, which are endowed by hundreds of millions of dollars, while most of the mechanisms of the Crispr system which were elucidated by her and Doudna came by way of "good old methods of biochemistry which have been around for 15 to 20 years." She wanted to claim her own narrative in science, and felt, at least a little bit, hijacked. "I took risks," Charpentier told me. "The most rewarding thing a scientist can have is their own story. This is a story that I carried on my shoulders convinced about the nature of the mechanism involved and the potential for exploitation with the aim to develop new anti-infective therapies or genetic tools."[94]

Just how the intellectual line of achievement is traced, and which advances were especially fundamental, is a sensitive and highly contentious debate. Sontheimer, now a molecular biologist at the RNA Therapeutics Institute at UMass Medical School, argues that the 2007 to 2008 advances by Barrangou and Horvath, van der Oost, and Marraffini and Sontheimer revealed the Crispr adaptive immunity pathway and its central features of RNA-guided DNA targeting, and also provided the point at which the potential for Crispr RNA-guided genome editing applications were first recognized and articulated. Several key mechanistic insights into Cas9 function – its ability to induce DNA breaks, its ability to be portable and reprogrammed, and its requirement for the tracrRNA by Charpentier, Doudna, Jinek, and Chylinski in 2012 – were then provided in 2010 and 2011. Sontheimer has argued the 2012 proofs of Cas9-catalyzed DNA cleavage by Doudna, Charpentier and Siksnys, and then the five genome-editing papers in January 2013 from Church, Doudna, Joung, Kim and Zhang, represented a second stage of "reduction-to-practice" advances in the technology.[95] This amounted to the few molecular tricks needed to make Crispr efficient enough to work in cells, as accomplished by Church and Zhang. As the old proverb goes, "It is a poor carpenter who blames his tools." Some argue the work prior to 2012 which uncovered the pathway is the Nobel quality work that made the later reduction to practice nearly inevitable. And, by January 2013, a virtual five-way tie of papers were published to establish it as a technology.

By 2014, even the editors of the journal *Nature* were praising Crispr as a kind of second coming of molecular biology, putting it repeatedly on their cover, once in March above a splashy front page cover stating "Seek and Destroy," drawing on the poetry of Metallica's James Hetfield. And it had staying power in the news outlets of all stripes and feathers, remaining a top story over successive years. In December 2015, *Scientific American* had declared it one of the top stories of the year. But many academics saw it as a runaway train. Earlier that year, a fertility center in Boston made a statement that it will begin editing human embryos and a group of scientists in China announced that they've already done this and published the results. The mood was becoming nervous. Ethicists were sounding alarm bells that we may be on the threshold of a Gattaca-like future. I was starting to feel some urgency to the situation. I asked David Baltimore to meet me in the lobby of the Cambridge Hyatt Regency.

Baltimore told me the National Academy of Sciences was organizing an Asilomar-like conference on advising policy, and possibly to suspend gene engineering in the germline, the genetic material that is heritable. In short if you edit any of the genetic material in the cells in your body, it stops in that generation, but if you edit genes in the embryo, the initial product of sperm and ovum, that is the heritable code that sticks with us for generations. In this case, scientists in the field wanted to call for a moratorium or block to the actual work, to make editing the germline actually illegal. But by now, the science was moving so fast. On the one hand, concerns of engineering babies for intelligence and athletic prowess were looming. At Asilomar, scientists were asking daunting questions, and they largely got the answers right, informing the direction of research in a way that was laissez faire and still maintained practical boundaries. "We didn't want the government involved then, we wanted to self-police," Baltimore told me. Today, the stakes are higher. Baltimore said that he supported a moratorium in 1974 because it allowed scientists to "get their ducks in a row" and functioned as a means of "self-policing." "We felt very strongly that we wanted to keep Congress out of it," he told me. The moratorium, and subsequent guidelines developed at NIH's Recombinant DNA Advisory Committee, allowed scientists to "change regulations as they are needed." This new meeting, he hoped, would allow them to do something similar, to generate a flexible regulatory framework, which can be adjusted if needed. "The difference this time is that once you start modifying the germline, the issue is how far you should go," Baltimore said. "I think the technology has to be stacked up against preimplantion genetic diagnosis (a means of selecting healthy embryos in vitro for parents with diseases that run in their families). The number of circumstances where you'd need to edit the germline is very few. I don't think we should do that (yet)," Baltimore said. "The issue is how well we understand the consequences."

In fact, many scientists were arguing that Crispr-Cas9 germline intervention was not "medically necessary" to stop diseases, since genetic screening could already do that. An in vitro fertility procedure costs about $20000 in the United States, and it adds about $4000 to do a genetic screening of an early stage clump of cells called a blastocyst to pick the healthiest cells for implantation. The Stanford legal expert Hank Greely has argued that the genetic variant for Huntington's is dominant and is typically inherited along with a functioning copy of the gene. Therefore, it follows a Mendelian line of inheritance, meaning that 50% of the male's offspring will inherit the deleterious copy of the gene. So instead of editing the dangerous copy of the gene, fertility experts could simply select an embryo equipped with the functioning copy. In the words of the journalist Antonio Regalado, a "man with Huntington's, for instance, could have his sperm used to fertilize a dozen of his partner's eggs. Half those embryos would not have the Huntington's gene, and those could be used to begin a pregnancy."[96] Edward Lanphier, CEO of Sangamo Biosciences, concurred, saying "You can do it. But there really isn't a medical reason. People say, well, we don't want children born with this, or born with that – but it's a completely false argument and a slippery slope toward much more unacceptable uses."[97]

In truth, edits to the germline could result in unexpected consequences, and even if we did create a highly beneficial genetic variant, one that, say, improves the focus or reduces the risk of major depression in newborn, the effect would almost surely not be lasting for future generations. The reason is that genetic variants work in the context of a genetic background, a single gene variant exerts its effects on traits by working in coordination with other genetic variants. The important thing to keep in mind is that genes get shuffled each new generation (due in part to a well-described mechanism called "crossing over") so genetic variants often don't get passed on *together*. Even if a new gene edit came into circulation, it would end up interacting with ever new genetic backgrounds of other genetic variants, and its effects on traits would likely be washed out, an effect that Francis Galton once called "regression to the mean." And yet, a major issue with Crispr-Cas9 is using it when the functions of the genome remain incompletely described. Even if responsible scientists impose strict guidelines, the Crispr protocol has been published, and the technology seems impossible to put back on a leash. Any time we use it in human cells, it is, in effect, an experiment, since we don't have a comprehensive understanding of the multiple effects that any single genetic variant can have.

On the other hand, genetic engineering was becoming safer by leaps and bounds. RJ Kirk's company Intrexon had developed a "gene switch" which enabled scientists to install a gene into a cell, and enable that gene to only come on once a patient took a pill. This put genes newly installed into cells under tight controls, promising to make gene therapy safer. Mulligan was developing a second version of a gene switch based on a self-splicing ribozyme, the kind that Doudna helped to pioneer in her early career. In the words of Jennifer Kahn, "Doudna made her name as a postdoctoral researcher by mapping the structure of a particular type of RNA known as a ribozyme: a molecule able to catalyze chemical reactions by twisting to bring different atoms in contact with one another." Tom Cech, who was Doudna's postdoctoral adviser, noted "she has an uncanny knack for picking the best experiments to answer a question," Cech says. "From an early age, she had this talent for solving very daunting problems. Her whole career, in some ways, was preparation for Crispr."[98] What makes the ribozyme provocative as a molecule is that some forms are "self-cleaving," meaning that they can snip and reassemble themselves in a process of self-organization. Some scientists, therefore, have suggested that it may be one of the basic molecules of life, and that DNA only emerged later as a "storage" mechanism, a more stable form of code that could house the code of heredity over generations. Mulligan, along with other colleagues, learned that he could make use of the self-cleaving ribozyme as a technology. By adding a bit of the self-cleaving code into a gene installed into a cell, that code in that gene would self-splice once it turned into a messenger RNA and therefore never turn into a protein. If a patient was given a pill to bind to that snippet of code, it could block the self-splicing mechanism, allowing the gene to be expressed and turn "on." And scientists appeared to be largely solving the problems of gene therapy treatments causing severe immune reactions or cancer conditions, not only with switches, but by swapping out elements of the viruses that are used to deliver genes into cells with subtler molecular forms that were far less likely to trigger adverse events in patients, such as the notorious "leukemia-like conditions."

Jamey Golliday, the Bubble Boy I met in Illinois, appeared to be healthy and recovered. And yet, the FDA has been "kind of scratching their heads" on how to evaluate gene therapies, Mulligan told me. "They're used to situations involving a conventional drug, where its toxicity can be measured, and where there are more patients and more statistics." Applications for gene therapy have continued to mount. In 1992, there were 35 applications for a gene therapy drug candidate, but in 2013, when I asked for numbers, the FDA was weighing 1200 applications. Still, the agency had yet to approve a gene therapy drug for the commercial market in the US. In 2013, the European Commission approved the first gene therapy drug in the western world. Dutch drugmaker uniQure began to market its Glybera for lipoprotein lipase deficiency. The scheme was to use an adeno-associated virus as a craft to pilot into the cells along with its cargo, a shiny new gene – in this case, a copy of a gene that builds lipoprotein lipase. Once inside a cell, the virus hid, covertly, while the cell's machinery published millions of copies of the new gene. The gene continued to be translated into functioning enzyme years after a single injection to the legs of a patient. The company soon held a secret meeting with the FDA regarding a path to market the first gene therapy drug in the US. Shortly thereafter, it signed a lease for a sparkling acre-sized plant in Lexington, Mass. At $1.6 million for single-shot gene therapy treatment, Glybera is "the most expensive drug in the world." "The idea is that Glybera is a one-time treatment," CEO Jörn Aldag told me. "If we look out five years, there should be tens approved, not hundreds" of gene therapy drugs, which provide a "routine treatment modality."

Despite 50 years of debate, gene therapy is on the verge of becoming an accepted "biologic" that is safely regulated. The FDA is expected to approve the first gene therapy treatment in the US by 2020. It will mean rescuing many very sick children, and it fulfills the promise of molecular biology, in effect, the collision of the discovery of DNA and establishment of robust public funding mechanisms through the NIH in the post-war era finally finds its ultimate success in regulated drugs that actually take effect at the molecular level of our DNA.

In fact, the NIH's RAC, which had been developed in the aftermath of Asilomar, was being phased out, and the FDA's Biologics Group was taking increasing responsibility for the regulation of human genetic engineering trials. But still, no laws exist at the federal level to explicitly forbid human cloning, or genetic engineering, in humans but gene therapy including Crispr-Cas9 is handled under existing medical drug development rules. It would be tough to regulate DNA when it is as ubiquitous as water. Many libertarians said they had the right, but others argued they have a "freedom from" genetic engineering, a right to protect the space of agricultural crops and engineered mosquitos and animals from biotech overlords who threatened to engineer all of nature. And biotech might soon provide us with a "gene as a commodity" for purposes that are not solely therapeutic. Editing and disrupting the *MC1R* gene can give your future child a shock of bright red hair. But disrupting this gene can also dispose you to a higher risk for melanoma. There are several genetic variants that are "risk factors" and provide a strong predisposition to disease, such as the e4 variant of the *APOE* gene, which increases risk for Alzheimer's disease. But the e4 allele exists at about a 25 percent frequency in the population, a surprisingly high frequency for a genetic variant which is perceived to be so risky. The reason that nature has not selected against it, may in part be explained by the fact that e4 helps in maintaining higher levels of Vitamin D, which many adults have trouble getting enough of from sunshine in northern climates[99] – my doctor recently told me to take Vitamin D supplements, for instance.

The gene *PCSK9* lowers LDL "bad cholesterol" and reduces the risk of heart attack. But it turns out that disruption of *PCSK9* might also contribute to a heightened risk for ischemic stroke, making it what geneticists call a "balanced polymorphism." Most cardiologists would like to see *PCSK9* gene expression levels trend down zero. But your neurologist might disagree, since it might dispose you to a higher risk for stroke.[100] The same dynamic is at play with the gene *CETP* which has a raft of single polymorphisms that can elevate the HDL, the so-called "good cholesterol," a situation that is endeared by cardiologists, but again, unfortunately, these genetic variants may alter your risk for stroke. Genetic variants in a gene that cause people to have sickle cell disease also provide protection against mosquito-borne malaria, and thus, many people in sub-Saharan Africa have at least one copy of the gene variant for sickle cell disease, since it also protects against malaria. A genetic variant may confer a risk for one type of phenotypic effect, but often may provide another genetic advantage. Similar tradeoffs are probably in play in regard to the larger brains that provide us with deep memories and higher order intelligence, but also dispose us to a higher risk for psychiatric disorders and existential despair. Myelination is a coating on the axons and improves the speed of synaptic connections between neurons, and it turns out that "late myelinating regions" of the evolutionarily newer parts of the brain, which receive these sheaths later in life are also those that break down the soonest and put us at risk for neurodegenerative disorders due to their high metal content.

By now, as Crispr-Cas9 was emerging, scientists were staking out their positions. Ed Lanphier, head of the powerful genome editing company Sangamo BioSciences was making halting statements, calling for reserve. Meanwhile, an English bioethicist named Julian Savulescu was arguing there wasn't anything that heretical about editing a human gene. Remember Derrick Rossi's hypothesis that "adducts" from a variety of sources, such as cigarette smoking, were riddling cells with mutations, and that those mutations may happen with high frequency in stem cells? Saveluscu and colleagues posted their opinion on a website saying "Smoking tobacco, for example, causes mutations in the DNA of sperm which are then be (sic) passed on to the next generation. Older fathers tend to pass more germline mutations on to their children than young fathers, meaning delaying paternity also increases the rate at which mutations accumulate in the human germline. The only difference is that these mutations are completely random, whereas gene editing is intentional. But if anything this should make editing more attractive. Random mutations are always indifferent to human happiness and flourishing, unlike intentional modifications. Any attempt to justify restrictions on gene editing needs to clearly explain why the risks associated with germline modifications are so great that they justify restrictions on potentially life-saving research, but do not justify restrictions of parental age, or the lifestyle habits of potential fathers."[101]

The more researchers probe our genome, the more it appears to be constantly undergoing structural rearrangements, snapping and repairing, cobbling back together like a patchworked yurt built in the wood, rather than a modern sky scraper with high fidelity to its blueprint. In the words of Stephen Jay Gould, biology is "a quirky mass of imperfections, working well enough... a jury-rigged set of adaptations built of curious parts made available by past histories in different contexts." Or, in the words of the English statistician George Box, "essentially, all models are wrong, but some are useful." The ability of the genome to reorganize and structurally rearrange itself defies intuition; it is organized chaos. Recall "double-strand breaks," widely considered the most disruptive kind of insult that can happen to our DNA. The MIT scientist Manolis Kellis showed that these breaks are not only a kind of damage, but can actually happen on purpose as part of a program to rapidly mobilize the expression of a suite of genes in the brain as a means for memory and learning.[102] And it's been known for decades that some immune system genes chaotically restructure their code to generate a stunning diversity of antibodies. In other words, breaks in our DNA happen as damage, but they also happen on purpose. The amazing thing is how frequently they happen. Cracks in a foundation, they remold and self-heal. The genome truly is a "living document."

"The human genome is not perfect," says John Harris, a bioethicist at Manchester University, in the UK. "It's ethically imperative to positively support this technology."[103] Genetic changes happen so often that it's hard to decipher the real instigators of our maladies. Matthew Porteus, of Stanford University, for instance, explained the needle-in-a-haystack problem of identifying a single point mutation that causes sickle cell disease. "In the 6 billion character, 1.1 million page, 'Book of Genome' there is a single typographical error that causes disease." Not so easy to positively identify. And while these "single nucleotide polymorphisms," are fairly common, it's exceedingly rare to find a single spelling mistake that causes a disease. Our biology is often equipped with more than one gene or structure that can substitute for a key function, a property called "degeneracy," and a gene that evolves for one function through the process of mutation can devolve into holding second, third or even fourth roles or functions. It begs the question, if genetic mutations are happening all the time, with such high frequency, and as blind or random effects, technologists argue, then it's not so wrong to make a mutational change using our own technology. Porteus notes each somatic cell that builds the bone, blood and tissues in our body undergoes about 20 double-strand breaks a day, and from one to ten mutations a day. Considering the hundreds of trillions of cells in our body, this results in an astounding one million mutations per second, occurring in any given person. No wonder 50 percent of us will get cancer. Rust never sleeps.

Germline cells that make sperm and eggs are more protected from molecular insults, but take on hundreds of mutations in our lives. As Steven Pinker noted, the problem is not so much that we can't engineer our genomes, as that genes have layered histories and function within a complex web of relationships. "Germline editing should be treated like any other medical procedure, weighing benefits against harms. It should not be banned out of a nebulous terror about tampering with a sacrosanct entity called 'the human germline' – a concept which is biological nonsense. We affect the genetic makeup of our offspring, and the species, every time we choose one sex partner over another. And each of us introduces dozens of mutations into our own germlines by exposing ourselves to everyday radiation and chemical mutagens. Genetic editing would be a droplet in the maelstrom of naturally churning genomes... The principal harm of germline editing is the risk of producing a sick or deformed child. Frankly, I suspect that this risk will always be unacceptable, so most of this discussion is moot. But suppose safety could be ensured. Should we fear the prospect of parents genetically enhancing their babies, the outcome the prohibitionists dread? This is highly unlikely – a relic of the early 1990s, when people thought there was 'a gene for' this or that talent."[104]

It's unlikely that we will engineer improvements to our intelligence or personality traits, but it may provide small protective advantages, and in some outlying instances, it will be used to treat very serious illnesses. As I continued researching and writing, the gravity of what was happening started to hit me. In interviewing more than 40 scientists, doctors and patients involved in gene engineering in humans, I started out writing a book that centered on themes, but ended up building one that was structured chronologically. This book starts out highly documented, sourcing key experiments, and breaks into a format that is less documented and based on real-time current events relayed through experience and conversation. Its format owes something to Benno Müller-Hill, who characterized the "two faces" of molecular biology. "In the textbooks, almost everything is solved and clear. Most claims are so self-evident that no proofs are given. Old, classical experiments disappear... The other face of molecular biology is seen at scientific conference or read in research issues"[105] and amounts to work that emerges out of our deficit in knowledge with implications that are not yet clear. Or take, as Robert Pogue Harrison suggested, the metaphor of "two angels," drawing on Paul Klee's painting rendered famous in Walter Benjamin's Theses on the Philosophy of History which depicts an "angel of history borne upward through the air on outspread wings, facing backward. In Benjamin's vision, all the angel sees are the accumulated ruins of the has-been." He goes on to suggest that "science flies on the wing of another kind of angel – the angel of neoteny – who weaves in and out of enfolded spaces, forever turning a corner or rounding a bend, entering or exiting a crease of the cosmos, such that his expectant, forward-looking gaze sees a new world it has seen countless times before, always as if for the first time."

"Although memory engenders the storm in paradise that draws both angels upward, the angel of neoteny sees what the counterpart cannot see."[106] This brushes up against the perennial problems in philosophy: whether truth lies in memory or body. Particulate nature has no history, as scientists say: it has a "Markov property" of "memorylessness," but there are human histories, and our legacies, which put upon us a burden to endure, to learn and to master, a kind of transgenerational ownership. As Harrison notes, we don't get to be creative or participate in the genius that is often characterized as "domain-altering innovation" until we comprehend and master the domains that pre-exist. Thus, he reminds us, that we begin to innovate by sinking down into our depths and the wealth of insights and resources that exist before us. "Timeless truths do not exist," but there exist "books so pregnant with meaning that they never finish saying what they have to say." Dante once met a 1300-year-old ghost named Virgil who showed him the only way up the mountain leads downward before it leads upward. "To inherit the future we must hold to another path than the one that leads straight toward its blinding light – a path that circles back and descends into the past, away from the entanglements of the present, before it breaks into the futures *vita nuova*." Technology is agnostic to human history, reshaping and redefining the modalities of work and life, opening up new frontiers, and that's why there is this tension, since it redefines the terrain of our legacy and "shifts its paradigms," to borrow a phrase from Thomas Kuhn, a kind of disruption that breaks rank with existing dogma, standards and practices. As the pioneering scientists Janet Mertz and Paul Berg commented, workable biotechnology "methods," such as Crispr-Cas9, are perhaps more important than a disruptive idea in that it is a tool or device. "Freeman Dyson contrasts what he called the 'Kuhnian'and 'Galisonian' views of the origins of scientific revolutions in a review of Peter Galison's book, Einstein's Clocks, Poincare's Maps: Empires of Time. In The Structure of Scientific Revolutions, Thomas Kuhn proposes that revolutionary breakthroughs in science are triggered primarily by ideas that, by their novelty, transform or replace the prevailing paradigm (Kuhn 1962). By contrast, Galison (2003) attributes such breakthroughs to new tools that, by their nature, make possible new approaches to formerly intractable problems. Galison also acknowledges that the application of existing tools in novel ways often provides the means to explore what was previously impossible."[107]

Likewise, the pioneering geneticist Alfred Hershey has been quoted as saying, "there is nothing more satisfying to me than developing a method. Ideas come and go, but a method lasts." Importantly, Crispr-Cas9 was an easy and highly efficient method, which came with standard protocols which would be widely distributed in a very short amount of time. Despite whether the methods or ideas are credited with initiating a lasting transition, the "old problems" of biology relate exclusively to gaining insight into its mechanisms, and shaping its populations through regulation of pregnancy, eugenics and care of the aging. Early on in the course of genetics, the problems of technology and control over our biology were intractable. In 1924, the Harvard geneticist William Castle quipped that "we are scarcely as yet in a position to do more than make ourselves ridiculous in this matter. We are no more in a position to control eugenics than the tides of the ocean." Castle's skepticism still prevails, or at least, it should. But now, the "new genetics" thrusts us over a new threshold and into an era where we might control and master our biology. It shifts the terrain. We begin to engage with a whole new set of fine-grained ethical problems, which cannot be entirely informed by our legacy. As the ethicist Jonathan Moreno writes, "The old politics of biology operated in the dark about the underlying mechanisms in question. The new politics of biology arise in the midst of a rapidly growing understanding of basic life processes, with seemingly limitless opportunities to direct individual and social change."[108]

In fact, the new politics are decades old. "It is important to note that this debate has happened before. Indeed, it has happened multiple times, in response to each incremental step toward the ability to create changes in the human genome that are inheritable down the generations," The Hinxton Group, an international consortium on stem cells, ethics and law, wrote in a well-regarded report. "While the ethical issues raised by this prospect remain unchanged, the context in which they now arise is dramatically different. In comparison with earlier techniques, modern genome editing technologies and Crispr-Cas9 in particular are not only very precise, but also easy, inexpensive, and, critically, very efficient... In addition, since the last round of debates, other areas of science and medicine have likewise advanced; for example, we can now sequence entire genomes quickly and inexpensively. Further, there is increased acceptance and use of techniques of assisted conception, which are likely to be required for the use of genome editing in human embryos. As a consequence, and especially given the recent experience with purported stem cell-based 'treatments' in unregulated clinics, there is serious concern that genome editing technologies might be used in reproductive contexts long before there are data sufficient to support such use, and before the international community has had the opportunity to weigh the benefits and harms of moving forward." Today, the stakes are higher, immediate and real. As Eric Lander defined the moment "it's hard to recall a revolution that has swept biology more swiftly than Crispr."

On or around the time of Asilomar, when the first restriction enzymes appeared on the scene and enabled scientists to splice genes, a legal ethicist named Peter Barton Hutt raised a curious, but beguilingly simple question. "Could these experiments be performed by a high school science teacher?" The increasing flexibility and ease of the Crispr-Cas9 system means that science is poised to exceed technically what it may not yet have grappled with emotionally and ethically. If scientists throughout the world are able to tamper with heritable code, some will probably do it. "Science has made us gods even before we are worthy of being men," wrote the scientist and philosopher Jean Rostand, 70 years ago. Today we face an emerging reality that technological feats are achieving an ease of application that will make these warnings salient, relevant and slightly surreal. We will rewrite our own genetic code. The genie is out of the bottle, and despite our best legal interventions and foresight, the "Hutt question" may prove to be the most relevant of our times. I thought about these issues for a long time, whether the ease-of-use of genome editing tools made it futile to try to regulate, or whether it made policy-setting more urgent. Finally, I decided to contact a legal expert, and I knew just who to contact, Peter Barton Hutt, who I found, 40 years after his initial comments, through a law firm in DC. His response did nothing to ease my mind. "The relative ease of gene editing makes the legal issues *more* important," he wrote to me in an email. "From the earliest days of recombinant DNA technology, it was clear to me both that this day would come and that it is impossible to ban/completely control any new scientific process. We are simply entering a new era where there is no precedent. Civilization will be confronting unknowable consequences."

2   The Gene Trade

It was an absolutely stunning surprise to us that something as strange as viruses carrying genes from one cell to another can happen.

–Joshua Lederberg[109]

In 1939, Ephraim Anderson enrolled in the British Army. He was posted to the Middle East. "That actually was a place I wanted to go to, because my father had been there in the First World War and we had family in what was then Palestine. And I wanted to have a look anyway. I'd been, shall we say, pestered by Zionists in one way or another since childhood, on the whole I haven't been a Zionist, but I was just curious to see what was going on. I was a Regimental Medical Officer and Field Ambulance, with, in fact, the Seventh Armored Division, the original 'Desert Rats.' I don't know whether you've heard of them..."[110]

It was decades later, in the 1970s, that he'd retell his story to Charles Weiner, a professor of history of science and technology at the Massachusetts Institute of Technology. Weiner was part of a team of journalists and historians who assembled an oral history on the mounting science of "recombinant DNA" that surfaced at that time, unleashing powerful new technology to engineer life. It resulted in nearly 100 boxes of audio and transcripts from scientists throughout the world, deposited in the archive collections at MIT, which I was now poring through, reading. There are strict rules in the archives. It is practically a detention center. A lamp is fixed to the table. No coffee. It's pin-drop silent. You can only use a pencil. Myles and Nora are archivists in great standing with me, but they're bluestockings, straight-laced about the permanent ink and coffee. I would read for four hours and then sneak out into the hallway and chug a coffee in about two minutes. My head would be spinning, and then I would go back in, and hit the next folder.

I already knew a few things. Anderson was born to Estonian-Jewish immigrants in a working-class area of Newcastle-upon-Tyne on the northeast coast of England. He won a scholarship to medical school and graduated at the age of 22, "sweeping up major prizes along the way." Growing up in the rough-and-tumble 1930s, he had "a great gift for rubbing folk up the wrong way. That he was brusque and, on occasions, downright rude was perhaps because he had to fight for everything," the Guardian newspaper had once said.[111] After five years of working as a physician, he joined the British Army, the Royal Medical Corps, traipsing through Cairo and Cyprus, tracking down the sources of diseases that wracked the military, notably, typhoid fever, while embedded with his legendary division. He would come to see firsthand how microbes put the slip on antibiotics. As once-potent antibiotics became feckless and ineffectual, there was an increasing appreciation that microbes had an ability to undergo "fast evolution," or "saltationism," to borrow a term from early debates on evolution, to gain resistance to drugs. Most people know that it's important to continue to take the full course of antibiotics, since a small number of infectious microbes may mutate and develop resistance to the antibiotic during its treatment course. Those rogue microbes may then promulgate through the population, while the antibiotic is less effective. But Anderson and peers would show this evolutionary arms race is even more pitched than that.

Microbes that mutate and develop resistance to an antibiotic can share or transfer some of their antibiotic resistant genes to weaker microbes in a feat called "gene transfer." And so, Anderson was one of the first scientists to sound a clarion call about the promiscuous use of antibiotics in agriculture and medicine, and how that might be undermining the few effective tools that doctors had, while escalating this arms race against infectious diseases, even giving rise to "super bugs," which were resistant to just about any form of antibiotic treatment. In the summer of 2015, I had been to a talk by Eric Lander, director of the Broad Institute, on his work drafting a report on antibiotic resistance for President Barack Obama. That's how persistent this problem is. I was newly alive to the debate on antibiotics, but it goes back at least to the 1940s. At that time, Anderson was in Cairo. He was trying to hold his medic unit together, keep instruments sterile, and investigate how infectious microbes cause disease. The Nazis were killing people, but so was infection.

"And, eventually, about the middle of the war, it was one of those coincidences," Anderson said. "We were short of disinfectant and I suddenly got the idea of making electrolytic hypochlorite, using old carbon battery anodes and common salt solution which was just about the only thing we had plenty of; we had plenty of salt, that is. And so, I made gallons and gallons and supplied units all around for a long distance with this stuff, and it was rather a joke, really. But the man who was at that time Deputy Assistant Director of Pathology, D.A.D.P., was in charge of the laboratory at what was called the 15th Scottish Hospital at Aguza, in Cairo. I had been talking to him about this; we were, at that time, at base. And I was doing calculations of chlorine content, and so on, with a man from the University of Giza – it used to be called Fuad el Awal, it means Fuad the First, University – but, in fact, it's now, I think, called Cairo University because they've dropped kings and things. And he was rather taken by this stunt that I'd been pulling of preparing unlimited quantities of disinfectant for virtually nothing. It was like Milton – I don't know whether you know what Milton is; it is, in fact, an electrolyzed saline solution which contains hypochlorite. It's the same sort of stuff. Whether it was the same strength or not I don't know. There's a limit to the concentration of chlorine you can get because of the instability of hypochlorite. But it was very useful stuff. It's very active."

The deputy assistant was so charmed by Anderson's feat of making disinfectant out of salt and old battery anodes, that he gave the 30 year old medic a chance to do more science. "And so he sent me a message saying they were proposing to start up a course in pathology and was I interested? And so, within a fortnight I was out of the unit and into the lab. I stayed in labs for the rest of the war, for about the last three years, or so. I remember, I saw the thing build up until there were over a million men; I came in '40 – to the Middle East – 1940. I saw it build up until there were over a million men there. And I saw it dwindle until the only relics of the British and other Allied Armies were the flapping sackcloth of the empty latrines, along the Canal. I saw that and I got a nostalgic effect; it was a pity to see that all we could leave behind was excreta and banners to mark the spot, so to speak.

During the war, once I got into lab work, I went to work in Jerusalem with a man called Saul Adler. Adler was a Leeds Jew, who was a great Zionist, a great linguist, a great man. He was a parasitologist, certainly one of the world's greatest. And, in fact, it was he who made the original observation that Kala-azar was carried by the sand fly, in the case of Mediterranean Kala-azar."[112]

Adler had set out plucking flies from animals, dissecting the flies to search for traces of parasite. "He showed me his very, very beautiful preparations, serial sections of the sand flies. Very remarkable; a work of art, you know, the way he'd done this. He was essentially a research man; his feet were not firmly on the ground until you thought they weren't, so to speak. He had a disconcerting way of suddenly showing that he was aware of what went on. In fact, I moved over to Cyprus as a pathologist to a hospital at one part of my career, and they had still, at that time, Kala-azar in Cyprus, and I got the government to invite Alder over. We had a hilarious set of excursions at night looking for sand flies in the Morphou Bay area which is now occupied by the Turks. And I shall never forget the sight of Adler with an inverted test tube and a torch; test tube in one hand, torch in the other, prowling over the immense body of a sleeping sow, to which about – I forget how many teats a sow has, but there was certainly a piglet hanging on to every one of them also fast asleep, and it was hilarious in the extreme to watch the way he was solemnly going over the body looking for a sand fly." Anderson describes the scene at nightfall. Adler was immersed in the pig, picking over its belly in search for a disease-carrying fly as the "stereotype of the scientist, totally unaware of the fact that it was a comic picture."

Morphou Bay is on the northerly side of the island of Cyprus, cast in the Mediterranean Sea, in a subtropical climate with 400 species of birds. Citadels stand at the foot of penetrating blue waters, a collision of ancient ruins and modern city ports, and above all, jutting out of sea level in the background, is Mount Olympus. The two scientists were plying the northern coast of Cyprus, conducting lab work in the day, and then stealing away at nightfall to collect sandflies from sleeping pigs and dogs. Kala-azar, black fever or dumdum fever, are common names for visceral leishmaniasis, a disease caused by a protozoan parasite. The sand fly would serve as a vector carrying the parasite from animal to human, causing a fever, weight loss, fatigue and anemia.

One Saturday night, they had dinner in the port city of Kyrenia at the Dome Hotel. As sky burst into a starlight ceiling, giving them a chance to break away, they slipped through the alleyways looking for flies. "One house we came to, there was a large man prone on the ground in front of the house door, and sitting on the step was a small boy. Now, I don't speak Greek, nor did Adler, but there were four of us in the party; one of the other two was a Greek scholar, in fact, an Englishman. And he said to the small boy, translating for us as he went:

'Who is this man lying here?'

The small boy said, 'He is my father.'

'Why is he like that?'

'He's drunk.'

'Does he do this often?'

'No, only every Saturday night.'

'And do you always look after him.'

'Yes, I do.'

"And, this was perfectly sober conversation. Anyway, we left the drunk. I remember, it was most extraordinary the way we managed to get ourselves into bedrooms at about half-past-eleven at night, without the people, apparently, thinking we were anything but slightly mad... We found our sand flies, all right. And we found the Leishmania. The reservoir on Cyprus is the dog. One of the British Government official's wives came to us with her dog and she said it wasn't well at all, and she'd heard that we were interested in sick dogs. And, true enough, it was absolutely stiff with *Leishmania donovani*."

Anderson carried out his stint in the Mediterranean as the jackbooted continent was tumbled in war. He had entered the Army as a medical doctor, and also became a captain, and then a major, and a graded pathologist. As the battlefront was surging with Panzer tanks, back in the United States, science was proceeding at an inexorable pace. Firstly, scientists were racing to understand how infectious diseases emerged and were transmitted in the human population. Secondly, scientists were driven by an interest to gain insight into manmade causes of damage to our biological blueprint, born from an emerging atomic program. Warren Weaver, a US scientist and polymath in the early 1930s "persuaded Alexander Hollaender, a highly regarded radiobiologist, to survey the literature and write a report for The Rockefeller Foundation on the biological effects of radiation," recounts the science historian Errol Friedberg in an essay. "In so doing, Hollaender evaluated close to 5000 papers in the field, an effort that lent important impetus to the establishment of federal financial support for radiation biology in the United States. During the Manhattan Project and the ultimate emergence of the atomic bomb, laboratories dedicated to radiation research were established in several parts of the country, with the primary objective of learning how individuals exposed to ionizing (and other types of) radiation might be protected... radiobiological research was indeed dominated by simple survival curves, graphs that quantitated the killing effects of exposure to radiation in different cells and tissues in multiple organisms. Although largely descriptive, such meager data generated many bold speculations."[113]

In 1941, working out of Stanford University, George Beadle and Edward Tatum used radiation in an experiment to show that genetic code or instructions for proteins was packaged in discrete units, allowing scientists to conceive of genes as discrete units in a cell.[114] Beadle and Tatum had shot the opening salvo.[115] Genetics was now more than a theory. It was a practice. Norman Horowitz, a collaborator, codified their work as the "one-gene–one-enzyme hypothesis," suggesting that each gene is represented in a single enzyme, which in turn affects a single step in a metabolic pathway. Horowitz recalled that "these experiments founded the science of what Beadle and Tatum called 'biochemical genetics.' In actuality they proved to be the opening gun in what became molecular genetics and all the developments that have followed from that."

Consensus did not yet exist on the nature of a "master template" of nature, and questions remained how such simple molecules could result in such a stunning array of proteins with swirling structures.[116] Proteins held countless functions, such as transmitting cellular signals; enzymes were action molecules that cut or activated other molecules as "substrates." And, antibodies came in an astounding array of structures to clasp and target a substrate, or antigen, on virtually any invading pathogen in the natural world, focusing the intensity of the immune system on a precise target. Because proteins are diverse, on the order of hundreds of thousands, antibodies on the order of one billion, many scientists had stuck with the prevailing dogma that enzymes, antibodies, and the like, *acquired* their shape and function by locking onto their target substrate, or antigen. In 1894, Emil Fisher, one of the great organic chemists, had offered just such a metaphor, suggesting that a substrate and enzyme worked as a "lock and key." An enzyme was therefore a sort of key which opened the lock of the substrate, by molding and taking its shape. The idea that biological features or structures were acquired, learned or educated, traced back further to Jean-Baptiste Lamarck. But, at the turn of the century, August Weismann had advanced his "germ plasm" theory, making the important distinction between "germ cells," later called "gametes," such as sperm and ovum which transmit heritable information, and "somatic cells" which build muscles, organs and bones. The insight was that people could acquire strength, intelligence, but also, say, cancer, during their lifetimes, such traits could be learned, strengthened or "instructed," but the acquisitions of these "somatic" features would not be passed on to future generations because the heritable code was transferred through a *separate* line of germ cells. Weismann (should have) buried the idea of the heritability of acquired traits. But Lamarckism would not go gently into that good night.

The stakes couldn't be higher as these competing ideas were coming to a head in the 1930s. As the scientist Benno Müller-Hill so pointedly noted, "In Germany, geneticists and the Nazis had presented a rather special anti-Semitic, Darwinian, anti-Lamarckian world view. According to them, human genetics determined the fate of humanity. In particular, the Nordic race, i.e., the race of which the Germans belonged, was superior. In contrast, the communists claimed that education (i.e. environment) is everything and that even plants and animals could be "educated." Their Soviet spokesman, Trofim Lysenko, claimed that Mendelian genetics was a fraud pushed by capitalists."[117]

The scholar Jonathan Moreno noted in the United States, that the founding fathers, a "group of scientists," were persuaded by "fallibilism," the principle that, "with the possible exceptions of logic and mathematics, no scientific account of the world of experience can achieve absolute precision." In the US, this created a climate of rationalizing the removal of the "unfit" for taxpayer benefit, and employed social engineering through tinkering with biology: eugenics. "Taken together, these possible results of policies unconstrained by fallibilism and excessive state identification with a certain biological philosophy were vividly illustrated by state-sanctioned sterilization in America and "scientifically" justified genocide in Germany. So, too, were they shown through the fraudulent claims initiated in the midst of the 1920s Soviet famine by the agronomist Trofim Lysenko. As Lysenko persuaded Communist authorities that acquired characteristics could be inherited, the result was the censure and death of hundreds of opponents, the cessation of scientific research on genetics, and the ultimate setback of Russian biology for generations."[118]

Daniel Kevles, a legal historian from New York University, has noted that although a hundred thousand people were sterilized in Nazi Germany, "long before that, sterilization of unfit occurred in Britain, Scandinavia, the United States; it could and *did* happen everywhere." This was the emergence of social Darwinism. In fact, the word "eugenics" was coined by Francis Galton, in Kelves words, based on the "ideal of improving the human race, getting rid of undesirables, and enjoyed the high professional authority of Charles B. Davenport, a eugenicist and its principle proponent at Cold Spring Harbor, with doctrines propagated by Irving Fisher, Thomas Hunt Morgan and Alexander Graham Bell, who widely popularized the cause in books to rid communities of alcoholism, pauperism." The eugenics movement was "energized by fear of degeneration of society by feeble minded people, who were responsible for a wide range of social problems, and in fact, threatened social stability. Poverty and criminality were attributed to bad genes, and concerns of immigrants of Europe, social fear and the costs of welfare." In 1926, the American Eugenics Society put up a display with lights at a fair that showed that every 15 seconds $100 goes to care for one of its citizens with "bad heredity."

"Negative eugenics" was a term that connoted the removal of biologically feeble genes from the population (think sterilizations or gas chambers). "Positive eugenics sought to promote socially good genes, manipulate their distribution in the population to create superior or healthy people," drawing on the legacy of the British polymath J.B.S. Haldane. In the United States, positive eugenics captured the imagination in the Fitter Family Contest in Texas. Exhibits appeared at the Kansas Free Fair in 1929. One poster pleaded for fair goers to do with their children at least as they did breeding their livestock. "How long are we Americans to be so careful for the pedigree of our pigs and chickens and cattle, and then leave the ancestry of our children to chance, or blind sentiment?" Another listed a litany of "feeblemindedness, epilepsy, criminality, insanity, alcoholism, pauperism" and stating frankly that "if all marriages were eugenic we could breed out most of this unfitness in three generations." It was a utilitarian argument. Alcoholism, disease and feeblemindedness were cost burdens to taxpayers. By 1924, in the United States of America of all places, two dozen states had enacted sterilization laws, which tended to work against lower income and minority groups, which came to a Federal level in the 1927 case Buck vs. Bell, a decision that has never been explicitly repudiated. Carrie Buck was a plaintiff in the case, as she was ordered to be sterilized while in prison. Oliver Wendell Holmes wrote in the decision, "it is better for all the world, if instead of waiting to execute degenerate offspring for crime, or to let them starve for the imbecility, society can prevent those who are manifestly unfit from continuing their kind... three generations of imbeciles are enough." In truth, Buck grew up a poor woman, and was raped at age 17 by the nephew of her foster patents. She became pregnant with a daughter named Vivian Dobbs, who turned out to be a student who scored in the middle of her class with good grades in reading and spelling.

But social and judicial leaders were becoming quite comfortable mining nature for a justification for eugenics and upholding a status quo. As Moreno quipped, people love putting things in boxes, they love order. Genetics gave them that. But it was a mere impression. As the nineteenth-century biologist T.H. Huxley put it, "nature is no school of virtue." The war emerged amid and between those boxes, the low-lying violence and tension between classes. There was, already, a nativist impulse within the Jewish community, which was defined as "Jewish exceptionalism." The Nazis also wanted to claim preferred status. As Slavoj Zizek wrote, "Was it not already Schoenberg who dismissed Nazi racism as a miserable imitation of the Jewish identity as the chosen people?" These impulses to draw on ethnic identity are subconscious even for discerning thinkers. As Steven Shapin[119] wrote in his incisive essay in the *Boston Review*, "Everybody knows that the prescriptive world of *ought* – the moral or the good – belongs to a different domain than the descriptive world of *is*." Shapin reminds us this "naturalistic fallacy" is no new insight. David Hume in the 1730s noted that "it was common for a writer to begin with 'ordinary ways of reasoning' – and then, all of the sudden, and without remarking on it, there would be an imperceptible change" and the author would move from writing about what is or is not to writing about what ought to be or ought not be. But the *is* and the *ought* belong to different orders; it is "altogether inconceivable," Hume noted, "that you could deduce the one from the other."[120]

Everyone knows this, of course, but our subconscious seems to press the issue of racism into reality. The conflation of genes and race with hygienic descriptions such as "clean," or moral descriptions such as "valued," seem to be wired into our mentalities, even in our "modern" era. In the spring of 2016, a television commercial for Qiaobi laundry detergent was regularly running in China, in which an Asian woman shoves a detergent pod into the mouth of a black man, and then tumbles him headfirst into a washing machine. After a cycle, she opens the machine, and to her pleasant surprise, a pale, smiling and rather handsome young Asian man emerges from the washing machine with a wink. The female consumer is delighted, and the message is clear: sexual preference for a mate who is akin to us drives our motivations far more than the conscious maxim of social equity and fairness. Racial cleansing is something that the female consumer prefers, not consciously, but subconsciously, through her choice in a mate. Qiaobi wants to let consumers know this is secretly OK. And, they hope you buy their washing detergent.

The idea that biology is somehow instructive to morality seems to be deeply wired in our thinking, although the philosophers noted that mechanisms of biology could not be used as a prescription for how to live into modernity with its nauseating freedom, or serve in an external locus of control. Biology provided for big brains with trusts of plasticity, but it also was not groundless or formless. Recall that Fisher had suggested such with his metaphor of an interlocking substrate and enzyme, and by extension, the antibody and antigen, working as a "lock and key." Enzymes were considered to be pliable material with a property of self-replication with both quantities and functions that could be "learned" or "instructed." Sol Spiegelman suggested some mechanism was "kicking on the self-replication of enzymes." The German biochemist Schoenheimer spoke of the "dynamic state of living matter." In the words of Benno Müller-Hill, "proteins seemed not to be stable, but in a process of constant turnover, new assembly and construction."[121] How did enzymes and antibodies go into production? "A tentative explanation was given by John Yudkin (Cambridge, England)..." who "proposed that enzymes folded round their substrates and that the speed of enzyme synthesis depended on substrate-assisted folding, i.e., the presence of the substrates. This theory – Yudkin called it the mass action theory – was generally accepted. Karl Landsteiner adapted it without quoting it, to explain antibody production. The great Linus Pauling used it too, without quoting it as part of his detailed explanation for the synthesis of specific antibodies. The concept was also called the *instructive theory.* The immunologists believed that possibly all antibodies had the same sequence but just folded differently upon stimulation by antigen. Thus one could visualize inducers as instructing a protein to fold in a specific manner to become catalytically active."[122]

But, *instructive theory* was soon dead. If Beadle and Tatum had shot the opening salvo, more research would soon riddle the theory to pieces. In 1943, Oswald Avery, along with physician colleagues Colin MacLeod and Maclyn McCarty, developed methods of chemical analysis that showed genes were built from a sticky macromolecule of sugary bases composed of carbon, hydrogen, nitrogen and phosphoric acid. This complex was deoxyribonucleic acid, or DNA.[123] Armed with new technologies to probe the microsphere, scientists were turning toward simpler forms of life. As the war churned on, James Watson (an American), Max Delbrück (a German) and Salvador Luria (an Italian, and a Sephardic Jew) had converged in New York City at the Cold Spring Harbor Laboratory as the "phage group." These scientists had come to believe that the study of a virus that infects a microbe – a bacteriophage, sometimes just called a "phage" – would provide fertile ground to study cells at a molecular level. The "Luria–Delbrück experiment," as it became known, showed that genetic variations in microbes must follow Darwinian, and not Lamarckian, principles. In short, mutations can occur randomly in microbes which bestow resistance to infection by phages, and natural selection can be used as a model to explain the development of such resistances. In other words, a trait such as resistance is not learned or acquired, but rather, it is engendered by mutations to a microbe's own genetic material. The chemical nature of genes was declared. Natural selection won its day in court. It had to be accepted, since its theory explained how microbes could develop pathogenic qualities and resistance to antibiotics. And developments in the field converged with a remarkable new political will to fund science.

That same year, a key political event happened when Franklin Delano Roosevelt issued a directive to his chief of wartime research, Dr. Vannevar Bush, telling him to find a way to continue federal funding of medical and scientific research after the war. Bush busily drafted a report to the president, which would be titled *Science the Endless Frontier*, which included soaring language about how the American West had largely been settled, but that "the frontier of science remains," and going so far as to insist that science was deeply intertwined with the tenets of democracy: "without scientific progress we could not have maintained our liberties against tyranny." This led to the nationalization of research, robust public funding through the National Institutes of Health, and the creation of the National Science Foundation. The identification of the chemical nature of genes was now coupled with a powerful national engine of finance to drive research, and it resulted in a florid expansion of work and a briskly expanding network of scientists.[124] Warren Weaver had christened the emerging field "molecular biology." Roosevelt died in office in spring 1945 of a cerebral hemorrhage. Harry Truman made use of the directive by repurposing wartime research labs, as he "designated these entities as national laboratories and placed them under the aegis of the newly created Atomic Energy Commission. In time, the laboratories became the breeding grounds for many early contributors to the emerging fields of DNA repair and mutagenesis."[125]

Beadle and Tatum had used radiation to determine that genes were discrete packets of information by showing that radiation damage could compromise an essential gene product in a bread mold, creating a dependency for an amino acid before the mold would grow again. The phage school would conduct similar experiments to show that other gene products were important for "cell maintenance" and "DNA repair," while compromising these gateway genes led to molecular breakdown and could help to explain the initiation of cancer. In Friedberg's words, "In time, a number of celebrated investigators interested primarily in understanding how genes function, including Max Delbrück, Salvador Luria, and Hermann Muller, originated experiments that, while continuing to make extensive use of survival curves, led to the discovery that the killing effects of exposure to ionizing radiation or UV light are profoundly influenced by the inactivation of certain genes. Thus, the notion of DNA repair was born."[126]

Bush's elevation of science as a potent source of purpose, industry and self-esteem in American life was not restricted to the new space industry, but also saw its articulation in newly surging biology and medical fields. It was then, more than ever, that innovation became institutionalized and officially anointed as a particular component of the American spirit. As Shapin wrote, science and scientists were in the midst of a long process of growing up that seemed to reach a decisive moment of organization, which was crystalized in the coupling of science with robust funding engines. Questions began to emerge whether scientists could retain their *Veritas* and give us the facts if they were boggled by money, biotech and winner-take-all grants. "Even after the Second World

War, and the increasing inclusion of American scientists in the materially comfortable middle classes, there were still researchers who expressed concerns about the rise of professionalism and the decline of scientific asceticism: "the 'true scientist,'" the cancer researcher Frederick S. Hammett reminded us in *Science*, is "only concerned with following his vocation." Even in the mid-1950s the physicist Karl Compton said of scientists in general, "I don't know of any other group that has less interest in monetary gain..."[127] But "by the end of the early twentieth century, scientists were increasingly employed by research laboratories attached to large industrial corporations and government establishments, often with ties to the military. From the 1940s, American sociologists were beginning to give accounts of something newly designated as 'the scientific community.'" And while the sociologist Robert Merton discerned in the "norms" of this community many of the values of a liberal, meritocratic and open society, he insisted that there is no "satisfactory evidence" that scientist are "recruited from the ranks of those who exhibit an unusual degree of moral integrity."[128] In conversation, beginning in the end of the twentieth century, science was regularly coupled with its mechanisms of production and modes of revenue "science and industry" or "science and technology." Legions of soldiers were returning home from the war, their spit-shine and elbow grease redirected to domestic goals, putting a man on the Moon, building highways, and curing cancer and infectious disease.

In 1945, the dust was settling from the war. Ephraim Anderson returned to civilian life. He found no special privilege. "Really, I suppose, I was being rehabilitated after six years of army life. It was a rude awakening to have to clean my own shoes and look after myself, cook my own food or pay for it, and so on, instead of being – well, I was a major when I left the Army and I had, of course, my own personal servant most of the war. Our creature comforts were looked after, insofar as it was possible, wherever we were, even when we were in the field. So, it was something to find that I had to stand on my own feet and to work for myself and, as I said, clean my own shoes; this was the ultimate indignity. And to beg for cigarettes, because I smoked in those days and they were in short supply; to go to the tobacconists who kept them under the counter for those prepared to pay more."

Anderson wouldn't have long to fret and beg for cigarettes. "When I got back I was pitch-forked into an investigation of a typhoid epidemic," he recalled. The work of the phage school was changing the way that epidemiologists tracked pathogens. Anderson had heard the term "phage type" bandied about, but admitted that at the time "I really didn't know what it meant." Phages, of course, are viruses that infect microbes. "Phage typing" was a means to track a specific strain of typhoid throughout a human population, simply by identifying the type of phage that infected the strain. If there were multiple typhoid carriers, and each of the samples had different phage types, it might mean to the epidemiologists that there were multiple infectious strains of typhoid on the loose in the population, and this lent more knowledge for their treatment.[129] "Well, they kept getting typhoid outbreaks, but they weren't the same phage type," Anderson recalled. This gave investigators a clue there might be various strains of microbe causing the outbreaks. And so, now a civilian scientist, Anderson set out to investigate the science of phage typing.

"When I got back from the Middle East, one of the first things I did was to ring up the man running this laboratory (in London), a man called Arthur Felix. Now Arthur Felix is a romance all to himself. Because he was born in Poland, was in the Austrian Army in the First World War, he was the co-originator of the Weil-Felix test for typhus, of which you may or may not have heard, I don't know, but this dates back to 1915."[130]

Felix "was a great Zionist. He went to Palestine after the First World War. He expected to get the Chair at the Hebrew University when it was founded, the Chair in Microbiology. It went instead to an American, because the Americans were putting far more money into the foundation of the university than anyone else and so they really owned the bigger vote. That was too much for Felix – so he packed his bags and came to England where he worked at the Lister Institute (in London) from about 1925." Felix discovered the Vi antigen, which led to Vi-typing, a way to classify a strain of salmonella typhoid by its type of antigen, or serotype. This was "a very important antigen, which he believed, at any rate, to be concerned with the virulence of typhoid" and was used to identify dangerous strains of the microbe.[131] "He was quite positive but then, Felix was quite a positive man."

Anderson wanted to talk to Felix about a new strategy for tracking infectious microbes: phage typing. Anderson recalled that "the only thing

I have to say is that Felix himself was not enthusiastic, at first, about it; he thought it was a waste of time. I telephoned Felix and asked if I could come up. And as I was later dumbfounded to realize, he said yes. Because he wouldn't allow... he was very German, in many ways; Prussian in his outlook, very rigid, unbending. To the last day of his association with me he never called me Anderson or Andy; I was Dr. Anderson and I had to call him Dr. Felix; he was very much the Herr Direktor, you see. But he said I could come." Anderson hinted that the phage might be mobile and that it might change properties of the bacteria, causing it to be pathogenic. To Felix, however, this was nonsense. He believed the phage was fixed in its nature. "Felix was a very dogmatic man; to him there was something about the phage-types which was almost holy. When I'd finished working here for a fortnight I said to him, I'd like to come and work here."

"And he said, 'I'm sorry, there is nothing more to be done in this subject. You have come too late. The whole thing is worked out.'"

But things were about to get fascinating, as scientists went crashing through an edifice. The logic had it that genes are only transferred in a linear line from generation to generation, in parent to offspring, but it was soon to be augmented with a new logic that genes could be transformed "horizontally" between species in the same generation in a vast network of gene exchange.

In 1946 and 1947, the French scientist Joshua Lederberg took a leave of absence to study with Edward Tatum at Yale University. The scientists showed that *Escherichia coli* could swap, or transfer, genetic material through a process called "conjugation" or "conjugal mating." The bacteria, it was later learned, did this by opening small portals, as one bacterium slipped a circular piece of DNA into a second bacterium.[132] In 1952, Lederberg gave the name "plasmids" to these circularized extrachromosomal genetic elements (their circular structure wouldn't be determined for another decade).[133] Further work by Ester Lederberg, published in conjunction with her husband, would show that plasmids, which were also called episomes to convey their situation of being free-floating circularized genetic constructs that were not part of a hardcoded chromosome, actually conveyed a "sex" or gender of bacteria. Yes, it's true. Bacteria have a gender. Ester Lederberg discovered one type of plasmid is called an F-factor, which means fertility factor.[134] A bacteria with an F-factor plasmid acts as a male donor cell, and a bacteria without an F-factor plasmid in most cases acts as a recipient cell. In what was a whirlwind year, Lederberg and

Norton Zinder also reported that genetic material could also be transferred from one strain of bacterium *Salmonella typhimurium* to another by using a phage as an intermediate step to transfer the material, a process called "transduction."[135] To do this, the phage could capture a gene from a microbe that it was infecting as a sort of cargo, and then install that gene into the next microbe that it infected. And this was not an anomaly. A couple of years later, Lederberg also showed that genes could be traded between *E. coli* through the proxy of a phage called *lambda*. And, on the other coast, in Seattle, a scientist named Victor Feenian showed that a dangerous gene from a phage could be popped into *C. diphtheriae*, thus transforming the microbe from an innocent non-virulent strain into a virulent strain that causes the toxic nerve-stunning disease diphtheria. In other words, a gene had been transferred from a virus to a bacterium. By the end of the decade, scientists in Japan would show that different species of bacteria were trading genes to confer antibiotic resistance.

In "generalized transduction," as a virus multiplies in a host cell of a bacterium, "random segments of the infected cell's DNA are also incorporated into newly formed virus particles in place of viral DNA," Janet Mertz wrote. If this phage-bacteria hybrid molecule enters a new bacterium it "recombines at low frequency with the cell's chromosome to become a permanent part of that cell's genetic makeup... In this way, any part of the genome of one *E. coli* strain can be transferred to the genome of another *E. coli* strain."[136] By comparison, "specialized transduction" occurs when lambda phage DNA integrates into the infected cell's chromosome, and bacterial DNA adjacent to the site of integration is excised and packaged into phage particles along with the viral DNA. The cellular DNA acquired by the phage can then be transferred to new hosts during subsequent rounds of infection." Scientists were newly alive to the idea that bacteria could use conjugal mating transduction to transfer genes between them to enable resistance to antibiotics, or swap any number of useful genes around the microsphere. Something very strange was happening in life. Evolution was known to occur in a linear progression through natural selection and dissent with modification, but it also now appeared that genetic material was being transferred between peers in the same generation. "Bacteria trade genes more frantically than a pit full of traders on the floor of the Chicago Mercantile Exchange," the iconoclast microbiologist Lynn Margulis would later note. "We find that the entire basic genome of *E. coli* is continually exchanged," the evolutionary biologist Purushottam Dixit quipped. A stunning new paradigm had emerged. Genes were passed, or transferred, not only from parents to offspring in a vertical line of evolution, but between peers of the same generation. It was called "horizontal gene transfer."

In 1952, Luria published a method called "host-induced modification of phage" in which the microbe could change the genetic code of the phage that infected it. Anderson found out about it when he went to a colloquium in Royaumont. The trouble was, he had figured this out five years earlier, and hadn't published it. "I was hopping mad because this was '52 and I had discovered in it '47." Consider that there are a number of types of salmonella (F1, F2, A, 29) each of which is infected by a unique phage. Anderson (and Luria) had shown that a phage could acquire properties from one type of microbe, and then when it moved on to a new host cell, transfer those properties to the second microbe it originally occupied. This research would fuel Anderson's belief that phage typing was highly dynamic, with phages which could transfer resistance or pathogenicity, or change or be changed by a host bacterium.

"There was an outbreak in '48, actually, which really gave me the key to the whole story," Anderson recalled. "Miss Isa Caughey, was an eighty-five-year-old lady living on the banks of a river not far from Glasgow. There was a typhoid outbreak. There was one sunny day, one year, in Scotland, and a whole bunch of – I think it was actually a Catholic Sunday School – something like eight hundred people, went out for an excursion to a place called Kilcreggan. It was a very hot day, and so they were thirsty and decided to drink water from the river. And they all lined up; and there were forty cases of typhoid. But some were infected with type F1 and some with F2 and some with both F1 and F2 –these are different types, but related. And, eventually, an investigation identified the carrier. She had a cottage by the river, she was eighty-five. This was '48; she had had typhoid in 1895; she'd been a carrier ever since. In 1926, her niece and niece's friend, who were staying with her, both went down with typhoid and the niece died. But it didn't connect. She (Isa) didn't know until '48, when she suddenly realized this. She was a very sensible, retired school-mistress; she must be long since dead. And the point about it was that I got to play with these two types, F1 and F2... Well, then Felix said to me, 'What are you doing, what do you think you're doing?' I said, 'I want to lysogenize (infect) F1 with the phage from F2.'[137] He said, 'What do you think, ha-ha, do you think you are going to change the phage-type?' I said, 'Well, it could be.'"

"A little later, he went off for a long weekend and while he was away I did this. And the phage turned (salmonella) F1 into F2; that was the first clue. And then we ran through the whole scheme and found a whole lot of examples. But the fact is that, when I'd just done this one set of experiments, it also changed the phage-type of Type A, which is the sort of archetype. So, when he came back from his long weekend he saw a sort of gleam in my eye and he said, 'What have you been up to?' So, I said, 'Well, I've changed F1 into F2 and the phage from F2 also changes Type A into 29.' So he said, 'Bring me your protocols.' The records, to him, were always 'protocols.' So I brought my protocols, which had been as fastidiously kept as he demanded. And for two hours he tried to break it down. And then he sat in that corner, he slumped down in the chair and he said to me, 'This is a terrible thing you've done.' You see, to him, as I told you, there was something holy about a phage-type. And to be able to change it at will, this rattled him. Anyway, he accommodated to that and we went off on a gay spree of changing types, and so on. And we bust the whole thing wide open..."

In 1954, Anderson had become director of a lab at the Public Health Laboratory Service,[138] gaining a high-ranking position which he would hold for the next two decades. "When I came here Felix said there were some things he wanted solving; he had ideas about phages and he wanted me to help him work out these ideas. And I have to say that his ideas were all wrong. This caused a sort of conflict between us. Because he was persuaded that phages were endogenous enzymes, auto-enzymes, of bacteria, and I was persuaded that they were viruses. And, well, they are viruses, to cut a long story very short, they are viruses. But I remember that toward the end of Felix's time here, I had to say to him, because we were at a crossroads, you see, and I said, 'I'm afraid I have to tell you, Dr. Felix, that I believe the phages are viruses.' And he said, 'If I had thought the phages were viruses, Dr. Anderson, I would never have worked on them; I believe they are auto-enzymes.' And so, that belief he held to the end of his days; he died in '56, two years later."

"That was finished in '56. That was published and I felt, as I said to a colleague at the time, I feel as if I've killed an old friend," Anderson recalled.

"There's nothing more to do on the phage-types."

Paul Berg had grown up in Brooklyn, Jewish, his father a clothing maker. At Western Reserve University in Cleveland, Ohio, he had been a student of Harland Wood, an industrious, bootstrapping scientist who once built a "water-cooled thermal diffusion column in a five-story abandoned elevator shaft" to generate his own isotopes for a biology experiment, and another time based on some second-hand knowledge from a physicist, "built a mass spectrophotometer from scratch."[139] But, after graduation, Berg initially declined Wood's offer to hook him up with some training at Washington University in St. Louis. "Much to his chagrin, I told him that I preferred not to live in St. Louis because of its vestiges of racial segregation and notoriously torrid summers; perhaps apocryphal, foreign consular officials were said to receive a "tropical pay bonus" during their assignment in St. Louis." Instead, Berg decided to spend a postdoctoral year working with Herman Kalckar in Copenhagen, Denmark. "Living in Taarbaek, a small upscale fishing village bordering on the King's private deer park on the outskirts of Copenhagen, was a welcome relief from 4 years in Cleveland and from my wife Millie's 4 years of nursing at the university's hospital. My daily commute to and from the institute and the bike ride home through the woods to our 'villa' provided the quiet time for preparing and thinking about the experiments of the day." Living next to the King's deer park, Berg was living on a $3600 stipend from the American Cancer Society, which by Danish standards, "might have been more than the King's allowance."

In 1953, the biochemist Arthur Kornberg decided to decamp to Washington University to rebuild the faltering microbiology department. Berg returned to the United States, and this time went with Kornberg, the two heading into the southern heat with no tropical pay bonus. In these post-war years, it was time to roll up the shirt sleeves and get back to work. The power of genetics was being unleased. That year, a seismic shock had rippled through the world. James Watson and Francis Crick showed, through dazzling deduction and splendid showmanship – building a colorful, larger than human-sized sculpture of the DNA molecule – that the basic molecule of DNA was wound in a helical form with two strands of the four nucleotides, adenine, guanine, cytosine and thymine, attached to one another to form a helical structure.[140] DNA is bound in a double helix, a curling ladder, whereby the steps are hydrogen bonds between adenine and thymine (while RNA swaps out uracil for thymine), or guanine and cytosine. Along the rails of the ladder, each nucleotide is bound along a phosphate backbone.[141] The mechanism of how cells and their DNA assembly were duplicated, but also how it gave rise to the vast species of RNA molecules that themselves turned into a stunning array of proteins, would begin to be unraveled. In the months that followed, for instance, Kornberg discovered an enzyme called DNA polymerase, which was responsible for replicating the DNA into more copies during cell division, a finding so integral to life that he'd win a Nobel Prize by the end of the decade. Berg and Kornberg were about to do some damage.

"It was a typical fall day in mid-November, 1953, when I arrived at Washington University Medical School to join Kornberg's laboratory," Berg wrote in a reflection. "Located at the top of an antiquated clinic building, the only way to reach the microbiology department was by passing down a long corridor lined with patients in various states of despair waiting their turn to see a doctor. The final ascent was via a somewhat 'ancient' elevator, which, after the sliding gate was secured, inched and lurched its way upward to the fourth floor. On my arrival, the shabbiness of the surroundings was plainly evident. The main corridor's bare bulb lighting, suspended from the unusually high ceilings characteristic of buildings of that vintage, could well have been installed when gas lights went out of fashion. It was hard to realize that that department had been where Sol Spiegelman and Al Hershey had helped usher in molecular biology and where some notable work in medical immunology had been done. However, Kornberg's enthusiasm at my arrival, his excitement about those who would follow, and the prospects for the soon to be completed renovations lessened the importance of the shabby surroundings. Kornberg's escorted tour of the laboratories that had been newly done over, including the one I was to work in, assured me that I had made the right choice for the second year of my postdoctoral fellowship. After settling on a place to live, I was ready to get to the laboratory."[142]

By 1955, Berg had made his mark, which to this day he calls his proudest feat. He discovered a "new kind of reaction which nobody knew about before, and which solved a major dilemma that had been concerning biochemists."[143] In short, a molecular fuel called ATP is attached to a protein side chain, such as a fatty acid or other compound containing a carboxyl group, to produce a molecule called acetyl adenylate; (this is a process called adenylylation, in Berg's words, "the first discovered of a general class of enzymatic reactions"). This molecule then undergoes a second reaction to produce a nucleotide and molecule called acetyl-CoA, a compound used in many biochemical reactions and an important entry molecule in the "Krebs cycle." The completion of this cycle results in the creation of more ATP and the precursors of amino acids; it was a key to understanding the metabolism of sugars into energy, and the synthesis of the building blocks of life.

In 1956, in what proved to be a stunningly productive early career, Berg co-discovered a molecule called transfer RNA, or tRNA, which turned out to be a critical molecule that enabled RNA to assemble, or translate, into protein.[144] In fact, an aminoacyl-tRNA is a new molecule created by "charging" or "loading" the tRNA with the amino acid.[145] "It seemed logical that the aminoacyl-RNA was somehow involved in the assembly of amino acids into proteins," Berg told me in an email. "It took other experiments to establish that each tRNA molecule had a single acceptor site." A one-to-one match between each amino acid and each tRNA "squared with Francis Crick's surmise that the aminoacyl tRNAs serve as 'adaptors' for matching amino acids to their cognate mRNA codons," in other words, the assembly of proteins.[146,147]

DNA provided instructions for proteins. The phage school would help to shed light on how it happened. Esther Lederberg, wife of Joshua Lederberg, had discovered the phage *lambda*, which infects the common bacteria *E. coli*. In fact, this model system – phage and microbe – would enable scientists to gain some of their first hints into how genetic instructions are transcribed into parts that build a cell's equipment and carry out its functions. Soon after phages insert their DNA into bacterial cells, the scientists noted, traces of RNA rapidly appear. Intriguingly, phage scientists noted, the molecular spelling of RNA molecules had an uncanny resemblance to that of DNA molecules, suggesting a relationship between RNA and DNA.[148]

Consider that *E. coli* makes an enzyme called beta galactosidase which breaks down lactose into two simple sugars, glucose and galactose, which it can then use as energy. Joshua Lederberg and colleagues inferred that there was some "inducing machinery," which differed from the enzyme that was expressed or induced. The lac system, or "lac operon" as it later became known, was a tightly controlled set of mechanics, a system of switches, which were turned on in order to enable a set of genes to begin to express their products into RNA and then into the enzymes. A conversation between the microbiologist Jacques Monod and the atomic physicist Leo Szilard[149] soon resulted in an elegant, famous experiment referred to simply as the "PaJaMo."[150]

Monod argued that the cell generated its own "internal inducer" or apparatus to turn on a set of genes, including beta galactosidase, to break down sugars. Szilard argued instead that a negative control mechanism was at work with a cell providing a repressor, while an "external inducer" of lactose triggered the lifting of this break, and the expression of the genes. "In September 1957, Monod gave a semi-private lecture of the lac system to a guest of the Institut Pasteur, Leo Szilard. It was known that some molecules worked as 'inducers' to turn on gene expression and some parts of the mechanism worked as a 'repressor' to control the system to keep it turned off. But how did it work? Monod ended his lecture with the question, how is the lac system controlled? 'By negative regulation of course,' was Szilard's immediate answer. Continuing on he explained that there are two modes of control, negative and positive control, and that negative control is easier to achieve than positive control. It is easier to inhibit the start of a reaction than to provoke its start."[151]

As an atomic physicist, Szilard was only thinking in terms of what made sense from the logic of initiating an atomic reaction. Monod came up with an experiment to test Szilard's hypothesis. He used "conjugal mating" of strains of bacteria with functioning and non-functioning lac systems to create new strains that had one functional set and one non-functional set of the critical genes, or operon, to express beta galactose, the enzyme which breaks down lactose into simple sugars the microbe can use, and another called permease, which allows more lactose into the cell. Most bacteria contain plasmids, circular rings of DNA which are free floating in the cells, and basically, two cells bump up against each other, and open pores in their membranes and these plasmids can move from one bacteria to another, transferring new DNA from the donor to recipient cell. Monod used this mating strategy to create hybrid bacteria with both functional and non-functional operons. The non-functional lac system was constitutive, meaning that those critical genes were on all the time, even in the absence of the lactose stimulus. He observed that the new hybrid strains synthesized beta galactose at a high rate, but after a half hour the expression of the enzyme plummeted. This showed that there was at least one copy of a functioning gene that repressed the system so it could exert a negative control. In terms of genetics, this showed that the repressor was *dominant*.

The experiments further showed that when an inducer molecule was added to the growth plate, it stopped the repressor and allowed the set of genes or operon including beta galactosidase and lactose permease to be expressed and break down lactose into simple sugars. Scientists would learn that microbes contain sets of genes that are turned on all together as an "operon" which are under the control of a single stimulus. Importantly, Monad and colleagues wrote up the first report which demonstrated that the machinery for expressing a gene into a product was separate from the gene.

In a 1957 paper, Francis Crick proposed what came to be known as the "central dogma," conjecturing that DNA is copied or transcribed into RNA, which in turn is translated into proteins. The PaJaMo experiments contributed to a new awakening that the central dogma was probably correct, and that DNA was transcribed into a mirror copy of RNA, an important intermediary molecule in the expression of a gene. By 1960, Jacob and Sydney Brenner named this vanishing molecule "messenger RNA."[152] In the meantime, Paul Berg was doing outstanding work, which would interlock with these findings, identifying, for instance, transfer RNA which was essential for turning RNA into protein.

Berg was working out of the microbiology department at Washington University, which was in stasis, while Stanford University, the institution of Beadle and Tatum, was rising as a preeminent place with no biochemistry or molecular biology department and needed one fast. In the spring of 1959, Berg, Kornberg, Dale Kaiser, Mel Cohn and David Hogness piled pipets and glassware into cars, hit the road, winding up in California and set up shop at Stanford. "There was nothing special about the drive west as we had done it many times before," Berg told me in an email. "We moved into the new labs in June of 1959 and were doing experiments by August and were teaching a novel biochemistry course in October." Samuel Weiss and Leonard Gladstone discovered RNA polymerase, a second component along with transfer RNA which was required to translate messenger RNA into protein; in 1960, Michael Chamberlain, a graduate student working in Berg's new lab at Stanford, isolated RNA polymerase, following the discovery of messenger RNA, only months beforehand. Chamberlain, and fellow graduate student Bill Wood then showed that "the product of the RNA polymerase reaction could serve as a template for the production of proteins," Berg told me. The polymerase transcribed DNA into messenger RNA, which provided the template needed for Berg's transfer RNA to assemble amino acids into protein.

Ephraim Anderson began collaborating with Naomi Datta on how bacteria transferred genetic material by trading plasmids, conjugal mating. Datta was a British geneticist, who, while working at Hammersmith Hospital, expanded upon the work of Lederberg, who had coined a new term, "microbiome." Datta would show that horizontal gene transfer was not only a quirky finding of interest, but a deadly weapon in action: antibiotic resistance could be transferred between bacteria.[153] In fact, Datta found bacteria were *learning* from us, adapting the information and trading this intelligence among their colonies. And each time we used an antibiotic, we escalated the evolutionary arms race. In 1959, there was a severe outbreak of *Salmonella typhimurium* phage-type 27. Datta found that 25 of 309 strains were drug-resistant, including eight that were now resistant to streptomycin, which had been used to treat the patients. Earlier cultures of the *Salmonella typhimurium* strains had not been drug-resistant; her conclusion: antibiotic resistance had been acquired through genetic mutations and shared though transfer of plasmids, a finding she repeatedly showed.[154,155]

In 1962, there was an outbreak of typhoid amongst more than 400 skiers in Zermatt, Switzerland. Anderson recalled, "I was the one who told the Swiss they had a typhoid epidemic – it's an ill wind, as they say; they asked me if I would supervise the preparation of a report on the outbreak for publication...which I did, and they asked me what I wanted to be paid for the supervision and I said, 'Nothing, it's a pleasure.' Sometime later, they sent me a letter saying 'Well, if you won't take any money, would you like a holiday in Switzerland with your family as long as you like wherever you like,' and I said it would be ungracious of me to refuse. So, we went to, just below St. Moritz, actually, a place called Celerina. That's why I say, it's an ill wind that blows nobody any good; some people got typhoid but we got a holiday. The Zermatt outbreak stopped my research in resistance, which I took up again toward the end of 63'. And it just so happens it was a critical moment. You know, there is so much serendipity in scientific research that without it we would never have gotten anywhere. Just the thing happening – over the years of '63 and '64 there was a blip in the incidence of typhimurium in man and animals; it was mostly in calves. And this was caused by one type which we called 29. Then, early in '64, it sort of paused. And then it took off: and from the middle of '64 onwards we had a raging outbreak in calves, with a lot of human cases. And the organism was resistant, first of all, to streptomycin and sulphonamides. After streptomycin and sulphonamides it was tetra-cycline; then ampicillin; and chloramphenicol, neomycin, kanamycin, furazolidone.[156] So, we got a whole lot of resistances. It was towards the end of '64 when we started our conjugation experiments with transferable resistance. What it showed us, in the end, was that there were what we now know to be plasmids."

Anderson showed that infectious microbes not only acquired resistance, but then amplified copies of those resistant genes in circular plasmids which were distributed to other microbes. "Whereas the other people found all their resistances transferred in a lump, ours were transferred in separate packets, or packages. Nobody thought of examining the organisms without selecting for drug resistance. But we did think of that. And the result was that we ended up with the knowledge that there were several types of R-factor,[157] that is, the plasmids; that one of them gave resistance to ampicillin, another one to streptomycin and sulphonamides, and that another one gave no resistance at all. It just transferred, silently. A very interesting business: and we called this thing the delta factor; it doesn't give resistance at all, it just transfers and helps resistances to transfer. But the organisms that carry it are drug-sensitive. And, if I ever want to be remembered for anything, it's for the test that I devised to spot which drug-sensitive organisms were carrying this transfer thing. . . I was right."

Now there were several types of plasmids, F-factor plasmids for fertil-ity, R-factor plasmids for resistance, delta-factor plasmids for change. Through various combinations, bacteria were able to mutate, and mate, and importantly they were able to trade resistance genes. Lederberg had also shown, the trading of genes throughout the microsphere also occurred through the skilled proxy of viruses. Anderson was alarmed, observing that antibiotic resistance was transferred "from organism to organism – you know, like a shuttlecock." In the 1960s and 1970s, Anderson would sound a clarion call of "an emerging worldwide danger from multiple drug-resistances in bacteria" due to the overuse of antibiotics and the promulgation of those treatments in agriculture, and he "eventually changed the views of doctors and governments," to the "fury of drug companies and many farmers. He argued that unless antibiotics were protected, medicine might lose its new 'miracle drugs' and find itself back with the problems of the 1930s. Although a pathogen nicknamed 'hospital staph' (now called methicillin-resistant *Staphylococcus aureus* or MRSA) and extremely resistant to a wide range of antibiotics was already emerging in medical wards, Anderson's work and arguments came under fierce attack, primarily from drug companies and most frequently outside Britain."[158]

Stanley Cohen, a Stanford University geneticist, in a review paper,[159] wrote that "after the development of antimicrobial agents in the 1940s, the notion was prevalent that these drugs would end infectious diseases caused by bacteria. Of course that did not happen, and the reason was the occurrence of antibiotic resistance. Investigations carried out primarily in laboratories in Japan and the United Kingdom in the early 1960s showed that antibiotic resistance in bacteria commonly is associated with the acquisition of genes – often multiple genes – capable of destroying antibiotics or otherwise interfering with their actions. The resistance properties commonly did not map genetically to the bacterial chromosomes, suggesting that the genes encoding resistance were located on separate elements (some had called them episomes) analogous to the fertility factor (F-factor) discovered earlier.[160] Like F-factors, resistance factors (R-factors) were capable of being transferred between bacteria by cell-to-cell contact..."[161,162] "The antibiotic-inactivating genes carried by resistance plasmids provide a biological advantage to host bacteria in populations exposed to antimicrobial drugs, and, in barely a decade after the introduction of antibiotics to treat human infections, R-plasmid-mediated multi-drug resistance had become a major medical problem as well as a scientific enigma."

"Importantly," Cohen wrote, "nothing was known about the genetic recombination mechanisms that had enabled the accumulation of multiple resistance genes on the same genetic element." The bacteriophage lambda was the "most extensively and competitively investigated bacteriophage of that era, but the role of R-plasmids in antibiotic resistance was being studied in only a small number of microbiology laboratories; I liked the prospect of working in what was still a quiet backwater of scientific research. Research in the burgeoning field of molecular biology during the 1960s focused on bacteriophages for an important reason:

a bacterial cell infected by a virus generates thousands of identical copies – clones – of a single infecting genome during the normal viral life cycle. Thus, phenotypic effects can be correlated with the results of biochemical analyses. I realized that elucidation of how resistance genes function and how R-plasmids evolve required a way to clone individual plasmid DNA molecules and to isolate the resistance genes."

Viruses can easily be evaluated and quantified as they slip between cells, but the plasmids were much more dark and mysterious. Indeed, it wasn't until the early 1960s, bacterial plasmids were predicted to exist as DNA circles.[163,164,165] Scientists needed to come up with mechanisms to clone, or replicate, plasmids and to cut them apart and map them, if they wanted to learn more about how they acquired and transferred resistances between bacteria. Cohen set out to "to assess changes in circle size associated with the gain or loss of resistance phenotypes or transferability." Stanley Falkow, whose work had "been instrumental in attracting me to plasmid biology, agreed to provide bacterial strains and plasmids for my initial experiments."[166]

Cohen arrived at Stanford in March 1968. The following year, Christine Miller, a newly hired laboratory technician, had purified an intact circular DNA of the large antibiotic resistance plasmid called R1. Along with Norman Davidson and his graduate student Phillip Sharp at Caltech, Cohen began using a new electron microscope-based "heteroduplex" analysis, and through these experiments, provided direct physical evidence that plasmid sequences known to transfer between bacteria had become "linked covalently to resistance genes to form large circles of R-plasmid DNA."[167] In other words, antibiotic resistance genes were naturally being recombined in the transportable plasmid vectors and shipping between bacteria. In addition, Sharp would also show that random insertions were leading to rearrangements of plasmid structure.

Scientists were learning how to remove and investigate plasmids, but they just did not yet know how to get them into bacteria. But a new procedure showed that *E. coli* cells treated with calcium ions could take up DNA of bacteriophage lambda or P22 or, even, plasmid DNA derived from a deleted variant of bacteriophage lambda that had transduced along with it some genes from *E. coli*. "Peter Lobban, a graduate student working with A. Dale Kaiser in the Stanford Department of Biochemistry, had begun using it to introduce phage P22 DNA into *Salmonella typhimurium*, a close relative of *E. coli*... if R-plasmid DNA could be taken up by *E. coli* even at low frequency, and if the antibiotic resistance genes carried by circular R-plasmid replicons were expressed in these cells, colonies of bacteria that acquire plasmids could be selected using culture media containing appropriate antibiotics."[168] In May 1972, Cohen and lab technician Annie Chang "began to break apart molecules of the large multi-drug resistance plasmids R6 and R6-5 using the mechanical shearing procedure."

Not long after, Cohen would come to collaborate with Herbert Boyer, who had such a pair of scissors, called *EcoRI*, which could cut plasmids at precise sites, which would allow them to recombine a new plasmid,which he named pSC101 (plasmid Stanley Cohen 101), recently isolated during his shearing experiments, with multiple antibiotic resistance genes. By doing this, scientists could alter a plasmid, introduce it to a bacteria, and then by introducing an antibiotic, decimate all of the bacteria that did not get transferred plasmid. Thus, they could select or isolate the cells that acquired the recombinant DNA.

Paul Berg, the Stanford scientist who'd deduced many of the basic machinery of gene regulation, initiated some of the first experiments that would become called "recombinant DNA." But alarms soon began to sound throughout the scientific community, some of them raised by Berg himself, that creating such antibiotic resistant strains of bacteria may lead to unintended consequences. Ephraim Anderson, who had sounded for antibiotic resistance, was now concerned that his clarion call was being muted by an even louder alarm, that this new recombinant DNA could result in a societal catastrophe, either through the splicing together of plasmids for several antibiotic resistant genes which would make an infectious outbreak impossible to stop, or by newly initiated experiments to splice together tumor viruses into bacteria that can grow in a human gut, altering microbes into potentially dangerous microbial species which might have new powers to transfer genes with oncogenic properties or trigger human cancers.

I had been reading this transcript and other scientific papers in the Special Sections Collection at MIT for about five hours, and it was clear that I was reaching a climatic point in the story. The journalist Charles Weiner interrupted Anderson in the transcript I had been reading.

Weiner asked, "Had you been aware of the research in recombinant DNA, the work that the Stanford people were doing?"

"Yes, yes. Oh, by hearsay. On the grapevine, you see; because I'm on that particular grapevine, anyway, the plasmid grapevine. So, I would naturally hear automatically by word of mouth or letter," Anderson said. "Well, I knew what Stan Cohen was doing. In fact, Stanley Cohen used one of our plasmids; he used the Ssu plasmid.[169] He hybridized that with the pSC101, using the *EcoRI* enzyme to open the plasmids. But, he's had that plasmid for quite a while. It goes under the name of RSF1010. That in itself has a history, because it (Ssu or RSF1010) was stolen from my laboratory by a Czechoslovak worker, who later on, claimed that he'd isolated it himself, and distributed it to a number of people. And then, eventually, he had even the gall to send it back to me as a discovery of his own. That's quite a story, because it's got cloak-and-dagger stuff in it which is quite comical. A burlesque of cloak-and-dagger, I mean. He wanted to establish a reputation. In fact, he did, in his own country; he holds a senior position there. He's a *persona non grata* in this one. He can't come here."

Once the technology worked, it immediately became a piece of technology to be fought for. Scientists could use plasmids and viruses to install newly engineered genes into cells. It had immediate applications for drug companies. For instance, rather than harvesting insulin from a pig, a company could add a gene for insulin to a microbe, isolate that microbe from other strains by including an additional drug-resistant marker, and then have that microbe produce many copies of the insulin protein. That is the power of recombinant DNA. Engineering the code of life was also perceived as a stunning new intrusion into nature that found parallels with nuclear programs. If nuclear physicists could unleash the power of the atom to destroy major cities, they could probably unleash the power of genetics to similar ends. I was simultaneously aware that this work had been initiated at the end of the 1960s and leading into the early 1970s and there was a deep distrust of the scientific community. People thought of scientists as manipulators of nature for the sake of power. A sharp awareness between scientific culture and nature was newly emerging.

In 1962, the theorist Thomas Kuhn published *The Structure of Scientific Revolutions*, suggesting that science itself was dogmatic, an apparatus of power. A full generation earlier the German socialist Max Weber had presented a lecture titled *Science as a Vocation*, delivered in Munich. As Steven Shapin wrote. "The world, Weber said, was

'disenchanted.' In principle, everything can be known by rational calculation; there is nothing that is not calculable. Scientists may have once
believed that they could show you the way to God, but not anymore... if
there is such a thing as the meaning of the world, there is no scientific
way to discover it... Aligning himself with Leo Tolstoy, (Weber) insisted
that science gives no answer to the question 'how to live' – or, as the
existentialists later liked to say, 'Everything has been figured out, except
how to live...' By the early 1960s, Thomas Kuhn's picture of 'normal
science' portrayed scientific activity not as an open-minded philosophical quest but as puzzle-solving – the extension and application of
existing paradigms. To the shock and indignation of some, Kuhn argued
that being a scientist involved obedience to 'dogma' and a narrowing of
perception. Scientists remained, of course, the most reliable knowledge
we had, but whatever moral authority might follow from regarding
science as uniquely free of prejudice was – for those persuaded by Kuhn –
no longer available."[170] In 1961, Dwight D. Eisenhower identified
the "military industrial complex" which was later codified by Senator
William Fulbright as the "military-industrial-academic complex."[171]
After Hiroshima and the Cold War, "Scientists had, for the most part,
given up asserting their moral superiority; now, many of them argued
that scientists should not be thought of as *worse* than anyone else.
Robert Oppenheimer worried that he had 'blood on his hands,'but many
other scientists insisted that Hiroshima was not their fault; they were
following democratically legitimate orders." Shapin noted that, "So
accepting that science, of course, cannot make you good is just an
acknowledgement of the world's disenchantment and of the massive
achievements of amoral modern science..." while there was a new
awareness that[172] "the tendency to think one could extend scientific
method everywhere and thereby solve problems of morality, value,
aesthetics, and social order – was just sloppy thinking."[173]

In contemporary life, this impulse that science *is* all the life of reason
is pervasive and residual in the dogma of "scientism," the disposition
that the scientific method can be applied to any phenomenon, and is
somehow even required to make judgements "official."[174,175] Oppenheimer was painfully aware of this when he concluded that "science is not
all of the life of reason; it is a part of it."

Recombinant DNA was not right or wrong. It was meaningful. Conversation was crackling on how it would be applied and who had the

right to do it. Many scientists were grappling with whether it could even be made to work. Anderson Continued, "Yes, so what I was saying was this: you can take a specific system, a particular system, and you can test it with everything you can think of and then you can say, with your hand on your heart, 'I cannot find any pathogenicity here. And if we want to use it for particular purposes, it seems to me it's perfectly safe.' And in the event, in time, you'll probably find that nothing happens, it's all right. But you can't generalize. Especially if you're working with things like viruses and oncogenic viruses, at that. How can you generalize? And at what point are you going to say, 'So okay, it's safe for man?' Where do you have to go before you can be satisfied it's safe for man? Well, in the event, I suppose, what people will do is gingerly to try the experiments and nothing will happen, and they'll get the hybrids and nothing will happen. And they'll do the experiments again and they'll go on and nothing will happen. And then they'll say, 'Well, it seems okay.' I can't see any other way of doing it, except that. You may be able to progressively relax your precautions as time goes on and it's shown that this is just a harmless lump of DNA which can, perhaps, fix nitrogen or whatever. I was talking about the things I think one could go on with... the nitrogen fixation plasmids."[176]

"But, by and large, I think that it's possibly safe."

"I don't even know whether it's going to be successful."

Weiner cut him off in the transcript. "...the Berg letter..." Paul Berg and colleagues had just written a splashy letter in *Science* that they could use restriction enzymes to cut and paste plasmids to create recombinant DNA; and, they accompanied that notice with a directive that nobody should be doing it until the effects of this stunning new technology could be evaluated.[177] The 1974 letter read: "Several groups of scientists are now planning to use this technology to create recombinant DNAs from a variety of other viral, animal, and bacterial sources. Although such experiments are likely to facilitate the solution of important theoretic and practical biological problems, they would also result in the creation of novel types of infectious DNA elements whose biological properties cannot be completely predicted in advance. There is serious concern that some of these artificial recombinant DNA molecules could prove biologically hazardous. One potential hazard in current experiments derives from the need to use a bacterium like *E. coli* to clone the recombinant DNA molecules and to amplify their number.

Strains of *E. coli* commonly reside in the human intestinal tract, and they are capable of exchanging genetic information with other types of bacteria, some of which are pathogenic to man."[178] If scientists spliced together bits of microbes and viruses, some of those hybrids might have cancer-causing or infectious properties and they could be exchanged and promulgated through the human population, since many common microbes reside in the human gut. It would be more than likely that anything that scientists did in the lab would leak into the wild. But, Anderson thought it a bit of pomp and circumstance for the Americans to be claiming a fait accompli and then sounding a clarion call.

"I was phoned up by *Nature*," Anderson explained.

"And they said, 'Have you seen this thing?'"

"So I said, 'Which thing?'"

'This letter from Berg, and so on. Would you be prepared to write about it?'

"So, I saw the thing and I said, 'Yes, all right.'"

"I thought that there'd been a certain, yes, éclat was the word I used, not in the letter, I mean I used it myself. There was too much éclat in the announcement. Tara! A fanfare."

Weiner: "You used the word 'pompous.'"

"Yes, I did," Anderson said.

"I wish it had been presented less pompously. Yes, I did. They were offended. They thought that I was getting at them. And I was, in a sense. Because I thought it was too conscious a gesture, thrusting yourself out bravely into the limelight and saying, 'We have done this, we think there are risks, we are stopping as from now on and we think everybody else should pause while a bunch of people whom we will choose will debate the evolution of satisfactory containment of hazards or decide, perhaps on unacceptability.' I don't know. This is the way I felt the thing had been worked. It was a little bit of American ballyhoo, I felt. I'm not saying I think so now. But at that time I thought, what a pompous way of saying it."

Berg's letter to *Science* had called for an immediate halt, a moratorium on recombinant DNA in the United States. In England, a group would convene a parallel process resulting in the "Ashby Report." "I thought the Ashby Report was a pretty sensible report," Anderson said. "It was much less diffuse in content than the Asilomar thing was. It was written by, shall we say, mature characters. There were a lot of youngsters at Asilomar. I don't mean that the young can't be terribly intelligent; but the young are rarely mature." Anderson's rebuttal was titled *Indiscriminate use of antibiotics has exerted more pressure on the bacterial population than could be wielded by all research workers in the world put together.* "It's very different to persuade them that people they may regard as being intolerably square may sometimes, you know – there's an old German saying, 'Soga rein blindes Huhn Findet auchmal ein Korn!' Even a blind chicken sometimes finds a grain of wheat! Perhaps the old boy knows a little something, sometimes."

3   Asilomar

The commercialization of molecular biology is the most stunning
ethical event in the history of science, and it has happened with
astonishing speed

–Michael Crichton[179]

David Baltimore is short, dressed in a sports jacket and has a reserve.
A former president of California Institute of Technology, he maintains a
lab as professor emeritus, where he is currently overseeing four projects in
gene therapy which have moved into clinical trials. I met him on May 1,
2015 at the Hyatt Regency Cambridge, MA. White blossoms were in
bloom on cherry trees standing along the banks of the Charles River,
some falling, and giving the morning a soft touch, as breeze carried
along the river, and the sunlight flittered, but was not yet harsh. He
was in Cambridge for a memorial service for colleague Herman Eisen,
an immunologist. "Did you ever publish with Eisen?" I asked. We moved
up an escalator. Baltimore paused, he didn't think so. As a virologist, he
had worked out of MIT in the 1970s, and was caught up in the hurried
moment of what became the recombinant DNA controversy, a jugger-
naut of new experiments and endless ethical conversations set on course
when colleague Paul Berg and his lab performed the first gene splicing
experiments. In 1974, Baltimore had co-signed the halting "Berg letter,"
which urged caution about proceeding into recombinant DNA. Now
there was a very similar letter, also appearing in *Science*, and also signed
by Berg and Baltimore, and including Jennifer Doudna, urging a timeout
in proceeding with Crispr-Cas9 genome editing soon after she and others
had invented it. Ephraim Anderson might have called it éclat.

Crispr-Cas9 had already become deployed by thousands of laboratories throughout the world to create new genetic variants in cell cultures
in vitro, or model organisms such as mice to evaluate the effects on the
organism. It could allow scientists to test virtually any hypothesis of
"forward genetics," meaning the effects that a gene variant has on a
phenotype, or observable trait. Scientists for decades had been performing gene edits on the somatic cells in our bodies, the cells that comprise

our blood, bones and tissues. Edits to those cells are not heritable. The germline, by contrast, is composed of sperm and egg cells, and editing those cells is to make a permanent alteration that will be carried forth in all generations. Crispr-Cas9 was the first tool that was fast and easy enough to use that ethicists warned it could now be used on heritable code, snipping and editing cells in human embryos and stopping diseases before they even happened. Inded, just months before, scientists at Sun Yat-Sen University in Guangzhou, China, reported they'd already done it to repair a flawed gene in human embryos that's responsible for a rare blood disorder, thalassemia. "CHINESE SCIENTISTS EDIT GENES OF HUMAN EMBRYOS, RAISING CONCERNS," wrote *The New York Times*. Marcy Darnovsky, director of the Center for Genetics and Society in Berkeley, CA, called for caution in an interview to National Public Radio. "This paper demonstrates the enormous safety risks that any such attempt would entail, and underlines the urgency of working to forestall other such efforts." Importantly, Darnovsky argued, "the social dangers of creating genetically modified human beings cannot be overstated."

The ethics of genome editing were already coming up hard against the principles of "first strike" in science, the incentive to be the first person to do something and establish a historical authority. The work of the Chinese researchers showed the system could cause unexpected mutations, or "off-target effects," which occur when Crispr-Cas9 edits a sequence that is identical or highly similar to the one it is designed for.[180] In a sea of three billion nucleotides that make up a human genome, a 20-base target can occur more than once.[181] But even as these reports were hitting the news, Keith Joung and colleagues at Massachusetts General Hospital were selecting new varieties of Cas9 from bacteria[182] that could hit a broader spectrum of targets in the human genome with higher precision.[183] Darnovsky's emphasis on "social dangers" implied an awakening that technical limitations were being overcome, and we'd better be ready to cowboy up and engage our democracy. The improved precision of genome editing technologies was emerging in lockstep with advancing laboratory techniques. The Cambridge biotech company OvaScience said it planned to use the system to correct genetic disorders in human eggs. The company, a few years old, was developing a new technology based on precursor cells or "immature egg cells found inside the protective ovarian lining."

Jonathan Tilly, chairman of the biology department at Northeastern University, first identified these stem cells, which exist in human ovaries and have the potential to develop into mature eggs, replenishing a woman's egg supply, once thought to be finite. Cara Mayfield, a company spokeswoman, confirmed at the time the company was planning to edit germline DNA to stop inherited disorders.[184]

In December 2013, OvaScience, which is based on the scientific work of Tilly, and Harvard geneticist David Sinclair, announced a $1.5 million joint venture with RJ Kirk's synthetic biology company Intrexon with objectives including gene-editing to eggs to "prevent the propagation" of human disease "in future generations." The destruction of human embryos was among the most contentious issues in bioethics, a cause celebre for activists, but few people could find reason to protest harm to precursor eggs, which had not yet been fertilized, or the wanton destruction of sperm, which live fast and die young. Indeed, germline editing could sidestep concerns about the destruction of human embryos by engineering parts upstream in the process. Such feats shifted the ethics to new concerns about the creation of genetically modified people, how society might accept them and also, in very simple terms, because any genetic variant we create is apt to have different effects in different people. As the journalist Antonio Regaldo remarked, "What was surprising to me was that OvaScience's research in 'crossing the germ line,' as critics of human engineering sometimes put it, has generated scarcely any notice… A Pew Research survey carried out last August found that 46 percent of adults approved of genetic modification of babies to reduce the risk of serious diseases. The same survey found that 83 percent said genetic modification to make a baby smarter would be 'taking medical advances too far.' Luhan Yang, a postdoc in Church's lab, which collaborated with Sinclair, explained the strategy to edit genetic variants that contribute to a risk for breast cancer, which runs in families. The researchers hoped to obtain, from a hospital in New York, the ovaries of a woman undergoing surgery for ovarian cancer caused by a mutation in a gene called *BRCA1*. Working with another Harvard laboratory, that of antiaging specialist Sinclair, they would extract immature egg cells that could be coaxed to grow and divide in the laboratory. Yang would use Crispr in these cells to correct the DNA of the *BRCA1* gene. They would try to create a viable egg without the genetic error that caused the woman's cancer."[185]

Baltimore, Berg and other leaders including Doudna, were calling for an informal and non-binding moratorium on applying gene editing to the germline and scrambling to set up a major conference on how and whether to institute one. Moratoria in the sciences are rare. One was related to nuclear fission, but that only affected a few atomic scientists who could actually do that work. The last one began as a "self-imposed moratorium" on cloning bits of virus that contained oncogenes, meaning that those viruses were thought to initiate a cancer in mammalian cells, and held from the fall of 1971 when the first gene splicing experiments were conducted until 1979, when the NIH finally changed its guidelines to lift the moratorium. It was Berg and Baltimore's *Science* letter, initiated the formal mechanisms of that moratorium through a process set into work at a meeting held at Asilomar, a rustic conference center on 100 acres of sand dunes that hammerheads into the Pacific Ocean on the Monterey Peninsula in Pacific Grove, CA. That conference drew 140 prominent scientists who batted about the effects of engineering life and was captured by a lone tape recorder set to turn on a desk in the open room. It was an effective example of self-policing, in the words of Stanford ethicist Hank Greely, "*undoubtedly*, the most famous story in modern scientific self-regulation." Things had come full circle. Crispr-Cas9 was shaking up the world. Baltimore had just participated in a similar dialog in January 24, 2015 in California at the Carneros Inn in Napa Valley. "It was a feeling of déjà vu," Baltimore told a reporter at the time. "These are monumental moments in the history of biomedical research. They don't happen every day."[186]

In a blog post at the Stanford Law Review, Greely recounted the discussion at Napa. "The conversation... was lively – and, for me at least, great fun. Well before the end of the day, a consensus seemed to be emerging, one part of which was to move from 'emerging' to 'written down.'"[187] Indeed, on March 19, 2015, *Science* published the historic letter *A Prudent Path Forward for Genomic Engineering and Germline Gene Modification*, which included a string of 18 authors (eight of whom attended Napa) including David Baltimore, Paul Berg, Alta Charo, George Church, George Daley, Jennifer Doudna, Ed Penhoet, Keith Yamamoto, Jonathan Weissman, Dana Carroll and Greely. It recommended steps taken to "strongly discourage...any attempts at germline genome modification for clinical application in humans, while societal, environmental, and ethical implications of such activity are discussed among scientific and governmental organizations."[188] It was the 1970s all over again, but it wasn't. We live in more potent times. Biotechnology is now a well-resourced apparatus for leveraging technology and marketing it. Sinclair was already peddling OvaScience to investors, telling them that we are approaching a new chapter in "how humans control their bodies," and would let parents determine "when and how they have children and how healthy those children are actually going to be..." not only using in vitro fertilization to conceive a child but "to have healthier children as well, if there is a genetic disease in their family..." For instance, Huntington's disease is caused by a genetic variant in a single gene, which can trigger a fatal brain condition in a descendant who inherits only one copy. Sinclair suggested his company could make a gene edit to the defect from an egg cell, before it was ever an embryo, noting OvaScience's vision was to "correct those mutations before we generate your child."[189] Darnovsky was quick to point out that *in vitro* techniques fall into a category of engineering, something much different from a medical procedure that is used to help a person who is already alive and struggling.

Greely cautioned that preimplantation genetic diagnosis, an in vitro genetic test, could accomplish the same results, since the mutation that causes Huntington's disease is passed on 50 percent of the time. Fertility doctors could simply select an embryo that did not have the genetic variant rather than edit one that did. In a blog post, Greely summed up the spirit of consensus at Napa that resulted in the *Science* directives. "I read that as clearly encompassing 'making babies' and to include 'making babies' for enhancement purposes as well as disease prevention purposes. The 'clinical application' there, I am confident, is in contradistinction to 'research uses,' not to 'non-clinical baby-making applications.' I think it just as clearly does not prohibit research on cells, cell lines and tissues, even cells, cell lines and tissues that *could* become part of the germline, such as human embryonic cell lines (hESCs), human induced pluripotent cell lines (hiPSCs), various more direct egg and sperm precursor cells, and even human eggs and sperm. To me, it is putting the modification into the germline of what is or is intended to become a living human being that is our focus."[190] But now, the National Academy of the Sciences was preparing a more formal organizational meeting, an "Asilomar-type" conference which was designed to recommend major policy issues, at the end of the year.

"We felt very strongly in 1975 that we wanted to keep Congress out of it, and regulate through self-policing," Baltimore told me. But, Crispr-Cas9 had now injected a new sense of urgency, harkening the spirit of the times 40 years ago, and throwing us into a dangerous, if brave, new world. It was having a stunning effect on research and biotech companies were in a clamor, grabbing funding and poised to treat rare blood and immune system disorders, some said, even cancers, by editing somatic cells. Labs now appeared ready and willing to move the technology into the germline to make a buck. "The number of circumstances where it is actually needed are very few," Baltimore told me, agreeing with Greely, that existing fertility procedures and genetic counseling could already enable us to evade telltale genetic defects in the germline. At the same time, Baltimore said, many of the concerns of moving power and politics into the genome may be overblown due to an old principle in genetics codified by Francis Galton called "regression to the mean." Each new generation that emerges involves a shuffling of versions of genes, or alleles, from a mother and father, so that the same genes rarely remain side-by-side. It's kind of like a kindergarten class that changes desks. The bad kids get broken up. The good ones do, too. And so if there is a group of genetic variants that cause problems when inherited together, they undergo this shuffling, or "crossing over," which by nature, breaks up the group.[191] The same thing goes if we engineer a genetic variant that provides a strong evolutionary advantage, since it will continue to undergo shuffling and get reassigned to cluster with other genes, each of which account for unique genetic backgrounds. "Could you make modifications to make a child smarter? Maybe, but those genes won't get passed on together and they will interact with different genetic backgrounds, so we can't really predict," Baltimore told me. Furthermore, any new genetic variant we create will have effects that are speculative at best, since it "hasn't gone through the process of natural selection."

Genes seldom work in isolation. Instead, they function in complex interplays which we scarcely understand; furthermore, a gene often has more than one function, so adding a new genetic variant may result in a desired effect, but it could also have three or four other unintended effects. There are logistical issues. Scientists can gainfully make gene edits to a small number of somatic cells in cases in which simply adding a functioning copy of a gene to a small number of cells can help to treat the disease. Those are cases, for instance, when a patient's cells are making either no or very low amounts of an enzyme and adding a functioning copy of that gene to even small numbers of cells can help the patient immensely. Glybera, the first gene therapy drug to go on sale in Europe is used to treat lipoprotein lipase deficiency; ornithine transcarbamylase deficiency was one of the first diseases to be attacked by gene therapy trials in the 1990s. These are both enzymes, and before this, doctors had to treat patients with enzyme replacement treatments doled out over a patient's lifetime. Now they might be treated in a single shot; indeed, Glybera is delivered as a shot to the leg. But some diseases, like the brain-wasting disease Huntington's, are hypothesized to be "dominant negative," meaning that a single dysfunctional copy of a gene can cause havoc on a person. In diseases like those, genome editing probably does no good unless every cell in an organ is correctly edited, and that's tough to do, since there are 37.2 trillion cells in a human body.[192] Those diseases may only be attacked through the germline. But for a mix of technical and moral issues, Baltimore was arguing that germline modification is something we might never want to do. And at the same time, he suggested the discussion could shift and change his opinions, in short, never say never. "We don't know what things will look like 20 years from now. We can always adapt."

Baltimore grew up in a Jewish family in New York and attended Swarthmore. His father was a woman's coat manufacturer, his brother a physician, his mother a psychologist, a teacher at St. Lawrence. "I don't know that much about Gestalt psychology, but that's how she views the world," he once said.[193] He credits a summer internship at Jackson Labs in Bar Harbor, Maine, with turning him on to the power of molecular biology, which was emerging as a new paradigm. Baltimore was enrolled in a Cold Spring Harbor internship when he met phage school pioneers Salvador Luria and Cy Leventhal. "They basically invited me to apply to MIT as a graduate student. That was the only place I applied; and they accepted me."[194] Once Baltimore got to MIT he started making a push to study animal viruses, believing that after so much had been accomplished by using phage to probe the cellular machinery of microbes, that animal viruses held the key to deciphering the mechanisms of mouse and human cells. That was a bit brash. Few people who were around to mentor him were working on these things. "And so, I remember going to Leventhal and saying 'Look – I think what I want to do is work with animal viruses.' You want to learn about higher cells, you use the viruses of higher cells. And Leventhal looked wisely at me and said, 'Yes, you know, I've thought of that, too.'"

Next, he went to Luria. "Why don't you spend the summer (the first summer of graduate school) learning about animal viruses? First of all, there's nobody here who knows anything about animal viruses. And second of all, there's a guy (James Darnell) coming in the fall, and so if you were interested, maybe you could work with him. So he sent me off for the summer to work with one of the few people who were doing animal virology in a quantitative way at the time. There were damn few people in 1961."[195] That summer, Baltimore took a course on animal virology at Cold Spring Harbor and met the virologist Philip I. Marcus,[196] who had been the first to culture HeLa cells while training with Theordore Puck at Colorado. Baltimore was planning to take the techniques and apply them back at MIT that fall. But when he finally ran into the edgy James Darnell that summer he "gave me a 'get-away-from-me answer.'"[197] "Luria felt very much that he'd let me down," Baltimore recalled, because Darnell was being avoidant, and there was no one else at MIT to mentor him on animal viruses. If not Darnell, he wanted to work with Richard Franklin at Rockefeller.[198] And so he went.

Baltimore found Rockefeller to be "a patrician institution, with coats and ties, and we ate in the Abbey, in the velvet lined room, with breakfast served by lovely ladies in their black and white uniforms." Baltimore was at Rockefeller only 18 months when he completed his thesis work. In 1963, he returned to MIT to work with Darnell for his training. "It was when I came to Darnell's lab that I learned how you did modern virology, because Darnell had already picked up the techniques and developed many of them himself, that allowed one to do experiments much more simply than Richard could ever do them."[199] In 1964 and 1965, he continued his work on virus replication with Jerry Hurwitz at the Albert Einstein College of Medicine, before being recruited by Renato Dulbecco to the newly established Salk Institute for Biological Studies, out in La Jolla, a suburb of San Diego. It was at Salk that Baltimore started to do some damage. He discovered that viral proteins could become cleaved into multiple parts, one of the tricks that scientists would come to call "post-translational modifications." "This

student and I found ourselves working on protein synthesis of polio virus
and we came up with the fact that there was a cleavage of one protein into
two, which at that point was unique. And we extended that over the time
after I came here to show that all the proteins were made from one long
polypeptide and that was pretty revolutionary at the time. I mean, that
gave me the sense that I could do new things, and come up with concepts.
I think that was the thing that really gave me the most self-confidence. It
was really a kind of new thing for virology and that was pretty good."[200]

Luria made a pitch to Baltimore to return to MIT and take a faculty
position. Baltimore's marriage had broken up, and he returned to MIT to
take the job in January 1968, bringing with him Mike Jacobson and Alice
Huang. He married Huang that fall. "At Salk there was a lot of griping at the
junior levels, in which I was involved some, about the powerlessness of
everybody there but when I came back to MIT my reaction was one of
relief. I just became a committed virologist, and have really been ever since.
I guess intellectually, I find it much more satisfying to work with a discrete
entity where the problem is small, than the enormous problem the cell
represents."[201] And that's when he makes his big breakthrough. RNA
polymerase is an enzyme that copies DNA into RNA at the level of
transcription. DNA polymerase copies DNA into more DNA and is used
for self-replication, or as Baltimore would discover, some forms of polymerase can copy RNA into DNA. When he made this discovery, his first
thought was to call Howard Temin, also a Swarthmore grad, who was
about five years older.

"Alice and I started working on a virus she developed for her thesis,
vesticular stomatitus virus. The virus particles had an RNA polymerase in
them, which was fairly unique. This was really quite striking. We published that, and then, in thinking about the extensions of that, it seemed
possible that one of the extensions was that there was a DNA polymerase
in RNA tumor viruses. And I got myself some RNA tumor viruses, which
I'd never worked on before, from NIH, and tried the assay, and after a
couple of days it worked. And so, I – well there's a long story in there.
I took off a week while I struck against the university and everybody else,
because the Cambodian invasion occurred the day after I made the
discovery."

In 1970, Baltimore isolated an enzyme of DNA polymerase, which
became known as reverse transcriptase, which proved to be the essential
component that enabled a RNA virus to return back into DNA. It upset
the "central dogma" of a transition of DNA to RNA to protein because no

one at the time thought that the RNA code could transition back into DNA, hence the "retro." "When we saw the lifecycle of the RNA virus involved integration of DNA, the implication was reverse transcriptase allowed for this, but did not prove it," Baltimore told me. "And then I got back to work and finished it up and wrote up a paper for *Nature* and sent it off, and then I called Howard Temin because I knew Howard was very interested in this. It's basically his hypothesis that led me to thinking about it... And I said, 'Howard, there's DNA polymerase in the virion of RNA tumor viruses,'and he said, 'Where'd you hear that?'And I said, I didn't hear it; I did it. And he said, 'You did it – I did it!'"[202]

Paul Berg was coming under the increasing opinion that it was necessary to transition the basic lessons from the bacteria to animal cells, if scientists were going to learn anything about the more complex cellular machinery that is useful to medicine. "In '65 I decided to work with animal cells. One of the top people in that field was a man named Renato Dulbecco, who has his labs down at the Salk Institute. I spent my sabbatical year there," Berg said.[203] Berg began collaborating with scientists who were studying a "lysogenic" virus that infects *E. coli* microbes. These viruses integrate into the host cell's nucleus or even its genome, and multiply along with the cell as an "obligate intercellular parasite." *E. coli* grows in the human gut, and this is one reason it has been a key microbe to study. What's more, Berg considered the relationship between the virus and microbe to be analogous to a virus that infects monkeys, simian virus 40, or SV40, a small DNA virus known for its ability to cause tumors in animals and eukaryote cells. A virus is essentially a "transposable genome," and if Berg could design an efficient way to transfer segments of genes attached to this virus into monkey or human cells, he could investigate their contributions to the basic mechanisms of cell machinery, and learn how individual genes affect cellular processes, even the circuitry of cancer. A new world of experiments laid in wait. Scientists could add any new gene to a cell and watch its effect. Berg, and one of his all-star students, Janet Mertz, would write in reflection "it seemed reasonable to consider whether a comparable virus-mediated gene-transfer system exists for mammalian cells. The small DNA viruses, polyoma and SV40, were deemed to be good candidates. It was already known that infection of cultured mouse cells with polyoma virus results in the production of infectious polyoma progeny and virus particles containing exclusively mouse DNA.

Importantly, the mouse DNA contained in these polyoma 'pseudovirions' is representative of the entire mouse genome. A similar finding was made with the related primate virus, SV40. However, in this case, some virus particles are produced in which host cellular DNA is covalently joined to the viral DNA. Might it be possible, we mused, that polyoma or SV40 could be used to transfer genes from one mammalian cell to another in much the same way that phage transfer genes among bacteria?"[204]

No one knew if "recombinant DNA" could be applied to "higher" eukaryotic cells. "During the 1960s, enormous progress was made in understanding the structure of genes and the mechanisms of their replication, expression, and regulation in prokaryotes and the viruses that infect them. However, largely unknown at the end of that decade was whether these findings were applicable to eukaryotes, i.e., organisms with an authentic nucleus, and, in particular, mammalian cells. The reason was that the experimental tools available at that time for exploring molecular and genetic properties of mammalian organisms were woefully inadequate for the task."[205]

Berg wanted to use recombinant DNA to investigate which components of a "tumor virus" can trigger a cancer in a human cell. "In early 1971, the American Cancer Society approved a grant application in which Berg proposed to develop the means for transducing foreign DNA into mammalian cells. In the proposal, he identified SV40 DNA as the vector because it can be taken up by rodent and primate cells, including human ones, where it can replicate to high copy number as an autonomous plasmid or integrate into the host cell's genome."[206] By adding or deleting parts of SV40 and adding them to a mammalian cell, scientists might learn which parts of the virus triggered a cell to take on properties of a cancer. In the transcript I had been reading at MIT, Berg recalled, "Now, if you've come from the field of molecular biology of microorganisms, what you have to recognize is that one of the most powerful tools in opening that system was the use of genetic techniques for analyzing both the viruses and the cells, and the ability to manipulate the genes of these cells, construct any assortment of genes that one wanted in order to study the consequences of that conformation, were very impressive... It was known that the SV40 chromosome integrates into the cellular chromosome, and when it transforms the cell, converts it into a tumor cell. If it can do that, and if you can now insert genes in the chromosome of SV40 and use the SV40's capability of integrating in the host chromosome, then you can also transport new genes in as well...Well, that turned out to be surprisingly easy."[207]

In 1971, members of Berg's lab had managed to splice into an SV40 genome an "operon," which is a suite of genes expressed together, in this case three genes, which enable E. coli to metabolize the sugar galactose (gal) along with a snippet of genes from the bacteriophage lambda that enables the DNA to replicate as a plasmid in E.coli; in effect, the lab had spliced together genes from a bacterium and a primate virus.

In a first step, Mertz, in collaboration with Douglas Berg, a postdoc in the A. Dale Kaiser lab and David Jackson, a postdoc in Berg's lab, isolated a "deleted variant (dv)" of the lambda phage that included an operon of three gal genes from E. coli that had been located directly adjacent to the site at which this virus had integrated into the bacterial genome.[208] In a second step, the scientists spliced this lambda-galactose hybrid, named λdvgal 120 into the DNA genome of SV40.[209] The second step in this process was quite tricky. To do it, Jackson used six different enzymes in a precise order to carry out a "terminal transferase tailing method" which would add artificial tails, or overhangs, a string of nucleotides, to the ends of double-stranded linear DNA molecules. To one of the DNAs, he added a "tail," or single string of adenosine (A) nucleotides, and to the other DNA he added a tail of thymidine (T) nucleotides. The tails of the two different DNA molecules hybridized together by natural hydrogen bonds. The SV40 and λdvgal 120 were covalently pasted together using some of these numerous enzymes to form circular DNA molecules that could, in theory, now enter a mammalian cell. In his 1972 PhD thesis, Peter Lobban, a student of Kaiser who was concurrently developing this method for joining together two DNA molecules, foresaw the prospect of inserting any foreign DNA, including from mammalian cells into newly spliced combinations, believing it would usher us into a new age of "genetic engineering."

"Thus, by the fall of 1971, the first chimeric recombinant DNA had been produced by sequentially using six enzymes with previously known properties," Mertz wrote. "Noteworthy is the fact that none of the individual procedures, manipulations, and reagents used to construct this recombinant DNA was novel; the novelty lay in the specific way in which they were used in combination."[210] Berg agreed to a "self-imposed moratorium" on putting the hybrid molecules into living cells in December 1971. In any case, these very first "recombinant" molecules constructed in a testtube could not have replicated in *E. coli* because a critical gene for their replication had been disrupted in the process.[211] It hardly mattered since the process was a bit of an art form to execute, a dizzyingly complicated protocol; as Mertz told me: "nobody outside of Stanford would likely have had access to all six of the enzymes needed to try to replicate their work or to use it to make their own hybrid DNAs."

In the summer of 1971, Mertz took a course in animal cells and viruses taught at the Cold Spring Harbor Laboratory by a microbiologist named Robert Pollack. During the course, Mertz mentioned to Pollack that her planned PhD thesis project was to map and identify the functions of the SV40 genes after replicating defective insertional mutants of SV40 in *E. coli*, once a postdoc in Berg's lab, David Jackson, had succeeded in developing a method for making SV40-$\lambda dvgal$ recombinant DNAs. Upon learning about Mertz' planned project, Pollack, a 31 year-old microbiologist, called up Berg and sent him to the woodshed. How could Berg knowingly splice together genes from SV40 and genes from a bacteriophage that infects a bacterium that naturally grows in the gut of humans? Simply, if their recombinant DNA expressed the oncogenes of this primate tumor virus after being put into *E. coli*, then Berg might-potentially place all humans, as well as primates and some other mammals, at heightened risk of cancer if this SV40-containing bacteria were to escape from the lab. After all, *E. coli* grow in human guts. You may be creating a "pre-Hiroshima condition," Pollack snapped. "No one should be permitted to do the first, most messy experiments in secret and present us all with a reprehensible and/or dangerous fait accompli at a press conference."

Berg was not caught completely unaware. He had dined at the house of Maxine Singer, a scientist who operated a lab at the NIH, along with dinner guest Leon Kass, who would write a major position paper that year arguing for caution and laying out the stakes of gene engineering. Singer and Kass had informed Berg of the rumor-mill that had started around his work, and how many scientists were pressing for caution in private conversations. Michael Crichton's terrifying science fiction novel *The Andromeda Strain* had been released two years earlier, and the film version hit cinemas nationwide in 1971, the same year that Berg revealed his stunning technical feat. Crichton's sci-fi thriller was about an extraterrestrial microbe on the loose that caused human blood to clot. And what if reality was stranger, if not more deadly, than fiction? Berg's splicing of genes from a cancer-causing virus and a microbe might result in an actual microbe strain which could emerge on the loose and trigger cancer throughout the population. The tempest over genetic engineering had only just begun. And Berg had crossed the threshold, introducing a means for genetic modification and launching a wave of deep debate within the scientific community, which he in part initiated by self-imposing a moratorium on genetic engineering.

In the spring of 1972, Mertz, in collaboration with Ron Davis, a new assistant professor in her department, discovered a simpler way to cut and paste genetic material. Importantly, their elegant method for recombining DNA molecules, using just a restriction enzyme followed by DNA ligase, fully preserved the functions of the genes that were spliced. It meant that they could be inserted into a bacterium which could carry on its growth and spread the spliced genes each time it replicated. It was also far easier to apply than the existing protocol requiring a half-dozen enzymes to engineer a gene splice, and they knew instantly that anyone could now create recombinant DNA. "The only reason I didn't do so was because of our self-imposed moratorium against cloning SV40. I presented this work in August 1972 at public talks held both in the Stanford Biochemistry Department and at a Cold Spring Harbor Laboratory meeting," Mertz told me.

But by now, Berg's lab had indeed put on a stunning display of splicing of genes from a bacterium and the virus SV40. The danger was that SV40 was known to induce cancers in some animals. And it had a notorious past. In the 1950s, the two competing polio vaccines, those made by Albert Sabin and Jonas Salk, were both found to be contaminated with SV40. Millions of people had already been inoculated with these contaminated vaccines before SV40 was discovered. Were some cancers in humans being triggered by the tainted polio virus vaccines? Sabin and Salk were stung by the horrible irony of putting the global population at risk of cancer.

An enzyme named *EcoRI* changed everything. Japanese researchers had been the first to notice the phenomenon of restriction enzymes at work in bacteria in the 1950s. In effect, phage yields can drop significantly when grown in some microbes, hence the virus' growth is "restricted," and for which they soon became termed "restriction enzymes." They are also more broadly termed "endonucleases" because they shred genetic material. The Swiss microbiologist Werner Arber and his student Daisy Dussoix carried out much of the research that showed that the DNA of restricted phage is enzymatically degraded by such restriction enzymes, demonstrating the mechanism.[212] Arber had spent time in the laboratories of Joshua Lederberg at Stanford and Luria at MIT, and during a 60-day stint in 1963 with Gunther Stent at the University of California in Berkeley, provided the first solid experimental evidence showing that the addition of tiny molecules called methyl groups, a process of so-called methylation, was required for the enzyme to function as tiny molecular scissors. In 1964, contributions from Bill Wood, Bob Yuan and Matthew Meselson would fully elucidate the mechanism. Scientists had learned to use these molecular scissors to cut DNA into specific small units and then learn the function of those units, or genes, by observing their effects on the cell. Silvia Arber, one of Werner Arber's two daughters, born in 1968, learned about it and asked her father to explain the concept of a "restriction enzyme," re-expressing the science in her own language as "the tale of the king and his servants."

In the words of 10-year-old Silvia, the molecular fairytale goes like this: "When I come to the laboratory of my father, I usually see some plates lying on the tables. These plates contain colonies of bacteria. These colonies remind me of a city with many inhabitants. In each bacterium there is a king. He is very long, but skinny. The king has many servants. These are thick and short, almost like balls. My father calls the king DNA, and the servants enzymes. The king is like a book, in which everything is noted on the work to be done by the servants. For us human beings these instructions of the king are a mystery. My father has discovered a servant who serves as a pair of scissors. If a foreign king invades a bacterium, this servant can cut him in small fragments, but he does not do any harm to his own king. Clever people use the servant with the scissors to find out the secrets of the kings. To do so, they collect many servants with scissors and put them onto a king, so that the king is cut into pieces. With the resulting little pieces it is much easier to investigate the secrets. For this reason my father received the Nobel Prize for the discovery of the servant with the scissors."[213]

Arber's restriction enzyme did not cleave DNA at a single location. In 1970, Thomas Kelly and Hamilton Smith had identified a restriction enzyme named *HindII* that did cut DNA at a single site.[214] Kathleen-Danna and Daniel Nathans then showed this enzyme cleaves DNA of the mammalian tumor virus SV40 into 11 unique fragments. Arber, Smith and Nathans would receive the 1978 Nobel Prize in Physiology or Medicine for these accomplishments. But there was an important limitation to the *HindII* restriction enzyme. It would cut leaving "blunt ends," meaning there was no overhang. "That is why folks assumed all restriction enzymes would cleave leaving blunt ends," Mertz told me.

Near the same time, Robert N. Yoshimori, working in the lab of Herbert Boyer at the University of California at San Francisco, had isolated from a microbe a restriction enzyme called *EcoRI* (pronounced "echo R one"), which others would soon show worked like scissors, cleaving DNA at a unique sequence.[215] Boyer was at Yale for a postdoc when he became "hooked on the restriction-modification thing. I was convinced that these were going to be very helpful enzymes at that time."[216,217] By the time he was at California, he had blown the lid off the field. Importantly, *EcoRI*, didn't require the addition of a methyl group, and made reliable, precise cuts to genetic material at specific sites. Boyer was soon passing out his molecular scissors, slipping a set to John Morrow in Berg's lab at Stanford. Through a set of elegant experiments in the spring of 1972, Mertz and Davis showed *EcoRI* was the first pair of tiny molecular scissors that could easily be used to create recombinant DNAs; importantly, unlike the other types of molecular scissors, it created "sticky" or "cohesive cuts" to the ends of its genetic target, meaning a double-strand break with an overhang of one of the strands left dangling.[218] Mertz's "sticky ends hypothesis" would have major implications, since it would allow for scientists to anneal together any two DNA molecules which had complementary dangling ends. Berg later commented: "It doesn't take a genius to figure out that if you can create artificial ends that are complementary to each other, the two DNA molecules will come together."[219]

"Boyer had assumed the *EcoRI* cleavage site would be blunt and was trying to sequence it using the Kelly & Smith protocol without success," Mertz said. "When I told him it was cohesive, not blunt, we then suggested how he could successfully sequence it, which he proceeded to do."[220] Morrow's thesis project was to find a restriction enzyme which could clip the SV40 DNA once at a unique site so he could open up the circular genome and have an endpoint. SV40 is a double-stranded DNA genome that is 5kbp long and is closed as a circle. By clipping it at a single spot, he could begin mapping components of the virus using an electron microscope. The first two enzymes Morrow tried did not clip the SV40 genome at a unique site, but when he tried *EcoRI*, it did clip the genome at a single reliable site.[221] Morrow had clipped open the circular DNA of the virus, turning it into a linear molecule. Mertz then tried to see if SV40 DNA linearized in this way retained any of its functions. She found that when she put the cleaved viral DNA into a monkey cell it was not only functional, but spun out baby viruses that were again circular. "To my initial surprise, these linear DNA molecules were infectious, producing progeny viral DNA genomes that were circles," Mertz told me. Based on her prior experiences working with phage lambda, she hypothesized that when EcoRI restriction enzyme cleaved the SV40 DNA it left cohesive ends. Some breaks in double-stranded DNA are blunt, meaning they result in a perpendicular clip, and some are cohesive, or "sticky," meaning they leave an overhang. If the break was cohesive, it would be possible that a DNA ligase, an enzyme in the cell, would be able to "ligate" or paste together the overhangs with high efficiency.

In 1956, Berg had discovered the first instance of adenylation, which it turns out is the same enzymatic mechanism that a DNA ligase uses to catalyze the covalent joining of DNA ends. Mertz obtained a DNA ligase, which had been purified from E coli., from Paul Modrich, another graduate student at Stanford (and winner of a Nobel Prize in 2015). She then incubated her EcoRI-cleaved SV40 DNA with this enzyme at low temperature in a test tube. She discovered that the ligase turned the linear DNAs back into circular ones. The first definitive proof that the EcoRI-generated ends were "sticky," came from Mertz and Davis showing that they hydrogen-bonded to form circles at refrigerator temperature, something blunt ends can't do.

Working together with Ronald Davis, a new assistant professor in the department, they then proved that EcoRI-generated ends were both sticky and identical in sequence by showing that lots of different EcoRI-generated ends could be annealed together by hydrogen bonding at refrigerator temperature even without adding ligase. With this finding in hand, Mertz then used EcoRI to clip two different DNAs into linear molecules with cohesive ends, mixed them together, and added the ligase to recombine them to create chimeric DNA molecules. "That is how we discovered that some restriction enzymes cleave DNA leaving cohesive ends that can be used to easily make recombinant DNAs at high efficiency," Mertz explained. Mertz and Ron Davis had pulled off the feat of splicing genes into SV40 using just EcoRI and a ligase, a surprisingly simple enzymatic method that was highly efficient.[222] They had radically simplified the process, turning it from a method that once took six enzymes into one that could be widely adopted for use in just about any biochemistry or molecular biology lab.

"Janet Mertz and Ron Davis did the first experiment which showed that you could take two different DNAs cut with the enzyme, mix them, and make hybrid molecules. They're never given credit for it, frankly, but in fact they did the first experiment which showed that you could make covalently joined hybrid molecules" in an efficient way that any appropriately skilled scientist could also readily perform, Berg said in an MIT archive transcript.[223] "I told Boyer about our discovery," Mertz said. "He then used this fact to rapidly determine the sequence of the *EcoRI*-generated ends, a project he had unsuccessfully been working on up until then because he (like everyone in the field) had been assuming restriction enzymes cleave leaving blunt ends. In order to not scoop him given we knew his project was to determine the *EcoRI* cleavage site and he had very generously provided us with enzyme, we waited to publish our findings in the same issue of *PNAS* as his, cross-referencing each other."[224] The moment was of historical importance and, not surprisingly, it was also a moment of controversy. Mertz's version of these events saw evidence in Sally Hughes' oral history project archived at UC-Berkeley.[225] Stanley Cohen claims Victorio Sgaramella, a postdoc in the genetics department at Stanford, independently discovered that *EcoRI*-cleaved DNA leaves cohesive ends, with Sgaramella publishing a paper in the same issue of *PNAS* in which the Mertz and Boyer papers appeared.[226,227]

Boyer and Cohen would soon collaborate, using *EcoRI* to combine genes from two different microbes, resulting in a single microbe that had acquired resistance to two different antibiotics. The experiment was legendary, conceived at a Waikiki Beach deli during a plasmid meeting in November 1972. Cohen had organized a meeting on plasmids with Tsotomu Watanabe and Donald Helinski, seeking to bring together Japanese and Americans, held at the University of Hawaii in Honolulu. "Don contacted me to suggest that Herb Boyer, whose work on the plasmid-encoded *EcoRI* enzyme he had just learned about, be added to the list of speakers," Cohen wrote in a reflection. "The actual collaboration began during a long walk near Honolulu's Waikiki Beach in search of a sandwich shop to have a late evening snack. Boyer and I were joined by Stanley Falkow, who recently had moved his laboratory to the University of Washington, Charles Brinton, a microbiologist from the University of Pittsburgh, and Charles's wife, Ginger. During that walk,

Herb and I discussed recent results from our laboratories. I described our experiments showing that *E. coli* could be transformed genetically with naked plasmid DNA, and our plasmid DNA shearing experiments, which had not yet been published, and Herb described the similarly unpublished sequencing data that he, Joe Hedgpeth, and Howard Goodman had obtained for the *Eco*RI cleavage site. As Herb and I talked, I realized that *Eco*RI was the missing ingredient needed for molecular analysis of antibiotic resistance plasmids. Large plasmids would be cut specifically and reproducibly by the enzyme, and this method of cleavage would surely be better than the haphazard mechanical shearing methods I had been using for fragmentation of plasmid DNA circles. Because *Eco*RI recognizes a six base pair sequence, cleavage sites on duplex DNA would be on average about 4,100 base pairs apart, and each of the DNA fragments produced would likely contain only a few genes...

Because of the asymmetry of cleavage of the *Eco*RI recognition sequence, the ends of the multiple plasmid DNA fragments generated by *Eco*RI would be complementary – and under the right conditions individual plasmid DNA fragments in the mixture could join to each other in different combinations... By the time we encountered a small delicatessen having an enticing window sign that read, 'Shalom,' in place of the ubiquitous 'Aloha,' we had decided to proceed collaboratively and agreed on the basic design of the project that our laboratories would jointly carry out. We would target the R6-5 plasmid, which Sharp, Davidson, and I had learned much about from heteroduplex analysis (a new microscope trick), and which Chang and I had been shearing using a mechanical stirring device and metal blades, in our initial experiments. A few minutes later, over warm corned beef sandwiches and cold beer, Herb and I sketched out an experimental plan on napkins taken from the dispenser at our table."[228]

Phillip Sharp, Bill Sugden and Joseph Sambrook had developed an agarose gel electrophoresis/DNA staining method which would allow experimental scientists to separate and visualize fragments of DNA generated by restriction enzymes. "This advance offered a hugely important addition to the centrifugation and heteroduplex methods we were using to analyze plasmids," Cohen recalled. "Data were analyzed at both places (Stanford and UCSF) and results were discussed between laboratories almost daily. I'd arrive in the laboratory early in the morning to look at the culture plates when colonies produced by cells plated late the previous evening were still tiny. I often wished that the bacteria would grow faster so that we could obtain results sooner. Annie lived in San Francisco and carried materials between Stanford and UCSF. We'd hurry to isolate plasmid DNA so that she could carry some of it to Herb's laboratory for gel analysis the next day. It was an extraordinarily exciting time for all of us."[229]

In these experiments the researchers chopped up an R6-5 plasmid from *E. coli* into fragments and created new recombinant plasmids, discovering that one of those plasmids expressed kanamycin resistance, but not the other resistance genes of R6-5. If such a plasmid included a resistance gene, then the recombinant molecule could be selected for by dosing a plate with the antibiotic. Only the spliced plasmid would survive and remain. But, it turns out, some of the spliced fragments that resulted from cutting up R6-5 lacked the critical sites which were necessary for a plasmid to undergo autonomous replication, meaning to copy itself. By comparison, the replicon pSC101, which Boyer and Annie Chang had previously isolated, carried a gene for tetracycline resistance and sites for replication.[230] To get one that is also resistant for kanamycin, the scientists spliced pSC101 with R6-5 DNA fragments that carried the kanamycin resistance gene, achieving an autonomously replicating plasmid resistant to both kanamycin and tetracycline, and introducing the resulting recombinant DNA molecules into bacteria.[231] In effect, the scientists have used *EcoRI* as molecular scissors to "recombine pSC101 with a segment of DNA from an *E. coli* plasmid that contained a different antibiotic resistance gene; the new plasmid could be propagated in *E. coli* where it expressed both antibiotic resistance properties."[232] Born was a single genetically engineered microbe with multiple antibiotic resistances.

This experiment demonstrated that genetic fragments from different plasmids could be spliced together to create a newly engineered plasmid, which could be shipped into new cells. This led scientists to begin to try to test "barriers to interspecies gene transfer." Cohen and colleagues would design experiments by using a 18-kb plasmid named pI258 that replicates autonomously in *Staphyloccus aureus*, and had been shown to carry a gene encoding resistance to penicillin. The researchers dared to see if they could splice these penicillin resistance genes into a plasmid for *E. coli*, creating a "chimeric" molecule from two different species. "Whether DNAs known to be highly disparate in nucleotide composition and taken from microbes as different as the Gram-positive coccus

S. aureus and the Gram-negative rod-shaped *E. coli* could be propagated as part of the same replicon and whether the staphylococcal gene would be expressed in the new host was questionable," Cohen wrote in a reflection. "The experiments themselves were not complicated and the results were conclusive. We... combined the DNA fragments, introduced the ligated mixture into calcium chloride-treated *E. coli*, and selected bacterial colonies that expressed both the ampicillin resistance of pI258 and the tetracycline resistance encoded by pSC101."[233,234] This chimeric plasmid propagated efficiently in *E. coli*, exhibiting the unique antibiotic resistance characteristics of both parental plasmids."[235]

If Berg's work had set off a tempest, Cohen's work showing that recombinant DNAs could, in fact, be replicated and expressed in bacteria provoked a typhoon. Berg's work had suggested that tumor viruses could be incorporated into bacteria that live in the human gut, raising the potential that genetic engineers could introduce and promulgate dangerous or new infectious agents, some which could possibly give us cancer. But Cohen's work raised the prospect of engendering new microbes that would be superbugs which might be impossible to stop and create a runaway rogue microbe resistant to multiple antibiotic drugs. "I heard, I guess from Paul on the phone, about what Stanley Cohen had actually done, which was at that time unpublished," Baltimore said. "I think Paul sent me a preprint of it. Then I knew we really had a problem."[236]

Boyer was the first to publicly present this research, doing so at a high-stakes meeting called the Gordon Conference held in New Hampshire in June 1973. It was during this conference that Morrow proposed to Boyer that they try to splice a gene for ribosomal RNA from *Xenopus laevis*, a South African clawed frog, into *E. coli* using Cohen's pSC101 with its antibiotic resistance gene that could be used as a selectable marker for presence of the plasmid in the bacteria. Morrow, while still a student in Berg's lab, collaborated with the Boyer and Cohen laboratories to show such a method could also be used to clone ribosomal DNA from *Xenopus laevis* into a plasmid to create many copies of this frog's gene.[237] This suggested that DNA from any source, quite likely even human DNA, could be replicated and expressed this way in bacteria: the cloning of DNA. In Cohen's words, "this plasmid (pSC101) contained a single site for the restriction enzyme EcoRI and a gene for tetracycline resistance. The restriction enzyme EcoRI was used to cut the frog DNA

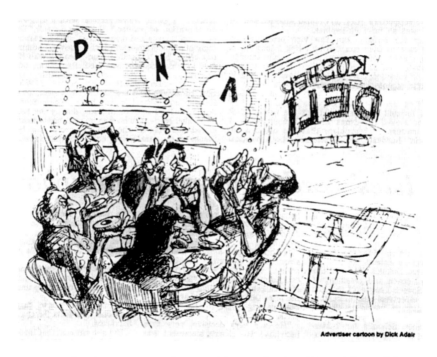

FIGURE 2   A cartoon accompanying an article reporting demolition of the Waikiki beach delicatessen where initial DNA cloning experiments were planned. Clockwise are Herbert Cohen (12 o'clock), Stanley Cohen, Ginger Brinton, Charles Brinton and Stanley Falkow. Cartoon by Dick Adair in the *Honolulu Advertiser* September 26, 1988.

into small segments. Next, the frog DNA fragments were combined with the plasmid, which had also been cleaved with EcoRI. The sticky ends of the DNA segments aligned themselves and were afterwards joined together using DNA ligase. The plasmids were then transferred into a strain of *E. coli* and plated onto a growth medium containing tetracycline."[238] The cells that incorporated the plasmid carrying the tetracycline resistance gene grew and formed colonies of bacteria. Some of these colonies consisted of cells that carried the frog ribosomal RNA gene. The scientists then tested the colonies that formed after growth for the presence of frog ribosomal RNA.[239] "The PNAS publications resulting from these pursuits generated considerable scientific excitement – and work aimed at repeating and extending the findings was undertaken almost immediately by other researchers. The papers also prompted a highly public controversy about potential hazards of "genetic tinkering," a decision by Stanford University and the University of

California to seek patents on the technology that Boyer and I had invented, and efforts by entrepreneurs and industry to implement DNA cloning methods for commercial purposes."

"The profound implication of this experiment was that DNA from any organism on the planet could probably be cloned and propagated in *E. coli*," Mertz said.[240] The gristmill was churning. Boyer got up at the conference and told the audience that these first scalable experiments in genetic engineering amounted to little more than a technical achievement, which was well controlled. Scientists had spliced together genes creating a new bug with multiple antibiotic resistances. That seemed provocative enough, and it was clear that scientists now had new powers that could be used for any gene splicing. After Boyer's closing comments, a scientist named Bill Sugden, a current colleague of Janet Mertz at UW-Madison, sounded loudly, and excitedly, the revelation that was on everyone's mind.

"Now we can combine any DNA."[241,242]

Shortly after the Gordon Conference, Maxine Singer, who had previously alerted Berg to the coming storm, and the scientist Dieter Söll of Yale, drafted an open letter to the National Academy of Sciences, or NAS, dated July 17, 1973. It began: "We are writing to you on behalf of a number of scientists, to comment on a matter of great concern..." Singer and Soll brought forth a rap sheet of concerns, most pressing that new strains of microbes could be created that inadvertently were highly pathogenic; if rDNA wasn't regulated, there was some outside chance that some unscrupulous scientist would engineer a microbe that was infectious and put the human race at risk. NAS president Philip Handler stepped forward a few days later to publically acknowledge the letter. Berg quickly organized a meeting in April 17, 1974, summoning Watson, Baltimore, Boyer, Cohen, Hogness, Bernard Davis, Daniel Nathans, Sherman Weissman, Richard Roblin and Norton Zinder to a roundtable at MIT. Watson was highly supportive of the call for caution and suggested a huddle of international scientists. At the meeting, Berg recalled Zinder saying, "If we had any guts at all, we'd tell people not to do these experiments."[243] The heads of the academy decided to play it conservatively. The NAS released a report on July 18, 1974 calling for a moratorium. In fact, moratoria in the sciences are exceedingly rare. Seldom had a regulatory body completely banned a set of scientific experiments. The only prior occurrence of a scientific moratorium in the US had related to work on experiments on nuclear fusion.

As Berg later wrote in a recollection, "Scientists around the world hotly debated the wisdom of our call for caution, and the press had a field day conjuring up fantastical 'what if ' scenarios. Yet the moratorium was universally observed in academic and industrial research centers. Meanwhile, the public seemed comforted by the fact that the freeze had been proposed by the very people who had helped to develop the technology."

"We also proposed an international conference at which scientists and appropriate experts could assess the risks of recombinant DNA technology and devise ways of reducing them. With the backing of the National Academy of Sciences and the National Institutes of Health, I and four others – David Baltimore, Sydney Brenner, Richard Roblin and Maxine Singer – drew up the agenda for the conference. Its main aim was to consider whether to lift the voluntary moratorium and, if so, what conditions to impose to ensure that the research could proceed safely."[244]

"I didn't like it," Philip Sharp recalled to me in his office in July 2014, of the moratorium on recombinant DNA. "It stopped experiments that I wanted to do." Sharp had been scooped up by James Watson at Cold Spring Harbor where he had done some outstanding work. Sharp was, at the time, one of the young guns eager to test the limits of the field. In 1974, he had been recruited to MIT by Luria, where he was working at MIT at the time of the moratorium. He had a set of experiments in mind on adenovirus. In rodents, adenovirus caused cancer if it was injected before their immune systems had time to develop. Sharp wanted to remove elements of the adenovirus and to determine which parts of it were oncogenic. But Berg co-authored a couple of papers with the other scientists who had been at the MIT roundtable, responding to the NAS letter, acceding to a moratorium in the field.[245] Science was moving fast, and nobody with any ambition wanted to slow down. In 1975, Baltimore was aged 37, on sabbatical at Rockefeller, when he became one of the youngest people to win the Nobel Prize. A reporter snapped a picture of his daughter (Laren) Teak, on his lap in a New York hotel room, before he came back up from New York for a press conference at MIT. "People with cameras a foot from your face... That battery of Nikons," Balti-more recalled. "I certainly didn't feel comfortable. I may have appeared at ease... The whole thing is a stereotype operation. What are you going to do with the money? And these kinds of things."

Baltimore was coming under increasing fire for his work with animal viruses, since they were suspected, and shown in some cases, to trigger cancer. If scientists continued engineering the viruses that can trigger cancers, using them to test basic cellular machinery, there was a sus-pected risk of inadvertently triggering a runaway pandemic. "I guess you couldn't be a newcomer to the field of tumor viruses, especially at MIT, and not feel the hot breath of worry. I mean, when I started working in tumor viruses, I had people down on my back almost immediately about whether it was safe to work with them, and wouldn't I give cancer to everybody who walked down the hall?" Baltimore said. "Paul briefed me about his contacts with people who were critical of his proposal... Some people had made wild accusations; others had been temperate. Paul and I took this seriously. Then the idea was that SV40 DNA in a bacterium could cause cancer and could be more dangerous than SV40 virus. We felt the probability of hazard was small, but could not argue that it was zero."

As tensions mounted, Berg soon organized 140 scientists for a meet-ing at Asilomar State Beach at California's Monterey Peninsula.[246,247] "Spiny grass and scraggly pines creep amid the arts-and-crafts buildings of the Asilomar Conference Grounds, 100 acres of dune where Califor-nia's Monterey Peninsula hammerheads into the Pacific. It's a rugged landscape, designed to inspire people to contemplate their evolving place on Earth," to summon the words of the journalist Amy Max-man.[248] The meeting drew superstars like Baltimore and Watson, and younger scientists like Sharp, who was 30 at the time. Asilomar "was on a plane way higher than anything I'd seen before," Sharp told me. "It was full of adrenaline."

Berg noted the debate contained "heated discussions," and major issues were containment of genetically engineered organisms and how to ensure that engineering new life, especially viruses and microbes, would not increase their pathogenic or oncogenic properties. "I was struck by how often scientists willingly acknowledged the risks in other's experiments but not in their own. (Sydney) Brenner repeatedly warned of the consequences of doing nothing, predicting that such apparently self-serving behavior would be publicly condemned and that government interference or even legislation would follow."[249] But, by all accounts, Sydney Brenner was a stable and solid presence at the meeting.

Waclaw Szybalski coined the term "synthetic biology" to describe the new engineering which would include synthesizing genes from different species. Those molecular tricks could have powerful consequences not only for inadvertently promulgating infectious diseases and cancers through a human population, but also opened up a new era for bio-warfare. As Baltimore described the state of play, "We could even play the game of scaring each other, with the underlying desire to come out being reasonable, but not knowing how to do that. And so you do it by the same way that scientists always come to agreements, which is by a process of advocacy and baiting, and whatever else."[250] A sole tape recorder was left to turn on the table in the open room, and the conference drew a few members of the press like Nicholas Wade and Mike Rogers from *Rolling Stone*. Watson and Joshua Lederberg were grandstanding, and taking up most of the time and attention. Lederberg was playing the role of obstructionist. He clearly wanted Congress to stay out and didn't want any intervention in his laboratory, and in Berg's recollection, "gave me the impression of a child who's being threatened to have his toys removed, and the whole theme of it very frankly, was sort of 'you've got to keep the feds out.'"[251]

A panel of plasmid scientists gave their assessments of the potential risks, and after a presentation, Watson, suddenly and erratically shifted his perspective to align with Lederberg, announcing that a moratorium wasn't needed at all. As Donald Frederickson recounted in his memoir, "Michael Rogers, the correspondent from *RollingStone*, later reported some sample reactions. Josh Lederberg rose to express grave concern about the danger of the panel's recommendations 'crystallizing into legislation'; Ephraim Anderson then demanded that the panel indicate, by a show of hands, which of its members 'had experience with the handling and disposal of pathogenetic organisms capable of causing epidemic *disease.*' When the panel members rather sheepishly admitted that they had all probably had too little, their tormentor added insult to injury by nipping away at the grammar and syntax of the report. Suddenly James Watson uttered a call for an end to the moratorium – moreover, 'without the kind of categorical restrictions called for in the plasmid report.' Rogers recalled that Maxine Singer was on her feet immediately to ask what had changed in the last six months to cause Watson to abandon the movement he had helped to launch."[252]

"What turned the debate around was the suggestion to assign a risk estimate to the different types of experiments envisaged, and to apply safety guidelines of varying stringency according to the degree of risk," Berg recalled. This system worked on two levels. The first was physical containment, whereby the degree of risk was matched with the type of laboratory facility required. So, experiments with little or no risk could be done on an open bench; those with some risk might require laminar flow hoods; a high risk might necessitate an airlock and a laboratory under negative pressure; whereas experiments using known human pathogens would be either prohibited or restricted to specialized facilities. Brenner suggested this should be supplemented with an additional, biological level of containment to minimize the damage should engineered organisms escape into the environment. Thus in cloning experiments that were judged to be of little or no risk, researchers could work on relatively innocuous organisms such as widely used lab strains of *E. coli* and *Bacillus subtilis*; riskier experiments would have to use bacteria that had been genetically modified so they could not survive outside the laboratory."[253] When all was said and done, some recombinant DNA research was allowed to proceed, but other work had a continuing moratorium until appropriate containment conditions could be decided. A draft document was created. Scientists broke out, "each one was sitting in a different part of the room writing a section, handing it on to the other guy, the other guy would rewrite it, then it would go back to a third person, and they would react. I've got all this junk, all these little notes and hand written versions of it, and 'this stinks' and 'this is lousy' and so I don't know," Berg wrote. "I just threw it all in my briefcase."

Watson, Francis Crick and Rosalind Franklin had described the structure of DNA, which was the molecular basis of heredity, just a couple of decades before. Now we could after that code. Scientists needed guidelines. And fast. "At the end of the meeting, Baltimore and four other molecular biologists stayed up all night writing a consensus statement. A few attendees fretted about the idea of modifications of the human 'germ line' – changes that would be passed on from one generation to the next – but most thought that was so far off as to be unrealistic."[254] Watson, who had expressed desire for caution and one of the scientists who sounded a clarion call for international intervention, now said he was not willing to institute any unnecessary safety procedures. "Jim sometimes says things because, I think, he's an enfant terrible, you know, and he has to say it to be different. But he eventually comes around," Berg said.

"Participants agreed on the final day of the conference that research should continue, but under stringent restrictions. The recommendations formed the basis of the official US Guidelines on Research Involving Recombinant DNA, first issued in July 1976. They have proved remarkably effective," Berg wrote. "First and foremost, I feel that scientists were able to gain the public's trust – something that is now much more difficult for researchers working in biotechnology. Because some 15% of the participants at Asilomar were from the media, the public was well informed about the deliberations, as well as the bickering, accusations, wavering views and ultimately the consensus."[255] Asilomar produced a number of guidelines to prohibit the following: cloning or recombinant DNA derived from highly pathogenic organisms; deliberate formation of recombinant DNA containing genes for the biosynthesis of toxins; deliberate creation of plant pathogens; widespread or controllable release into the environment of any organism containing a recombinant DNA molecule unless a series of controlled tests leave no reasonable doubt of safety; transfer of drug-resistance traits to an organism if they could compromise the use of a drug to control disease agents in medicine or agriculture. In addition, the Asilomar group recommended that "at this time" large-scale experiments (more than 10 liters in culture) with rDNA not be carried out. The draft guidelines were presented to NIH's Director's Advisory Committee, or DAC, in 1976, which would be the first move toward adopting the rules into a new body at the NIH to take up expressly these concerns. It was called the Recombinant DNA Advisory Committee, or RAC. Opinions on rDNA were wide-ranging, if minutes from the first DAC meeting are any testament. Robert Sinsheimer spoke in dissent: "The research we are talking about at this meeting marks the advent of a whole new era, the real turning of the corner in biological research... what we are doing is almost certainly irreversible." Susan Wright, also spoke in dissent: "Many of the claimed benefits seem dubious, the risks seem relatively clear." In a mood of caution, Charles Madansky suggested: "to me there are... no pressing social benefits to be gained from this research." And yet, others were leaning favorably. Peter Barton Hutt suggested the science of gene splicing superseded the precept of "do no harm" as "this may be [a case] where inaction could be of greater detriment to the public than action." Balti-more also cited a medical justification for the "potential for manufac-ture of biologicals" and a "potential for understanding the complicated diseases that arise from the malfunction of cells." Some comments were perplexed. Peter Hutt: "Could these experiments be done by a high school teacher?"

Barbara Ackerman had previously been mayor and was sitting on the nine-member city council in Cambridge in the spring of 1976. On May 28, a three-hour public meeting is held at Harvard. "I had watched *The Andromeda Strain* on television one night. It was on the late show. And the next morning at eight o'clock, Ruth [Hubbard] Wald called me up, whom I've known since the peace movement. As a matter of fact, she gave me a very clear picture of the issue." George and Ruth Wald were local activists and wanted to put a halt to gene modification, and they weren't alone. In Baltimore's words, George Wald had a "relatively naïve but honest fear of specific dangers. A civil libertarian, he understands the need of intellectual freedom, a man who understands, in fact, the dangers in legislation, and has spoken out, for minimal legislation." Sinsheimer had philosophical views against the techniques. And then there was "Science for the People," a watchdog group, "and that I believe, is quite ideological in orientation." One of their fears "is the danger of genetic research because genetic research can show, or can imply, that the differences between people are genetic differences, not environmental differences." At the time Jim Watson, once adamant that he didn't want gene engineering going on at this time, now thought the caution was overblown. Ackerman recalled the meeting at Harvard; she was "enthralled. The people's whose lifework was involved were not yet as exasperated as they became later, except for James Watson, who was very exasperated. He walked up and down and shouting – I think he shouted, 'Rubbish!' Or 'Nonsense!' And making a lot of unintelligible noise."

"At the end of the meeting, I got up and said that I wasn't clear whether this was a matter of public interest or not, but I just wanted to register my presence. But I remember saying to her [Ruth Wald] that morning 'what difference does it make what we do? How can you stop them from doing it?'"

The Boston Phoenix carried an article on June 8, 1976 entitled 'Bio-hazards at Harvard,' which basically blew up the issue around town. "The reservation that I have is that by lending our prestige to what was the NAS letter – or whatever it's called – we may have so dramatized the issue that we made it possible for a lot of things to happen that wouldn't have happened," Baltimore recalled. "I think it's at least arguable that the Phoenix article, and the local notoriety, the involvement of Science for the People (a watchdog group), maybe even George Wald's (local activist) involvement at all, might not have occurred had it not been for Paul Berg, Jim Watson, and me and the other people who signed that letter. And that, I think, is a serious problem. I mean, that's not a problem of logic, it's a problem, again, in sociobiology. As it stood, Jon King (an objector) was able to say – he has said, over and over again, 'I didn't raise the problem.' And 'if such a prestigious group raised the problem, there much be a real problem to be raised'. And it's an argument you can't counter. I don't think we could have avoided doing what we did, given how things developed; it would have been irresponsible to do anything else. But I really am sorry that we provided that opening."

Cambridge was the first place recombinant DNA had been taken up in a major way in a city government. "Anybody who has any concept of genes and meddling with genes finds it a fascinating subject, and is afraid of it. I think there is an automatic human terror at that concept of dealing with this right, that it belongs to God, in many people's minds," Ackerman recalled. "It was getting headlines, and called 'dangerous' and that's an unfortunate by product. I had other people who said, 'Look, they're going to be doing it. They must be in the most danger. If they want to do it, it's probably safe.' I realized more students were for it than against it. There are some scientists who are going to be careless and others who are going to be careful. You know whenever anybody called me up and said, 'Why don't you trust me?' Maybe I do trust him, but maybe I don't trust the other one." And then, there were opponents in people like Jonathan King who said, "We're meddling with things we shouldn't meddle with. I went and visited a guy at MIT, [David] Botstein. He said, 'I've been driving for two and a half days. I've driven day and night without stopping from Iowa, because I'm afraid you're going to stop me from doing my experiment.'" Ackerman was fielding opinions from every direction, but she wasn't convinced that the city had the right to enforce policy and limitations on the scientists, recalling "I'm mulling whether it was a city council matter." But, at the time, Alfred Vellucci was mayor. He was categorically against genetic modification, and as Ackerman later recalled, he decided he *did* have the authority to take up the issue. "Oh, he always makes everything a city council matter."

The Washington Post on July 2, 1976 carried an editorial that summed up the draft guidelines forged at Asilomar. "Not everyone is happy with the guidelines. Some scientists feel it is idiocy to attempt the curbing of scientific pursuits. Others believe that all experiments that might lead to genetic manipulation should be prohibited. The guidelines steer a narrow, but apparently safe course between these extremes. In the end they only extend the age-old medical admonition of *primum non nocere* – first of all, do no harm to a new frontier of potential discovery. The prognosis is good." And yet, not everyone was convinced. What would follow were debates in local townships and state assemblies throughout the US as the public came to terms with what was happening. As then-NIH Chief Donald Fredrickson noted, local bureaucracy did not always have the scientific literacy to take on these powerful issues, and were often left to "stumble on the stones of Gregor Mendel's Garden." But not everyone thought kindly of this sort of elitism. That summer Vellucci pushed for local intervention in lieu of federal bans. As Vellucci put it, "I don't think these scientists are thinking about mankind at all. I think they're getting the thrills and excitement and the passion to dig in and keep digging to see what the hell they can do."[256]

The council established a flimsy oversight committee and never achieved the votes for a ban on all recombinant DNA research. "We had legal counsel," Baltimore said. "Woulsey, from MIT's firm, met with us occasionally. And it was clear the City Council had no authority to do what they were doing and could only really do something on their own authority if they had a public health hazard, and in which case, it could be evaluated on the basis of whether there really was a public danger or not. We had little choice except to bring on a court battle. And that first of all we weren't sure we would win a court battle, and it would be disastrous to lose it, absolutely disastrous. But you know, we decided, you know, somebody's got to get to Barbara Ackermann and talk to her, or David Clem (another council member). And my next-door neighbor happened to have run David Clem's campaign, Dan O'Connell. So I met with David over there and talked to him in some length, and actually had some very long sessions. . . Luria (and Sharp) took them (activists and council members) through labs at MIT. . . Vellucci came here once. Salvy got very annoyed with me because they were dealing with each other on a kind of buddy-buddy Italian basis and I stuck my nose in. I'm sure it had no effect."

Capitalists soon pounced. Sharp and Walter Gilbert founded the company Biogen in 1978, which would go on to claim the first patents for rDNA in Cambridge. Sharp wanted to clone insulin by using rDNA techniques, essentially as a means to scale up a drug. To date, insulin had largely been isolated from pigs, a costly and limiting process to make a drug. A faster way to produce the drug was now in sight. At the same time, Herbert Boyer founded Genentech, and in 1978, in collaboration with Eli Lilly (which had been producing insulin since 1923) he produced synthetic insulin by using rDNA techniques to add the gene for insulin to a microbe.[257] The microbe could then be grown up, producing lots of the human protein. Boyer's fortune would largely rest on the "Boyer–Cohen" patent for recombinant DNA based on *EcoRI*, and was the first major biotech patent, first filed in November 1974. Biogen, on the East Coast, and Genetech, on the West Coast, would go to battle to see who would bring an effective insulin drug to market as the first major accomplishment of rDNA.

Victor McElheny had written an upbeat article in May 1974 for *The New York Times*, Cohen recalls, which was read by "Niels Reimers, whose job as Director of the Office of Technology Licensing at Stanford was to help fund the university's academic programs by promoting the licensing of inventions made at the university. The day after the article appeared, I received a telephone call from Reimers indicating that he wanted to discuss patenting the technology that Boyer and I had invented. My first reaction was quite negative. Could findings of basic research funded by the public be patented, and should they be? I told him that our work depended on years of fundamental research on plasmid biology by many laboratories and on properties of DNA, DNA ligase, and restriction enzymes that had been discovered by others. And would a patent adversely affect advancement of the science? Reimers pointed out that prior knowledge is a pillar for every invention and that a well-honed legal process determines whether a particular advance is novel and patentable, as well as the validity of the inventorship claimed in the application. He explained that only commercial entities would pay royalties, that a patent would not impede noncommercial use of DNA cloning methods, and that funds received by Stanford and UCSF would aid research programs at these institutions. I discussed Reimer's proposal with Herb, and together we agreed to let our universities proceed with applications for patents that eventually had 461 licensees before their expiration in 1997. Reimers' oral history is a source of further information about the events that led to these patents."[258] Boyer and Cohen's patent was filed as a method for making and replicating recombinant DNAs. Who deserves the credit for coming up with this technique is a matter of contention. Mertz and Davis had completed their *EcoRI* work "five months before the famous conservation at a deli in Hawaii where Stan Cohen claims to have had his 'eureka moment' on how to make R-factor recombinants," Mertz argued to me in an email. Mertz and Davis published their paper in the prestigious journal *PNAS* the same month as the Hawaii meeting, which "described in detail a protocol for making recombinant DNAs using EcoRI and DNA ligase. Suddenly, there was a method that just about any biochemist or molecular biologist could use to readily generate recombinant DNAs at high efficiency. As best I know, Boyer and Cohen easily did so their first try by simply following my published protocol," Mertz told me. "Herb Boyer had read a preprint of our paper so he could publish his paper on the sequence of the *EcoRI* cleavage site back-to-back with our paper with our citing each other. Boyer told Cohen about our paper. Cohen likely also knew about our findings from conversations and talks held at Stanford.

Mertz and Davis, while working in Paul Berg's lab, had been the first to show that *EcoRI* could be used for recombinant DNA techniques, but did not apply for a patent. As Mertz told me in an email, Boyer and Cohen "deserve much credit for demonstrating that all of the theory and methods developed by the Stanford biochemists could actually work in practice for cloning recombinant DNAs. However, patents are supposed to be based upon conception of ideas and development of methods, all of which were done by folks in the Stanford biochemistry department before Boyer and Cohen had their first idea for making and cloning recombinants in November, 1972. Thus, the Boyer–Cohen patents should never have issued, i.e., they were not valid because the ideas and methods of their invention had been made by others and were already in the public domain at the time of the first patent filing in November, 1974." In 2010, Mertz and Berg published an account of the events. "I purposely waited until all of the Boyer–Cohen patents had expired before writing about these events because, having obtained my Ph.D. from Stanford, I didn't feel that I wanted to undercut Stanford's ability to make money from their recombinant DNA patents. In 20-20 hindsight, it's my belief that patents on the ideas and methods for making recombinant DNAs and cloning them with plasmid and virus vectors should have been filed by Stanford two years earlier with (Peter) Lobban, Berg, (David) Jackson, me, and others listed as co-inventors, with additional patents filed later that included Cohen, Boyer, Morrow, and other Berg lab members after they documented utilities. Then, all of these patents would have been valid. As it was, nobody seriously considered patenting this stuff prior to 1974 and, by then, it was really too late. The US Patent Examiner originally rejected all claims on the 1974 patent application in view of Mertz & Davis 1972. That was a correct decision. Cohen proceeded to publish reviews about this early history which, as far as I am concerned, contain numerous 'sins of omission', half-truths and, even, some outright lies. I'm guessing he did so, in part, to justify the validity of the Boyer–Cohen patents, i.e., he had to downplay the importance of all of the 'prior art' from the Berg lab, including claiming (incorrectly) that the recombinant DNAs I had made would not have been clonable. With these patents being finally issued in 1980, he continued to write numerous review articles proclaiming himself as the father of recombinant DNA and cloning, leading to his obtaining numerous honors and awards (other than the Nobel) in addition to lots of money from these patents. By keeping silent on the questionable validity of the Boyer–Cohen patents, (Peter) Lobban, (John) Morrow, and I lost a huge amount in terms of the fame and positive effects on one's career that should have gone to us for our major discoveries. Lobban and Morrow became so disenchanted with academic research that they dropped out of the field. Lobban became an engineer working in biotech companies.Morrow became a practicing physician." Cohen declined to comment.

Sharp would proceed with his research, and continued to operate his lab at MIT. He had met a young scientist named Richard C. Mulligan, who was completing his PhD in Paul Berg's lab at Stanford University, where he was doing amazing work. "Richard was a special young guy," Sharp told me. "He was such a gifted experimentalist." Sharp wanted Mulligan back at MIT, and he spoke to Baltimore about it. The two organized an impromptu situation to make it work, splitting the money and lab space. Mulligan would be a postdoc for Baltimore, but operate out of Sharp's work bench. "It was a unique position. We'd pay for his workspace and he'd be independent," Baltimore told me. "He was clearly one of the brightest and most effective people of his generation."

In 1979, while a student in Berg's lab, Mulligan managed to delete helical coils of SV40 and insert a rabbit gene for beta-globin, and infected a plate of monkey cells with this recombinant genome. Globins are spherical glob-like proteins that are soluble in the blood, and include immunoglobulin and hemoglobin. Beta-globin carries iron in the blood. In effect, he had put a rabbit gene into a monkey cell, opening the door for what was next, putting a human gene into a cloning vector.[259] He had crossed a rubicon into a fertile new field of therapeutics. Scientists began to wonder whether they could get to the very root of a disease by replacing a malfunctioning gene with a functioning copy. Baltimore had mastered retrovirus and although Berg had performed his early experiments on SV40, Baltimore was tilting Mulligan to experiment with retrovirus.

"Retrovirus was a better bet for technical reasons," Baltimore told me. "Once he saw that, and understood the basic machinery, he set the field in motion." During those twilight years in the late 1970s, working with two powerhouses of twentieth-century biology, Mulligan would prove his mettle, going far beyond the expectations of his mentors.

In 1978, Stephen King released *The Stand*, the most adored novel he would ever write. The novel begins on a remote US army base where a weaponized strain of influenza nicknamed "Captain Trips" is acciden-tally released. The base goes into lockdown, but a security malfunction enables a foot soldier named Charles Campion to escape, which triggers a pandemic of apocalyptic proportions that kills off 99.4 percent of the human population. "There is no *moral* to *The Stand*, no 'We'd better learn or we'll probably destroy the whole damned planet next time,'" King later noted in his memoir *On Writing*. But by now, even if the public was still enamored by the idea of unleashing a genetically modi-fied organism, scientists had a grasp on how to self-police themselves. Parts of the moratorium called for in Berg's *Science* letter were lifted after Asilomar, but other parts were only gradually lifted over the years. By 1979, revisions to the initial, conservative guidelines proposed at Asilomar were being made, and becoming more precise and relaxed. What was just years before an intense firestorm of debate now seemed, to some, to amount to little more than Kabuki Theater. Even Maxine Singer, the one-time whip-cracker who pressed for a moratorium, was now suggesting that the guidelines were not being eased quickly enough. The RAC, she said, was holding up science and was beginning to resem-ble a "ponderous" regulator agency. And the courts would side with industry. The debate on the legality of patenting DNA was symbolically resolved with the June 1980 US Supreme Court ruling on Diamond vs. Chakrabarty, a landmark 5–4 decision, which involved a patent for a genetically engineered microbe which could break down crude oil in the case of a spill, allowing patenting of life-forms, in the words of the majority opinion, "anything under the sun, that is made by man."

The Boyer–Cohen patent claims were thusly validated in 1980, and an apparatus began to accelerate the privatization of science. In 1980, the Bayh–Dole Act was passed to permit universities and small businesses to claim patent rights using federal funds, galvanizing the public–private partnership and giving rise to "tech transfer," whereby academics could land patents with government funds and license to business. Mertz and Berg described the disruption. "The sociology among most US life scientists prior to the 1970s was to eschew patents, believing that they would restrict the free flow of information and reagents and impede the pace of discovery. However, that reticence disappeared in November, 1974 when Stanford University and the University of California at San Francisco jointly filed a United States patent application citing their respective faculty members, Stanley Cohen and Herbert Boyer, as the sole inventors of the recombinant DNA technology. Their claims to commercial ownership of the techniques for cloning all possible DNAs, in all possible vectors, joined in all possible ways, in all possible organisms were dubious, presumptuous, and hubristic. Nevertheless, these claims, only slightly modified, were eventually approved in 1980 by the U.S. Patent Office (Cohen and Boyer 1980). By employing what proved to be very wise terms regarding licensing and royalties, the two universities collectively garnered nearly $300 million in revenues during the life of this and two other related patents... Cohen, Boyer, and their respective university departments each received shares of the income from the 'Cohen–Boyer patents,' while the institutions' shares were used to support university-wide research and education. In retrospect, Stanford's and UCSF's action set in motion an escalating cascade of patent claims by universities covering their faculties' respective discoveries that continues to this day. The emergence of the biotechnology industry followed naturally from the encouragement of academic scientists to patent their research discoveries and to explore their newly discovered entrepreneurial instincts."[260]

"Especially striking was the rapidity with which the new technologies took hold and dominated research into many different biological problems. Today, recombinant DNA technology has altered the ways both questions are formulated and solutions are sought. Scientists now routinely isolate genes from any organism on our planet, alive or dead. The construction of new variants of genes, chromosomes, and viruses has become standard practice in research laboratories. Only science fiction one-half century ago, the introduction of new genes into microbes, plants, and animals, including humans, is a common occurrence. The tools of recombinant DNA greatly expedite sequencing of the genomes of humans and numerous other species. Along with these advances have come astonishing improvements in medical diagnoses, prognoses, and therapies."

In 1980, Paul Berg won the Nobel for his work on recombinant DNA. He would share his prize with Frederick Sanger and Walter Gilbert, who mentored a promising young student, George Church, for creating a means for direct sequencing of DNA. And yet, the drama anticipated by Asilomar was not over. That year a professor of medicine at UCLA named Martin Cline made an unauthorized attempt to use recombinant techniques in living human patients, one in Italy and one in Israël. He was attempting to treat a rare blood disorder that afflicted both patients. When the news got out, NIH chief Donald Fredrickson acted swiftly, barring his funding for three years. Cline was forced to resign from his department and chairmanship. But the genie was out of the bottle. Just two years later, a game-changing technique for installing new genes into living human cells burst onto the scene.

4　We Can Play God in that Cell

> Like artists, creative scientists must occasionally be able to live in a world out of joint, elsewhere I have described that necessity as "the essential tension" implicit in scientific research.
>
> –Thomas Kuhn

Richard Mulligan had been at a gas station when his assistant called on his cell phone. The billionaire investor Carl Icahn was on the office line, his assistant said. "He's important right?" Mulligan was returning from Martha's Vineyard and said "yes" and took the call. Icahn had cold-called Mulligan, tapping him as an expert to participate in an effort to gain board seats at the floundering ImClone Systems. In 2009, this relationship with Icahn thrust Mulligan into efforts to obtain seats on the board of Biogen Idec, "in order to try to improve the management," of that company, a process which became, as Mulligan acknowledged, "brutal." It was a pitched battle that resulted in Mulligan and Icahn's shark ally Alex Denner grabbing seats on Biogen's board. In another subsequent proxy fight, the Icahn group went after Genzyme Corp, efforts which resulted in the appointment of a designee onto their board, and ultimately the sale of Genzyme to Sanofi. Biogen had been the same company that Mulligan's mentor, Phil Sharp, had co-founded in 1978. As the longest standing member of the board, Sharp stepped down. Mulligan had become everything that Sharp and Baltimore believed he would become. Now he was taking over their companies. "Now, there's a colorful guy," Baltimore had prepared me.

By now, Mulligan was traipsing back and forth between New York City, handling his funds job, and Boston, where he maintained a lab as a virologist at Harvard and an endowed chair as the Mallinckrodt Professor of Genetics. In 2012, Denner started a hedge fund called Sarissa Capital and Mulligan would begin to plunge most of his energies into that fund. Not too much later than that he became Emeritus, the ordinary next door neighbor of the Harvard geneticist George Q. Daley. But, to be sure, he is tough to catch. He's usually in New York City, and when I first emailed him to set up an interview it was very touch and go, and we set a date for months in advance. He was in his late 50s. He was also very tall, with a commanding presence, but he could be especially gallant. When he whisked me into his office around midday, he asked his secretary to fetch lunch and she scribbled down his order, disappearing without complaint. Now it was just him and me, walled in by colorful bookshelves of medical texts.

Not only is Mulligan linked to a billionaire jet-set, he is also the father of modern gene therapy. He first became interested in gene transfer technology and gene therapy as an undergraduate in Alexander Rich's lab at Massachusetts Institute of Technology in the early 1970s. Rich was trying to insert elements of SV40, the same virus that Paul Berg had been toying with in his first gene splice, into eukaryotic cells (the kind that include human cells) to investigate signals that control the expression of genes. Imagine the tempest that Berg had stoked, and consider those debates moving into the realm of "man engineering man." It was inevitable that gene splicing would be transferred to the landscape of human cells. Mulligan marveled at what was to come, "I was struck at the time as to how sophisticated SV40 appeared to be with regard to its interactions with different kinds of cells and its strategies for achieving viral gene expression, and wondered whether viruses such as SV40 might be able to be engineered to transfer and express foreign genes in cells."[261] Those foreign genes might be from bacteria or even be other human genes. Mulligan went on to be accepted to the PhD program at Stanford University and gained a hard-won place in Paul Berg's lab, where he worked alongside Steve Goff, continuing studies begun by Morrow and Mertz toward understanding how SV40 infects, replicates and destroys its host cell, in other words, to elucidate the viral life cycle.

If they could break apart and classify components of viruses that infected human cells, they could certainly use them to get genes into people. Mulligan remembers Paul Berg's enthusiasm. "Paul was a truly magnificent mentor. He made us all feel that we were doing the most important and most exciting scientific work in the world. I have never forgotten how motivating a PI's enthusiasm for one's work can be for individuals in the lab."[262] During that time, the lab conducted key experiments with recombinant SV40 viral vectors, meaning that they sewed up bits of code for genes of interest into the code of the virus, turning it into "transportable genome" that could carry whatever bit of code they wanted into a cell, which in total was recombinant DNA or a recombinant virus. A notable achievement was getting a recombinant virus to code for human beta-globin, a gene that is defective in genetic blood disorders such as sickle-cell disease and beta thalassemia. Once installed into cells, it resulted in the expression of an authentic human protein.

Importantly, gene transfer technology would be useful for diseases just like this, whereby a small amount of supplementary gene could ameliorate the condition, whereas it would be less practical for diseases where even small numbers of cells in the human body with the mutation could trigger a disease, since it's almost impossible to remove or correct a risky mutation in every cell in an organ or body, say, for example, mutations that predispose risk for cancer. One cannot remove all the dangerous mutations, but one can add a supplement gene. This much was known. A second feat came when the lab showed that it could add a gene for a bacterial enzyme analogous to a human enzyme, to human fibroblast cells (those that produce connective tissue), to get them to produce an enzyme deficient in patients with the inherited Lesch–Nyhan syndrome, a serious metabolic defect in cells. "Although a very primitive 'gene therapy experiment,' I can well remember heated discussions within the department with my fellow students about that simple study." But, Mulligan admits, "I had become convinced of the power of viral vectors for gene transfer and their likely utility in gene therapy."[263]

Mulligan left Berg's lab at Stanford after graduation and returned to MIT where he was offered a unique position to be an independent postdoctoral fellow under the wing of David Baltimore while working out of the lab space of Phil Sharp. Not long after he started his postdoc, Baltimore approached Mulligan, asking him to become a faculty member at the Whitehead Institute for Biomedical Research, a new institute that Baltimore had founded and which was to be established at MIT. But, Whitehead would not open for a couple of years. In the meantime, Salvador Luria offered Mulligan a job at MIT, where he would begin to settle down, working with a strong group of young investigators including Andy Chess and David Altshuler. His work would progress fast and furiously. Baltimore began to nudge Mulligan into the use of retroviruses, which he had been dutifully studying. In the lifecycle of SV40, the virus infects a host cell, replicates, and then bursts the cell. By contrast, a retrovirus stably integrates into the genome of a cell, where it can become a permanent fixture. Mulligan became convinced that retrovirus was the best tool to use. He began to genuinely believe it could be used for "gene transfer" to get new genes into a human cell. It was something that had already been happening in nature. Since the 1950s, scientists had been observing that the trading of high-functioning genes in microbial genomes. Horizontal gene transfer works either through the trading of plasmids, or conjugation, or through the skilled proxy of viruses, as Norton Zinder and Joshua Lederberg had so elegantly shown. When viruses integrate into genomes they sometimes pick up fragments of the host genome, and "download" these bits of code like a cassette. And if those viruses move on to another organism, they can then "upload" the cassette from the first species to this new species. While most evolution is vertical with genetic material being based from parents to offspring, horizontal gene transfer, or HGT, happens between peers of the same generation. By the 1980s, a scientist named Michael Syvanen was promulgating the theory that HGT was not a fringe effect, but a major driver that shaped the history of life. The "tree of life" and its vertical line of transmitting code down through the generations had been complicated by evidence of a horizontal line, a "web" in the tree. If humans could download some of this "shareware" code, Mulligan and colleagues came to believe it could ameliorate diseases by installing working copies of new genes. What emerged through these discussions was "artificial horizontal gene transfer." Scientists began popping new genes into chromosomes like a cassette tape, and those genes would express protein products. The systems used to install new genes became simply known as "expression cassettes."

In 1981, Mulligan won the MacArthur "genius" Prize for his work on artificial horizontal gene transfer, the mechanism for installing new genes into humans. As I talked to him in his office, I learned how he came to hook up with the Masters of the Universe, how he became part Wall Street aggressor, part delicate virologist who would change the landscape of medicine – what he did with the money from MacArthur, "spent it," he shrugged – and how he engineered the first gene therapy tool. It all started with a virus. Mulligan's key contribution to medicine was to engineer a retrovirus into a tool for gene therapy. Retroviruses begin as RNA and then get transcribed back into DNA in order to incorporate into a genome, thus reversing the normal order of DNA to RNA to protein. Hence their name is defined by their function to proceed backward, or "retro." Once such a virus burrows its way into a genome like a pest, it becomes a "provirus." In essence, Mulligan gutted these retroviruses and turned them into stripped-down delivery vehicles that he could throw any cargo into – and that includes genes that he wanted to deliver to the human genome. This was the recombinant virus, a virus construct carrying the cargo of a human gene.

"The science has been there for a long time," Mulligan told me, speaking to headlines in the 2010s on the renaissance of gene therapy. "The technology developed really quickly way back then. It developed at the clip I anticipated. It's not simply the result of recent advancements." Mulligan sketched me a picture of a retrovirus he engineered for human use on a scrap of paper (Figure 3). Rectangles signified Long Terminal Repeats, the regions in the virus that included promoters or enhancers, code that attracts transcription factors, or proteins, which turn on the expression of genes. This jumble of shapes was a picture of the very *first* carriage, the Model-T of gene therapy vehicles.

In 1986, Mark Matfield, writing for *New Scientist*, explained the status of gene therapy and how the workings of retrovirus set the stage for a revolution in those years. "Many inherited diseases are caused by a defect in a single gene. In gene therapy, the idea is to replace the defective gene with a cloned copy of the normal gene. In some inherited diseases, the defective gene is not expressed at all, whereas in others, the gene expresses a defective or inappropriate function. The expression of the cloned, normal gene should restore normal function. Scientists have introduced cloned genes into mammalian cells for several years, but the techniques they used usually killed most of the cells. Moreover, the cloned genes were only incorporated into, at best, one cell in every 100000. In those cells, several hundred copies of the cloned gene would integrate (insert themselves) into the chromosomal DNA. The techniques were thus quite inappropriate for gene therapy. The new vectors for introducing cloned genes into mammalian cells are based on retroviruses. Retroviruses can exist in two forms – either as the free virus or, in infected cells, as an integrated provirus (which consists solely of the genetic material of the virus). The DNA provirus integrates into the cellular chromosomes at random. At each end of the integrated provirus is a multi-functional DNA element called the LTR (long terminal repeat). LTRs control the expression of the genes on the provirus and their integration into chromosomes of the host cell. Between the two

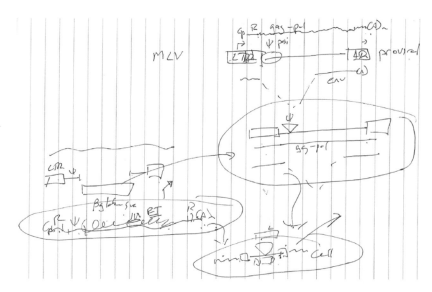

FIGURE 3 The "Model T of Gene Therapy." This is the picture that Mulligan drew for me in his office in the spring of 2013 of the first cloning system he developed circa 1981. He developed cloning systems with a retrovirus called murine leukemia virus (MLV) that infects mouse cells, and then later, an analog system from a retrovirus that infects human cells. Normally, a retrovirus enters the cell and incorporates into the genome as a parasite. Note that Mulligan used a triangle (at center) to show me that he added or removed an element called *psi* from the virus genome. It turns out that *psi* is needed for an envelope to form around the virus to allow it to repackage. A virus is essentially a "transportable genome" and by adding the *psi* element to the virus along with a "passenger gene" and gutting the rest of the virus, he created a recombinant virus vector, which could transport any human gene he wanted into a cell. But this recombinant virus could not replicate on its own. In a second step, he created a cell line that expressed the apparatus critical to replicating a virus, except that he deleted *psi*. Once he infected that cell line with his recombinant virus, it sensed the *psi* signal, and made many copies of the recombinant virus which included code of a human gene, but not code that it could use to again replicate itself. His cell line was now spitting out clones of recombinant virus, which he could use to infect other mouse or human cells, where it would install and put down its luggage, and never travel again. He had developed the very first carriage that could make a trip into a human cell and install a new gene. Once there, it would stay put.

LTRs are the genes that encode the proteins of the viral coat and an enzyme called reverse transcriptase."[264] In fact, retrovirus carries three major genes: *gag*, which builds basic infrastructure, *pol*, or polymerase, which builds an "RNA-dependent DNA polymerase," most often just called "reverse transcriptase," an enzyme which won Mulligan's mentor

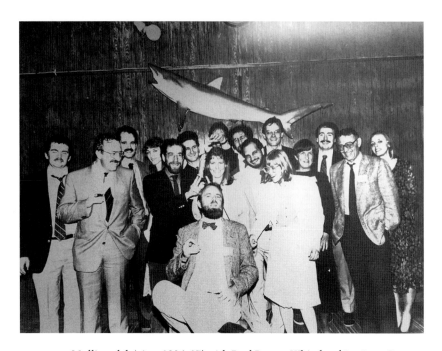

FIGURE 4 Mulligan lab (circa 1986–87) with Paul Berg at Whitehead Institute Retreat at the Chatham Bars Inn, Chatham, Massachusetts. Seated: Richard Mulligan. First row: Brad Guild, Pierre Lehn, Dan Silver, Heidi Stuhlmann, Jim Barsoum, Lisa Spain, Mary Collins and Paul Berg. Second row: Jeff Morgan, Cori Bargmann (Weinbergh lab), Olivier Danos, Paul Robbins, Mitch Finer, James Wilson, Doros Platika and Elaine Dzierzak.

Baltimore, the Nobel Prize. In effect, the reverse transcription enzyme copies the RNA virus into DNA that can incorporate into a genome; pol also includes code to build an enzyme called integrase which makes "double-strand breaks" to hack into a host genome. It is machinery to turn RNA back into DNA and to incorporate it into the genome of a cell, where it becomes a "provirus." After it is integrated in a chromosome, it can be expressed and packaged, turning into free virus, or more baby viruses, once again. A gene called *psi* is important in its ability to repackage into more copies of free, infectious viral particles, and a gene called *env*, or envelope, enables the packaged virus to make contact with a receptor on new cells to enable uptake of the virus particle.

The trick that Mulligan pulled was to tinker with a small bit of code, termed *"psi"* that was responsible for packaging the virus genome, enabling it to turn into an infectious virus particle and leap to another cell. He found that if he deleted a part of the *psi* element, the virus particles could install into the genome of the host cell, but, he told me, they would be "incapable of being further transmitted to new cells."

Mulligan's cloning system is complicated, but it helped me once I started thinking of it as a "two-component system." In a first step, Mulligan and his colleagues "cloned the provirus of a mouse retrovirus. Then they removed all the retroviral genes, leaving just the two LTRs, and the *psi* sequence. They then cloned a bacterial gene, called *neo*, into the remaining provirus 'backbone.' The *neo* gene is a bacterial antibiotic gene which is often used to test new vector systems. The resulting recombinant retrovirus contains all the DNA signals required for it to be packaged into the virus, infect a cell, be converted into DNA and integrate into the cell's chromosomes. However, because it no longer has any retroviral genes, the recombinant retrovirus could not make the enzymes required to achieve all this, resulting in a 'recombinant virus' which was 'an infectious, but not replication-competent vector particle.'[265]" Mulligan now had a recombinant virus vector – and he could insert any human gene into such a vector – but since it was not "replication-competent," he needed a cell line to replicate or "clone" his recombinant virus.

In a second step, he created a cell line that could clone or make many copies of his recombinant virus. "Mulligan took another provirus from a different mouse retrovirus and removed the *psi* sequence. He introduced the resulting provirus into a mouse cell line, where it integrated into the chromosomal DNA. This *psi*-deficient provirus was transcribed to the RNA copy and produced all the normal proteins and enzymes but, because it lacked the *psi* sequence, the RNA copies could not be packaged into the viral coats. These cells, called Psi-2 cells, normally produced no virus at all but, when Mulligan infected them with his recombinant retrovirus vector, the cells packaged the vector into the retroviral coats. The Psi-2 cells then started to produce retrovirus that contains the *neo* gene, but no retrovirus genes. Mulligan then used these recombinant retrovirus to infect other mouse cells, where they would integrate into the new cell's chromosomes, still carrying the bacterial *neo* gene. The infected cells could not produce any virus because they did not have the *psi*-less 'helper' virus to produce the proteins and enzymes required. Once integrated as a provirus, the recombinant retrovirus was stuck in the chromosomes and could only act like any other gene.

The great advantage of this system is that most of the cells infected with the recombinant retrovirus vector end up with a single copy of the provirus integrated stably into the chromosomal DNA. Also, once integrated, the genes carried on the retroviral vector are expressed under the control of the LTR. Mulligan and his colleagues have used their recombinant retrovirus vector carrying the bacterial *neo* gene to infect bone marrow cells from mice. They injected the marrow cells into mice which had all their bone marrow destroyed by radiation. When they examined the new bone marrow in these mice, they found that all the marrow cells contained the *neo* gene on the integrated retrovirus vector and that the gene was expressed in all these cells. This breakthrough paves the way for full scale gene therapy. Several serious inherited diseases, such as Lesch–Nyhan syndrome and severe immunodeficiency disease, result from the inactivation of genes normally expressed in the bone marrow cells. Such diseases would be ideal candidates for gene therapy."[266]

In Mulligan's own words, a new viral vector including a new gene he wanted to introduce was "capable of entering cells and integrating into chromosomal DNA, but did not carry into the cells the genetic material of the virus that could lead to further propagation of the recombinant genome to other cells." He had developed the first tool for genetic engineering in humans. He could control its range, and use it to publish "transcripts," or copies, of the gene he installed. "There were these 'gosh-oh-golly moments' that this could really work," Mulligan told me.

In 1982, the FDA approved the first synthetic human insulin, a recombinant technology that involved putting a human gene for insulin into a microbe, whereby the protein could be "scaled up" for mass production. Sharp and Gilbert had launched Biogen to add a complete gene to the microbe, while Boyer at Genentech had built an insulin gene from scratch from its individual nucleotides. Boyer's approach became dominant in the industry. The FDA license for the first drug built by rDNA techniques went to Genentech, which was strengthened due to its partnership with Eli Lilly, the company which first scaled up insulin in the 1920s. Just a decade after Berg spliced the first gene, a major rDNA drug had come onto the scene with dramatic benefits. In fact, there were many instances of drugs being prescribed as "replacement therapies," including not only insulin, but a raft of "enzyme deficiency disorders." In these cases, the drug did not exist to treat symptoms or intervene in a pathway, it simply worked to supplement or replace a key protein that was missing. Biotech was newly alive to the idea that they could install a human gene into their patients in one simple move, eliminating the need to give them a lifetime supply of a drug.

In November that year, the President's Commission on Bioethics released a report entitled *Splicing Life* in which the commission sought to de-dramatize the dangers posed by "human genetic engineering" by pointing to similarities between gene transfer for therapeutic reasons, on the one hand, and traditional drugs and biologics, on the other. But as gene engineering surged in the minds of biotech entrepreneurs, journalists were finding plenty of grist for the mill. "Doomsday: Tinkering with Life," the cover of *Time* magazine had read. "The Frankenstein Patent," *Rolling Stone* had admonished. But, the government was now siding with proponents who were arguing that recombinant DNA wasn't a stunning intrusion into nature, but simply a tool that could be regulated in the context of traditional biologics, such as vaccines. After all, the first vaccines also got off to a dodgy start, when some viruses cultivated in horses to treat patients for diphtheria, accidentally ended up killing some of those patients since they were tainted with tetanus. This led to the passage of the Biological Control Act of 1902, establishing standards and protocols for testing the safety of vaccines. Vaccines were now safely regulated. The government was coming to believe that gene engineering could also be regulated by tight protocols.

By this time, Mulligan had shown that he could engineer a virus called murine leukemia virus, or MLV, an expression cassette, by which he would splice a new gene into MLV and put it into a mouse. The next logical step was to engineer a retrovirus, which has the ability to work as a pilot, that carries a passenger gene directly into a human cell, as a tool for gene therapy. The President's Commission was backing human engineering. Mulligan would use his MacArthur prize to develop the technology into a humanized version.

In the coming years at MIT, Mulligan's lab would work on retrovirus and lentivirus to install genes into cells. Much of his work focused on using gene transfer technology to install human beta-hemoglobin into red blood cells, but his studies also focused on targeting specific cell types, including bone-marrow-derived hematopoietic stem cells (which give rise not only to red blood cells, but also to white blood cells of the immune system), fibroblasts (connective tissue) and keratinocytes (skin cells), hepatocytes (liver cells), endothelial cells (which build vessels and tissues) and T-lymphocytes (a type of mature immune cell, in short, T-cells). One of Mulligan's postdoctoral students, Jim Wilson began to focus on hepatocytes. Jeff Morgan was working with keratinocytes. Ihor Lemischka and David A. Williams were focusing on T-cells to treat a number of rare immune system diseases. The hematopoietic cells that build red and white blood cells became a promising first strike target because they could be more easily removed from the body.

Bone marrow is a soft sponge in the cavity of the bones which includes the precursors for white blood cells, including T-cells. If it could be extracted, it could be treated with gene transfer technology outside the body, or "ex vivo," and then returned to the body. "An obvious approach to the treatment of such diseases would be to "remove bone marrow, which includes white blood cells and the precursors to immune cells, and use a virus to transfer a new gene into those cells, and then add the bone marrow "back into a patient via a bone marrow transplantation."[267] It wasn't long before they put the techniques on stunning display.

Mulligan recalled in a reflection that, "In 1984, we published the first report of the transduction of reconstituting hematopoietic stem cells using replication deficient retroviral vectors." In other words, they put a new gene into a precursor cell that could go on to become a red or white blood cell. "The result was huge for us, as it clearly indicated the feasibility of developing ex vivo gene therapies for diseases including hematopoietic stem cells. The study simulated all our subsequent studies over the next decade focused on the development of gene therapies for different inherited diseases of the blood, including SCID, beta-thalassemia, and Wiskott–Aldrich syndrome."

Mulligan had invented the first efficient tool for "gene trapping," whereby a recombinant virus would install at a fairly random place in a genome. This would often be useful enough because it meant that somewhere in a sea of billions of nucleotides and thousands of genes, a new gene was added, at least, someplace. It was contrasted with another new technology that was coming out around the same time, so-called "gene targeting," a concept largely connected to the scientists Mario Capecchi and Klaus Rajewsky. Gene targeting would allow lab scientists to swap out a gene at a specific address in the genome. A sort of renaissance in technology was emerging. This gene targeting would emerge along with basic insights into DNA repair mechanisms, drawing on the concepts of cellular maintenance and repair.

Biotechnology had been instigated in the late 1960s with the discovery of restriction enzymes, which were first identified in microbes and had a function as a nuclease, meaning they could chop up strings of nucleic acids such as RNA or DNA. These molecular scissors would allow a bacterium to defend itself against foreign genomes which were invading it, in other words, viruses. But there was a second reason a cell would want to clip DNA: that would be to clip its own DNA! The way it would do that would be through a special kind of endonuclease, which could excise or resect sections of DNA which were mismatched, compromised or broken. Emerging insights into these repair mechanisms would lead to a second surge in biotechnology. The story is old school.

In 1931, Barbara McClintock made use of the electron microscope to show that recombination events were happening each time a cell divides, swapping versions of the same gene, with subtle variations in code and function. Indeed, a gene can come in multiple versions. In this process of "crossing over," each member in a pair of sister chromatid, or alleles, tilts in a comical sort of way like a tree bending a branch down, and swaps a version of the same gene with its complement chromosome. Cells used this mechanism to recombine alleles as a means to create "heterogeneity," so a single chromosome does not become stale in its partnerships as it is passed down through the ages. It *mingles*. And this mingling implores new genetic relationships to form. It's largely health promoting: we want diverse immune systems, for instance, which is why we go outside our families.

To do this, chromosomes create double-strand breaks, but then heal back together again, after trading parts with other chromosomes. This mechanism would be termed "homologous recombination," and is effected each time a germ cell divides. In somatic cells, the pathway is evoked as "homology-directed repair," and has a function in DNA repair. The genome is not a static document, but a living one. It has its ways to cut and paste its own document into new arrangements.

In the late 1960s, Richard Setlow, Philip Hanawalt and Paul Howard-Flanders had demonstrated that *E. coli* mutants had lost their ability to generate snippets of DNA enriched for "photoproducts," genetic defects which are caused due to exposure to UV light. One such type of a photoproduct is a "pyrimidine dimer," which forms when a pyrimidine base buckles and forms a covalent bond with a neighboring pyrimidine, resulting in a kind of bump in the genetic code. This finding led to an appreciation that the creation of such dimers may initiate programs of cell death, or halt cellular replication, until these genes carry out a microscopic repair by clipping out these dimers through an apparatus called "excision repair." Setlow and colleague Bill Carrier "showed that when cells are incubated after exposure to UV light, covalently joined pyrimidines, referred to as pyrimidine dimers, known photoproducts in DNA, appear in the acid-soluble fraction of DNA. Setlow correctly postulated that the appearance of acid-soluble pyrimidine dimers reflects their removal from DNA by enzyme-mediated excision."[268]

Errol Friedberg and Mutsuo Sekiguchi, and Lawrence Grossman then identified other such repair enzymes that helped to clip out these small buckling errors in a bacterium's DNA code, one of which was found, surprisingly, in a phage. Scientists were alive to the idea that there are several types of small errors that can occur in DNA. Pyrimidine dimers are a buckle between two neighboring bases on a single strand of DNA; molecular debris called "adducts" is caused by sediments such as nitrogen and toxins such as benzo[a]pyrene from smoking, and *alkylation* or the attachment of molecules such as methylation groups, can compromise a nucleic acid through the settling of molecular debris on the DNA template; oxidation and hydrolysis are chemical processes which can break a covalent bond to release a single nucleotide base, breaking from the DNA backbone; a *mismatch*, a kind of spelling mistake in which the wrong DNA base is stitched into place in a newly forming DNA strand.

Tomas Lindahl, a Swedish biochemist who worked out of the United Kingdom came to believe that spontaneous breaking of covalent bonds in DNA almost certainly occurs regularly and "this led him to the cogent conclusion that DNA repair enzymes yet to be discovered may have evolved to cope with such damage," Friedberg wrote. In fact, bonds break in a process of hydrolysis, in which a special process called deaminase, can involve the spontaneous change of a cytosine into uracil nucleotide. Lindahl proceeded to discover "a novel pathway by which the inappropriate base uracil is removed from DNA as the free base" which was "mediated by a class of enzymes that Lindahl designated

DNA glycosylases because they sever the glycosylic bond linking particular types of damaged or inappropriate bases (such as uracil) to the sugar phosphate backbone of DNA, thereby releasing a free base..."

In fact, "the loss of a free base, such as uracil, naturally leaves a new type of damage in the genome... which must undergo further repair to fully restore genetic integrity," wrote Friedberg, who, while training with Dave Goldthwait in the Department of Biochemistry at Case Western Reserve, identified this "DNA repair enzyme subsequently shown to be involved in the repair of sites of base loss."[269,270,271] In subsequent years, multiple other DNA glycosylases were discovered across many species. Lindahl was also the first to purify a DNA ligase in a mammalian cell, which has a pasting action, and he also discovered a class of enzymes called methyltransferases, which add or remove a methyl group to a nucleotide base in a process called alkylation. The DNA glycosylase worked as "base excision repair" to snip out a damaged base, but yet another pathway was engaged to snip out a base which was not damaged but improperly matched up during replication and named "mismatch repair." "I therefore suggested that it would be appropriate to recognize three distinct types of excision repair," Friedberg wrote. "Hence, the terms 'nucleotide excision repair,' during which, entire nucleotides, typically oligonucleotide fragments ~20 nucleotides in length, are excised, and 'base excision repair' during which, free bases are excised, were introduced to complement the established term 'mismatch excision repair,' which addresses the excision of mismatched bases typically generated as errors during... replication."

In the 1970s, Friedberg joined the faculty at Stanford, where he began studying the budding yeast *Saccharomyces cerevisiae*, where trainees in his lab and elsewhere would identify *RAD* family genes which had a role in excision repair of damaged DNA. Friedberg then took a chair at the University of Texas Southwestern Medical School in Dallas, Texas. The function of one of these yeast genes, called *RAD3*, "remained a mystery until a providential visit to my laboratory in the early 1990s by Roger Kornberg from Stanford... Roger informed me that his laboratory had recently isolated a large transcription factor." One of the subunits of this transcription factor, named *TFIIH*, was the same size as repair protein Rad3, raising the prospect that they were one and the same. "My ears perked up immediately," Friedberg recalled. The discovery prompted further studies with the Kornberg laboratory, postdoctoral fellow John Feaver and others that all the subunits of yeast *TFIIH* are required for both transcription initiation and excision repair in yeast... Roger and I hypothesized that yeast (and possibly other eukaryotes) may contain distinct multi-protein complexes that share multiple polypeptides and function as 'transcriptomes' or as 'repairosomes.'"[272,273,274,275,276,277,278] The insight was that DNA repair and copy mechanisms of the cell are inextricably linked. This makes sense because a cell would want to halt any copying if there was an error.

"Because DNA damage is, in general, a stochastic process, the DNA replication, transcription, and/or recombination machineries may encounter sites of damage before they are repaired. To cope with the deleterious effects of such encounters, cells have evolved a series of biological responses that I designated DNA damage tolerance mechanisms. As the term suggests, DNA damage tolerance allows cells to overcome the potentially lethal effects of blocked replication (and possibly blocked transcription) until a time when the damage is removed."

In fact, some repair mechanisms were found to be initiated by DNA polymerase, the enzyme which has a role in copying the genetic material during cell division. Paul Modrich would contribute work to describe "mismatch repair" which works as a copy editor to prevent errors as the polymerase replicates the DNA during cell division.[279]

DNA repair mechanisms had amounted to machinery which carries out microscopic genome surgeries, but did not yet account for how a cell might respond to one of the most catastrophic events, a "double-strand break," which is a complete snapping of the double helix. In 1980 some of the first clues would emerge of an apparatus to repair such a catastrophic break, which was called "non-homologous end joining," or NHEJ.[280,281,282] The apparatus relies on a ligase to paste back together two broken ends of DNA, and is a cobbled repair which can result in deleted, inverted or even patchwork code. In many events, the repair can be quite accurate, especially if small overhangs, or "micro-homologies," exist between two overhangs to help to guide the repair. But often it is a hazardous, makeshift repair, patching a broken double helix with whatever spare part is available. But there is an even tidier repair mechanism.

In 1983, Jack Szostak at Harvard University and colleagues presented a model now known as the DSBR pathway, which would help to elucidate the mechanism now called "homologous directed repair." RecA is a "recombinase" family of enzymes including the *RAD* genes, which bind to DNA and begin a "resection," sometimes called "chew back," to degrade a strand to expose a longer single stranded overhang which can be used as a template for repair. Non-homologous end joining (NHEJ) is a default repair mechanism, but chew back of a few nucleotides can commit the cell to homology-directed repair. Scientists swiftly found a use for these repair mechanisms as a technology.

In the late 1970s, Rudolf Jaenisch, now an MIT biologist and another founder of the Whitehead Institute, had created the first gene-modified mice using a recombinase. By the late 1980s, Mario Capecchi, a protégé of Jim Watson, was at work with colleagues Martin Evans and Oliver Smithies making use of "homologous recombination," or "homology-directed repair," for the purposes of gene targeting. If the genome had innate means to cut and patch itself, Capecchi realized it could be leveraged as a technology to remove or insert new genes on purpose. He introduced DNA molecules to a cell, and found that a small fraction of the time those added bits of code would incorporate into chromosomes at the *exact* site of the gene he had introduced. He decided to try to add a scrap of code, introduce it as a molecule to mouse cells. Sure enough, a chromosome swapped its functioning gene for the malfunctioning gene that he introduced in a feat of homology-directed repair.

The patchwork repair that was going on in chromosomes was an effect of a response to cases of the worst type of DNA damage: a double-strand break. In these cases, chromosomes that broke at random could be patched back up in a repair by similar bio-available genetic spare parts[283] and intriguingly, this repair pathway appeared related to "crossing over" applied to introduce more variation to offspring.[284] Capecchi's stroke of insight was to introduce scraps of code to compromise gene function after a repair, and thus, it was a means to "knock out" genes, and even create a "knock-out mouse," a mouse strain with one or more specific genes that were rendered non-functional. It was a slick new way to engineer mice and would bestow profound insights to basic science. Mulligan's tools would be useless if scientists did not elucidate gene functions, since they would not know which genes to replace or correct. By knocking out a single gene, and watching its effect on a cell or organism, researchers could elucidate the function of many genes. They could develop disease models in mice; for instance, a model could be created for severe combined immunodeficiency, or SCID, a mouse with a failed immune system.

At the same time, another astonishing technology emerged on the scene, the "Cre-Lox recombination" system. The Cre enzyme (which stands for "causes recombination" and is technically a pair of molecular scissors called a recombinase) seeks and cuts the *Lox* site in a phage. Scientists learned to situate two Lox sites anywhere in a mammalian cell and then deploy the Cre enzyme to snip out the genetic region in between the two sites. Scientists quickly learned that they could invert or organize two Lox sequences in many series in order to knock out genes, or rearrange genomes to order. Not long after, the German scientist Klaus Rajewsky would advance the system to a whole new level by putting it into embryonic stem cells and putting the Cre enzyme under control of his own promoters which was called "conditional gene targeting." Rajewsky used engineering tricks to get the Cre enzyme to be expressed only in some cells in mice; for instance, only in liver cells under the control of an external stimulus such as interferon. Therefore he had a way to target and compromise genes at certain times in embryo or growth development, or knock out genes only in some specific cells or tissue, say knock out a gene only in the liver or only in a neuron of a living mouse. Capecchi, and then Rajewsky, revolutionized the field of mouse genetics, because they allowed scientists to knock out any gene in a mouse and watch its effect, which led to designer mouse lines. But these rough and ready tools of gene targeting would never be efficient to use for gene transfer in humans. A gene would integrate only a small fraction of the time into a mouse chromosome and scientists had to spend a lot of mouse embryonic stem cells before they got it right so that they could grow up a "mouse line." But by now, Mulligan, a newly crowned MacArthur Fellow, had developed the first efficient cloning system to use viruses to transport genes into human cells. His strategy was to wire a human gene into a gutted virus, amplify many copies of this recombinant virus in a cell line, and then use those clones as a therapeutic to dose the cells of a human patient. The clones of recombinant virus would no longer replicate in the cells of the patient, but would be permanently installed at a random location. It wasn't as precise as "gene targeting," but it was more efficient, and more apt to succeed in humans.

Mulligan's gene trapping system put a gene at a random location in a chromosome. Questions remained whether the viruses would insert near genes governing the cell cycle. If it installed near a "proto-oncogene," which sends a signal for cell division, or a "tumor-suppressor" gene, which puts the breaks on cell division, it could be dire. Tripping those circuits could result in uncontrolled cell growth, a cancer. Scientists expected to avoid these genes. But, after all, murine leukemia virus, or MLV, which Mulligan had initially started working on, by its very name caused cancer. It was an "oncovirus." The scientists could not be sure that this engineered retrovirus would not do the same in human patients. Mulligan had been sitting on the RAC at the National Institutes of Health, reviewing a proposal by French Anderson to conduct human trials in gene therapy. So far in animal trials, no instances of cancers were reported. But Mulligan recalls that Dr. Anderson's team was not that good at actually getting viruses into cells, so it would not be surprising if there were very few instances of viruses transforming cells into cancerous states. Gene therapy was poised for its first human trials. It wouldn't go forward in complete confidence. The scientists knew that mutagenesis could be a problem. "French Anderson wanted to do some things," which were "somewhat premature in my opinion," Mulligan told me.

Anderson had been a scientist at the NIH where he was investigating mechanisms to repair defective genes. His efforts to date had been fruitless. When Mulligan finally published his methods in 1984, showing he could use an engineered retrovirus to insert new genes in human cells, Anderson jumped all over it. He began filing applications for a trial. He was denied in his first few attempts, but finally gained approval from the Human Gene Therapy Subcommittee at his home institution. On September 14, 1990, he led a team for the first approved gene therapy treatment, on a four-year-old girl named Ashanti DeSilva. She was born with a rare genetic disease called severe combined immune deficiency (SCID). There are several forms of SCID in humans, some of which are X-linked, meaning they occur due to mutations in genes on the X chromosome. Other forms of SCID are derived from genes on other chromosomes. DeSilva had a form called ADA-SCID; it was due to an inborn error in a gene on chromosome 20 that builds an enzyme called adenosine deaminase, which is necessary for a working immune system. Based on technologies such as SCID mice, researchers and doctors knew how to locate the genes which might cause the disease, and therefore which genes could be replaced to restore her immune system. Dusty Miller at the Fred Hutchinson Research Center in Seattle engineered a retrovirus and spliced it to a functioning copy of the ADA gene. Anderson's team extracted white blood cells from DeSilva and dispatched the viruses into a plate of her cells. The cells were then returned to her bloodstream. DeSilva was not cured through the procedure, and it only worked for a few months. But the treatment appeared safe, and due to this fact alone, it had an effect of boosting support for the fledgling field. SCIDs children are often sick, and always in grave peril, since even common colds could bring them to the brink of death. They can never have friends. They can never lead normal lives, vulnerable to any passing germ. Unless they make it through bone marrow transplants and a series of tricky hurdles, many of them don't make it out of childhood. The scientific consensus supported experimental gene therapy for children who'd virtually run out of luck. Anderson's team showed it could safely be done.

French Anderson's key insight was that immuno-compromised children could be treated by simply inserting a gene that builds a protein that they were missing. If such a patch were made, their immune systems would begin to work again. This was the case whenever immune systems failed due to an enzyme, or an immune system signal called a cytokine, or a receptor, such as interleukin 2, or IL-2 gamma receptor.

But, the insight that the immune system could fail also immediately led to beliefs that it could also be bolstered or amped up to go on the attack against cancer, as an appreciation was building within the cancer community that tumors evolved ways to knock down the body's immune system surveillance so as to avoid the immune system's rejection of cancer. "Another area of interest that our (Mulligan) lab pursued for many years involved the notion that gene transfer technology might be used to enhance the capacity of the immune system to recognize and kill tumor cells."[285] Glenn Dranoff (a postdoc in the Mulligan lab) initiated studies with Drew Pardoll and colleagues at Johns Hopkins School of Medicine, and the group began working to see if they could express different immunoregulatory gene products within tumor cells as a means to elicit anti-tumor immunity. The idea was to create a "cancer vaccine," whereby tumor cells engineered by viruses to express specific gene products could be delivered as a shot that would strengthen the immune system in its bid to fight the cancer. The scientists tried adding a number of genes, including one for an immune system gene called granulocyte-macrophage colony stimulating factor. In the meantime, David Nathan lured Mulligan to Harvard.

In 1996, Mulligan moved his lab to Harvard Medical School and became a Howard Hughes Medical Institute Investigator. At Harvard,

Mulligan also started the Harvard Gene Therapy Initiative. Anderson had shown gene therapy was safe in humans, and the technology appeared to be poised to transform medicine as we know it as it began entering its first trials. As French Anderson told *Time* magazine, "Physicians will simply treat patients by injecting a snippet of DNA and send them home cured." An article in *Discover* magazine titled "The Ultimate Medicine," informed us that "Genetic surgeons can now go into your cell and fix those genes with an unlikely scalpel: a virus." In the same article, Mulligan declared "We can use gene transfer to make a cell do whatever we want. We can play God in that cell."

Major regulatory bodies in Europe and the US were taking notice, approving the first gene therapy trials. At first, gene therapy seemed to be a fait accompli. Scientists were pulling off what seemed to be small miracles. They were reprograming genes and treating some rare diseases in a single shot. A gene therapy trial for X-SCID was orchestrated in France and England in the late 1990s. In those trials, scientists would try to install a gene for IL-2 gamma receptor, which was on the X chromosome, and which receives a signal for IL-2 cytokine from another immune cell.[286] By 2000, 18 of 20 children in the trials had been successfully treated for X-SCID, introducing a new gene that their immune systems lacked. But then, unexpectedly, and suddenly, everything went terribly wrong. Five of those patients developed "leukemia-like conditions." The viruses used to transport new genes were equipped with powerful switches (LTRs) which could dial up the volume on a gene it landed next to. In several cases, the viruses landed near a gene called *LMO2*, which controls cell division, and forced that gene into a constantly "on" position. It's a situation that geneticists called "constitutive" expression; and it was catastrophic. It wasn't a complete surprise since viruses are dependent on cells for replication, and they benefit from triggering cellular replication programs. "In those cases, very rare integration events occurred where therapeutic genes sent into patients' bodies in a convoy of viral vectors leaped into installation spots in the wrong spots in the genome, in fact, resulting in leukemia in some patients," the genome editing pioneer Dana Carroll told me.

These early gene therapy studies involved the insertion of a gene, along with some other fancy molecular equipment, including code that would produce a signal for poly-adenylation, which is a group of molecules that cap the ends of an RNA molecule and keep it from rapidly degrading. It also included a promoter, which turns on the gene so it can be expressed. But, a virus also has its own sort of promoter region, which is an extremely strong promoter that causes its code to be expressed at levels that are very high, and far above the "host range," the levels at which normal human genes are expressed.

In the years that followed, Mulligan's one-time student, David A. Williams, and others would engineer retrovirus to remove its LTR and install other weaker promoters from the genomes of woodchucks, cows, mice and other animals, to cause newly transferred genes to be expressed at a level that is similar to the levels that they naturally occur in human cells. If scientists ever wanted to turn genes on and off at specific times, especially if they wanted to add genes for IL-2 or other more dangerous cytokines such as IL-12, to use them as booster signals to fight cancer, they'd have to establish tight controls on the genes they installed, since those cytokines can fire up immune networks into overdrive, leading to a collapse in blood pressure, breathing arrest, life-threatening fevers and even organ failure. One of the lessons learned at the time was that scientists would inevitably need to put controls and switches on the genes they installed in gene therapy, to control their expression. A second lesson learned was that they'd have to be very careful about which viruses or constructs they used to get new genes into cells, since some viruses have "immunogenic properties," meaning they can trigger a violent immune system response.

Jim Wilson, a protégé of Mulligan, had been working out of the University of Pennsylvania. As the gene therapy trials were slamming to a halt in Europe, he was preparing to lead the first major gene therapy trial in the US. In 1999, 18-year-old Jesse Gelsinger was enrolled in his trial. Gelsinger had an inborn metabolic error called ornithine transcar-bamylase (OTC) deficiency syndrome, a condition that appears in one in 40000 people. The gene is on the X chromosome, meaning that males only have one copy; if it malfunctions, there is no second copy to supplement it. The *OTC* gene builds an enzyme that ships free nitrogen molecules out of the body as a component of urea in urine. Insufficiency of the enzyme results in excess nitrogen building up and binding with hydrogen molecules to form ammonia. Not good. A build-up of ammo-nia in the blood harms the nervous system. Patients with this disorder are candidates for gene therapy, since adding a supplemental gene can complete a pathway and revive their health. Mulligan and Wilson talked about which type of vector to use. Red flags had been thrown around retrovirus for its role in driving leukemia-like conditions in Europe. Wilson decided to select adenovirus for the trial. It wouldn't drive a cancer condition, but it was known to be "immunogenic," meaning it could stoke an immune reaction that was dire. Indeed, if a safer biologic had been used to treat Jesse Gelsinger, he might be alive today.

Instead, Gelsinger died in the grips of a "cytokine storm," the result of a cascade of cytokines, a catastrophic breakdown in the communication signals of his immune system. Innate immune cells and T-cells recognize antigens, or badges, on viruses and can kick up an overwhelming inflammatory response. This is usually controlled by feedback loops, but in the case of dosing a patient with a huge viral load, sometimes the feedback system can be overwhelmed. In a cytokine storm, the immune system goes haywire and cracks up, like a network going down. It can lead to collapse of blood pressure, heart attack and breathing arrest, and it's characterized by a sweet, sickly cloying odor. Despite the high-tech tools scientists had used to install a new gene in Gelsinger's liver cells, it was the ancient forces of the immune system's wrath that upended the tactic. As Moses said of the Pharaoh's chariots, they promptly "sank as lead in mighty waters."

Wilson told me in an email that he believes Gelsinger was infected with a similar virus as a child. "Our leading hypothesis is that some aspect of immune memory to a natural infection with an adenovirus" led to adverse reactions when the virus was introduced a second time. But despite his hindsight, he had to deal with incredible grief as the whole field, public, major media and the weight of the federal government came crashing down on his shoulders. Questions emerged about his choice of tool – adenovirus was known to be immunogenic, and other viruses, such as adeno-associated virus, might have been a safer bet. The FDA came forth with a rap sheet of complaints, accusing his team of failing to report liver damage in two patients who were treated before Gelsinger. And Gelsinger's ammonia levels had bounced up to a range above normal before the procedure, making the treatment unsafe. Most incriminating, the Penn researchers failed to promptly report to the FDA that 2 of 11 monkeys died in trials prior to the human trail.

A scientist named Bruce Levine had arrived on campus at Penn months before, and was budding with ideas on how to use new gene therapy tools to treat cancer; as a counter-strategy to chemotherapy, he was among a number of young guns poised to usher in a new age of "immunotherapy." Levine was a faculty member in Wilson's department, but his work would be placed on temporary hold as adverse events in early gene therapy trials sent the scientific community reeling.

Time magazine published a provocative cover story soon after Gelsinger's death called "Human Guinea Pigs." "Imagine everywhere we go, people say, oh yeah, Penn, that is where the gene therapy accident happened," Levine told me. "It was horrendously frustrating." It put the brakes on the program, sidelining Wilson's career, for a time, which was in its own way, a misfortune. "Jim Wilson has done tremendous work to advance gene therapy," Levine reminded me. But more than the effort to triage negative press, and keep their fledgling program afloat, the scientists struggled with their own internal grief and sadness at a singular death, and the heartache of a family. "Remember," Levine chastened me, "this was a tragic event." Even after Gelsinger's death, many in the field wanted to push on. Claudia Mickelson, then chair of NIH's RAC, stood steadfast, telling CNN, "We have no interest in stopping gene therapy. None whatsoever." The FDA felt otherwise. The agency suspended Penn's gene therapy program, among the largest in the country, on January 21, 2000.

In his landmark 1962 book, *The Structure of Scientific Revolutions*, Thomas Kuhn noted that science does not progress entirely in a linear step-wise fashion, but sometimes becomes broadsided by challenges, which cause it to shift its standards and practices, indeed, its entire paradigms. "Mopping up operations are what engage most scientists throughout their careers. They constitute what I am here calling normal science," Kuhn wrote. New ideas emerge to challenge the orthodoxy in a "pre-paradigm period" that is at first dismissed as nonsense and antithetical, and a little bit radical. At first, new ideas are briskly dismissed. "The pre-paradigm period, in particular, is regularly marked by frequent and deep debates over legitimate methods, problems, and standards of solution, though these serve rather to define schools than to produce agreement... Normal scientific research is directed to the articulation of those phenomenon and theories that the paradigm already supplies. Normal science for example, often suppresses fundamental novelties because they are necessarily subversive of its basic commitments." This was precisely what was happening with the field of genetic engineering as it was having deep and extensive impacts on basic research, while broadsiding the NIH and FDA with debates on its technical aspects, standards and practices, and how to model its governance and oversight. It was poised to upend the very way that modern medicine is practiced. Once a new technology such as this comes into practice, and its traction becomes irrefutable, Kuhn says we enter a "crisis phase," whereby we deal with serious upheaval and cope with how to incorporate new changes that are thrust upon us, and the scientific community was coping with an "essential tension" implicit in research. These changes to the foundations of a field can be so abrupt and upending that many scientists subconsciously refuse to adopt them, leading to Kuhn's characterization of revolution as the "Invisibility of Revolutions."

In the 1990s, it was pre-paradigm. Gene therapy was still, in a way, fighting against impossibility. Mulligan noted that Wilson's team broke several rules in that trial. When I pressed Mulligan about it, his voice flattened into a soft-spoken tone, clear with a hint of terse urgency. "They broke the rules," he said, gesturing with an opening of his hands as if he had nothing left to conceal. "They broke the rules."

The FDA had almost wanted to see gene therapy succeed, and had been perhaps as close to advocating as the agency ever came. The FDA recognized the persistent expression of a gene was more advantageous than the transient expression of a drug which had to be taken throughout a lifetime. "The FDA is not supposed to advocate, but was quite supportive of Jim's trial before the tragic event occurred," Mulligan told me. Gelsinger's death had a "chilling effect on the field."

Not much later, a young French patient, one of the five who had come down with a leukemia-like condition in the X-SCID gene therapy trials, died at Necker-Enfants Malades Hospital (Paris Children's Hospital). The FDA, watching what was happening in Europe, slammed down a hold on all trials in January 2003. The X-SCID death was like an uppercut, following the Gelsinger event, a hit to the chin, sending the entire field staggering. The field was thrown into deep retrenchment. "I have no doubt that the death of Jesse Gelsinger is going to lead to nothing but a cautious, go-slow approach," ethicist Arthur Caplan of the University of Pennsylvania told *The Los Angeles Times*. "As a society, we're more nervous about genetics" than about any other form of medical therapy. Jim Wilson would spend much of the remainder of his career actively investigating how features of a virus can trip up an immune system and whip it up into cytokine storms and initiate adverse events in patients. He would write a compelling and difficult review article a decade later called "Lessons Learned," as part of a legal settlement, which called upon his responsibility to inventory the errors, and there were numerous missteps in the clinical trial. Wilson would emerge again as a scientific adviser to a gene therapy company called REGENXBIO, Inc., which uses a safer adeno-associated virus. In short, scientists had learned two important lessons. One was that they'd have to develop new ways to temper the immune system's highly reactive and unpredictable response to gene therapy; a second was they'd have to find a way to tone down the triggers on the viruses, so that they wouldn't dial up gene expression in human patients and start cancers. To Mulligan and Wilson, the deaths were a deeply personal blow. And yet, the field would pivot on these lessons. It was a brook of fire through which we had to pass.

5　Modern Prometheus

Man is not going to wait passively for millions of years before evolution offers him a better brain.

　　　　　　　　　　　　–Romanian chemist Corneliu E. Giurgea

In the 1987 film *Innerspace*, Martin Short was cast as a hypochondriac and a weakling of sorts, until he was injected with a serum containing a miniature submarine piloted by Dennis Quaid, who was cast as a manly type of figure who introduces an element of chutzpah. The film won an Oscar, which, depending on who you talk to, is either surprising or unsurprising. Darian Leader, the British man of letters, in his 1996 expose "Why do women write more letters than they post?" even used the film as a basis for a foray into literary and film analysis. "The pilot of the submarine is by no means a wimp and the tension between pilot and host organism provides much of the film's humour. But what matters here is less the fact that the sub is piloted by an authentic 'hero' than that something symbolic, a product of science, has been incorporated into the body. To be a man means to have a body plus something symbolic, something which is not ultimately human."

Hollywood was capitalizing on an emerging zeitgeist, which was seeded by the first experiments in gene splicing and the recombinant viruses which had begun to be used to engineer human cells, potent technology developed a few years earlier, which began leaking into our subconscious. Not only would we be able to engineer our own biology, but we were entering a startling new era of the "gene as a commodity," whereby many of the elements of technology might be sold to us. The coming debate of moving genetic engineering into man had begun to take hold a decade before, as people began to weigh the consequences of being part synthetic. In 1970, Princeton theologian Paul Ramsey wrote the book *Fabricated Man: The Ethics of Genetic Control*. In the words of Jonathan Moreno, "Ramsey saw the prospect of genetic manipulation as one more potential case of the dehumanization of modern medicine, of the tendency to turn physicians into body mechanics. Genetic power could take the objectification of human beings to the extreme: if human beings are given the power to modify others as objects, they may come to see those they manipulate as mere objects. 'Man as a manipulator is too much of a God; as object too much of a machine.' ... any artificial intervention in the process of procreation violates that part of man that is essentially human."

In 1974, by contrast, the Christian ethicist Joseph Fletcher published *The Ethics of Genetic Control: Ending Reproductive Roulette*, which as Moreno describes, became the counter-position. "For Fletcher, on the other hand, to be civilized means precisely to be artificial. Fletcher held that, rather than become tyrannized by 'reproductive roulette,' we should control our biology... It is precisely because men are sapient that they can control their biology... Beyond any precedent we are now in a position to change not only the social and environmental conditions of mankind but even man himself, by this very stuff."[287]

The Fletcher–Ramsey debate became crystallized on the silver screen in the 1982 film *Blade Runner*, which is based on the sci-fi novel by Philip K. Dick, *Do Androids Dream of Electric Sheep?* Set in the year 2020, *Blade Runner* imagines a world in which a group of enslaved replicants (genetically engineered human-like creatures) revolted on another planet. Designed to live only a few years, they came to Earth to find a way to extend their life span, while the hero, Rick Deckard (Harrison Ford), must hunt them down and kill them. The film also includes a side plot with a character named Sebastian, a "gene engineer," who is a delicate man of age 25 whose shortening lifespan humbles him, and who finds himself in a large empty shell of a building, making the most of his considerable talents by creating automata companions.

Cinemas would begin cashing in on films such as *Jurassic Park* and *Gattaca*. As to the shift in the cinematic landscape, the ethicist George Annas noted at the time, "We could use our technology to explore outerspace with robots, but our current fascination is with inner space. Instead of expanding our minds and our perspective as a species by pondering the mysteries of outerspace with its possibilities of other intelligent life forms, we are turning inward, and contemplating ourselves on the microscopic levels. The new biology, perhaps better described as the new genetics or the 'genetics age,' suggests a biology-based immortality alternative to a digital brain in a body of metal and plastic: changing and 'enhancing' our human capabilities by altering our genes at the molecular levels." This abstraction of genetic engineering in literature and its projection onto the silver screen helped to distinguish the gap between the descriptive life of science and the conceptual right to do it. But as the new millennium approached, things were about to get surreal, as people began to mine our genetics for expansion of our biological limits. Marcy Darnovsky recently suggested we are approaching a "radical rupture from the past, where we will begin to take novelists' and film-makers' scenarios seriously." The new "genetics age" is upon us, and while armchair thought experiments abound on whether anyone would really try this, someone had.

"Repoxygen is hard to get. Please give me new instructions soon so that I can order the product before Christmas." Thomas Springstein, a track coach for the German national team, wrote an email to a Dutch doctor seeking "black market Repoxygen" for his Olympic runners. It was the first documented attempt at "gene doping," revealed (only later) in emails and documents in a 2006 court case. Oxford BioMedica, a publically traded Oxford, England company, had been making gene therapy drugs for diseases such as retinopathy and neuropathy, but the company also had a new drug for anemia, called Repoxygen. The drug uses lentivirus to deliver an *EPO* gene, which builds erythropoietin (Epo), a hormone that controls red blood cell production. Anemic patients are dosed with a supplemental copy of *EPO* as a therapy. Indeed, *EPO* alters a property called VO_2max, the oxygen-carrying capacity and catalytic turnover of oxygen, so it could also provide an extra boost for endurance athletes. Athletes who process oxygen at the most efficient rate are the ones who hike for miles into the mountains, swim channels and skip to victory in marathons. Consider a natural wonder. Eero Antero Mäntyranta, a Nordic skier and seven-time Olympic medalist, was one of the most astounding athletes Finland ever produced. Mäntyranta also has primary familial and congenital polycythemia (PFCP) which causes an increase in oxygen-processing efficiency due to a mutation in the gene that builds the erythropoietin receptor. The mutation was identified in a DNA study on 200 members of his family, and reported to increase up to 50 percent the oxygen-carrying capacity of his blood, a huge advantage when skiing for endurance in Scandinavia. Shouldn't we all be entitled to such a natural fluke through the addition of a genetic edit, and if so, what would that do to our sense of legend and wonder?

Although genetic enhancement isn't illegal, it is banned in sports by the World Anti-Doping Code. It is unclear whether Springstein ever obtained Repoxygen. The court slapped him with a 16-month suspended jail sentence for supplying various doping products to a minor, and the athletes he supplied were banned from competition. However, phrases such as black market "gene doping" and "performance enhancing gene" had entered the lexicon, and it appeared plausible that within decades an unstoppable black market would emerge where athletes or any person with the cash could order a gene. Illicit gene doping may put pressure on athletes to alter their genetic code, and may someday lead to the shattering of world records as well as a new realm of super athletes. A drug such as Repoxygen may even be used for genetic enhancement in a way that is permitted, for instance, in high-altitude climbing, where athletes suffer from low-oxygen climates in the "Death Zone."

The mutation in the gene for the *EPO* receptor that the Mäntyranta family carried not only provided a competitive boost, but it was technically a manageable health condition, since the family has thicker blood. In fact, *EPO* dosing could cause a number of health risks. A couple of decades before, scientists had tried to add extra copies of *EPO* to monkeys and baboons, but their red blood cell counts doubled in just two months. The animals' blood became so thick it had to be regularly diluted to prevent their hearts from failing. Steve Gullans, a venture capitalist and former Harvard Medical School professor, wrote a commentary piece in *Nature* called "Genetically enhanced Olympics are coming," suggesting that many athletes would almost certainly be willing to take such risks. "If someone else is carrying the *EPOR* receptor that I don't have, why shouldn't I be able to give it to myself to play on an equal playing field?" he wrote me, playing a bit of devil's advocate. "Doing things to our own bodies seems to be something many people are willing to do. Gene doping is an area of uncertainty in terms of legal and moral structures. Not sure who is the thought leader in this space. There is still too much concern about safety to do any enhancement, I believe. Once the safety issue is overcome in the minds of everyone, all bets are off."

But, time and again, scientists were finding, when they created a genetic variant, an advantage is coupled with a new disadvantage. As Jon Gordon noted in a 1999 paper a "spectacular failed attempt at enhancement resulted from efforts to increase muscle mass in cattle. When expressed in mice, the avian *C-SKI* gene, the cellular counterpart of the retroviral *V-SKI* oncogene, caused the mice to build massive muscles. This prompted efforts to produce cattle expressing a *C-SKI* transgene.

When gene transfer was accomplished, the transgenic calf initially exhibited muscle hypertrophy,[288] but muscle degeneration and wasting soon followed. Unable to stand, the debilitated animal was killed."[289]

Other times, scientists seemed to pull off the impossible. In 1999, a University of Pennsylvannia scientist named H. Lee Sweeney wired an extra copy of a growth factor gene called *IGF-1* into mice, while colleague Nadia Rosenthal built on his work to create a new line of super strong mice with big muscles, or "Schwarzenegger mice," which turned out to grow 20 to 50 percent bigger than normal mice. A separate group of researchers had shown they could alter the gene for a protein called PPAR-delta, a master regulator of numerous genes, to create a "Marathon mouse," which could run an incredible 5900 feet before quitting, staying up on a treadmill for an hour longer and far surpassing the 2950 feet that is the invisible "wall" where most normal mice fell off their treadmills into a spinning ball.

There are hints we might be able to use gene engineering to bestow to us superhuman powers. In her 2015 article in *Bloomberg*, Caroline Chen documented the case of Timothy Dreyer, a 25 year old, who has a diagnosis of sclerosteosis, which gives him super-dense bones, due to a mutation in a gene called *SOST*, which renders its protein product nonfunctional and therefore fails to put the brakes on bone growth. Only about 100 people in the world have this condition. According to Chen, "Dreyer, who lives in Johannesburg, was 21 months old when his parents noticed a sudden facial paralysis. Doctors first diagnosed him with palsy. Then X-rays revealed excessive bone formation in his skull..." Chen went on to explain that the drug company Amgen believed the genetic mutation could be useful to counter osteoporosis, a condition of bone loss.[290] The researchers who were studying this genetic mutation quickly saw the potential for drug applications, seeking out more such cases. "In 2010, Socrates Papapoulos, a professor of medicine at the Leiden University Medical Center in the Netherlands, visited an isolated Dutch community where much of the population had overgrown skulls and abnormally large bones. At a town meeting, he asked if anyone had been in a major car accident. One man raised his hand. He said, 'I was crossing the street with my brother, and a Mercedes was coming, and I didn't have time to move,' Papapoulos says. "And I said, 'What happened?' and he said, 'You should have seen the Mercedes.'"[291]

There is also evidence that engineering new traits is harder than it looks. Nexia Biotechnologies Ltd of Canada had a plan to wind spider-silk proteins into a super-strong fabric called "biosteel." The spiders could not be coaxed to spin webs on command, so hoping to extract silk proteins, they put the spider gene into the goats. The transgenic goats amplified the gene into proteins that were extracted from their milk, and electrospun into threads that Nexia want to use to create bullet-proof material. But the company never was able to replicate the tensile strength or incredible properties of spider silk. The dynamics of spider web-making largely remain a mystery. Nexia sold its remaining assets to the Canadian government. Gareth McKinley, a mechanical engineer at MIT, told me at the time that Nexia had gone bust in its quest to copy the spider's elegant web-spinning, its remaining assets amounting to "a herd of goats." In many cases, engineering in new traits would require a coordinated understanding of tens, if not hundreds of genes.

Stuart Kauffman got it right in his book *The Origins of Order* when he wrote that "evolution is not just chance caught on the wing." It is "not just tinkering of the ad hoc, of bricolage, of contraption. It is emergent order honored and honed by selection." Kauffman showed that emergent order is not as simple as plugging in a new gene, or making an edit to a gene. It is an entire system that is highly evolved and tightly regulated. Biological networks are not the same as computer networks. Biology is often regulated by feedback loops, so enhancement depends not just on altering a gene, but its regulatory controls. Selective breeding in dogs or cattle, for instance, involves the inheritance of thousands of genes in a suite that can corroborate to enhance a trait. Seldom can changes to a single gene stably improve a network.[292]

Furthermore, as Jon Gordon noted in his 1999 paper "Genetic Enhancement in Humans," genes often interact in complex and unpredictable ways with other genes. A gene often has three or four different functions, so altering a single gene may have three or four effects.[293] The breast cancer *BRCA1* gene is not only a classic tumor suppressor or "caretaker gene," repairing catastrophic double-strand breaks in the genome, but it also has a job in controlling the cell cycle in the timing and development of embryos, and has been shown to interact with 70 different other genes. It also contains a "zinc finger domain," meaning that it functions as a transcription factor that switches on tens or hundreds of genes. Any given genetic variant may be connected with a known risk or effect, but it may have three or four other effects. To engineer new systems would require a complete, schematic analysis of an entire network, not just a single gene. The list goes on. A gene that builds a protein named "protein S" is a blood coagulant, but it was recently shown to have a critical role in regulation of the immune system.

Scientists have gotten used to appealing to "Ockham's Razor," which states roughly, that "entities must not be multiplied beyond necessity."[294] The main idea is that debates often become trapped within their own circles of concepts and logic. To get to the truth of the matter, and circumvent those traps, it is best to reduce an argument back down to its slimmest of explanations. Once the genome was cracked, geneticists throughout the world were appealing to the Razor, suggesting that gene functions must be simplified, that we must not impose categories on them. If the Razor is correct, then a gene should exist for the slimmest and sparsest of purposes, nothing more.[295] But it turned out that genes have a long and layered history, and often have multiple functions. Francis Crick cautioned that "while Ockham's razor is a useful tool in the physical sciences, it can be a very dangerous implement in biology. It is thus very rash to use simplicity and elegance as a guide in biological research." Not only do many genes have a multiple functions, but the opposite is also true: multiple biological codes or parts can plug in and fill the same key function, an idea that was codified as the principle of "degeneracy." Many three-nucleotide sequences that make up a three-nucleotide codon can code for the same amino acid. Many unique sensors in a cell can trigger an innate immune response. New synapses can patch a connection, where other synaptic connections are lost. Biology is robust against a breakdown. That is difficult to mimic.

"People often ask, can't we banish all disease alleles from the Earth, to give people the best genome?" Eric Lander has said. One reason why not is explained by the multiple functions that a single gene may have. Often when a genetic variant poses a risk, it also provides an advantage, a tradeoff that's known as a balanced polymorphism. Genetic variants in a suite of genes including MC1R, which emerged a million years ago, and variants in a suite of genes which emerged as recently as 8000 years ago, can contribute to light skin color, which is helpful for Northern Europeans who need to absorb more Vitamin D.[296] But engineering a genetic variant into *MC1R* to give your child a shock of red hair and a summertime breakout of freckles would also dispose them to a heightened risk for melanoma. Fast-twitch muscle fibers due to a variant in the gene *ACTN3* may give you an advantage in racquetball, but such a genetic variant might be less than optimal if you were humping your backpack along the Appalachian Trail. Even so, some variants seemingly confer little benefit. Classic Mendelian, or single gene diseases, such as cystic fibrosis or Tay–Sachs disease have clear lines on inheritance persisting through human history, often with extreme disadvantages.

If Darwin's theory of natural selection is correct, if the "survival of the fittest" pruned the sickly branches from the tree of life, then after millions of years it would seem like disease-related genes would have been selected out of our hominid species, leaving questions as to why inborn diseases stay with us. One reason is that diseases can occur as *de novo*, meaning that new mutations can occur in the germline and cause the disease. But that doesn't explain why some rare diseases occur at relatively stable rates through history. It took a British mathematician named G. H. Hardy to propose an intelligent answer. In a 1908 paper, Hardy interjected himself into the debate, demonstrating with some fairly elementary math that rare alleles may remain in circulation in the population, despite assumptions in the body of literature that these disease-associated versions of genes would be selected out of existence. In fact, recessive diseases that are lethal can maintain a stable frequency in the population since a parent who carries only one copy of the deleterious gene may sustain a minor or perhaps unnoticeable affect. This is precisely the situation with the recessive disease cystic fibrosis, where 4 percent of European Caucasians carry one of two rare alleles for the disease, unbeknownst to them. It's only cases where male and female carriers get tangled up romantically, that a child is born with the lung-clogging disease. Hardy–Weinberg equilibrium became a paradigm concept in genetics and was a reliable mathematical model when looking at family trees, and enabled medical geneticists to develop a simple box test called the Punnett square which could predict the frequencies of babies being born with congenital diseases based on the family history. But there is a catch. The frequencies of rare versions of genes will remain constant from generation to generation only in the absence of evolutionary influences, which include natural selection, mutation, genetic drift and gene flow, as populations circulate into other populations, in short, everything that actually happens in life.

"By the 1930s, we discovered simple Mendelian diseases, and that led to the discovery of inheritance patterns, that if there were some genetic loci that were being passed forward, that the genetics causes couldn't be too far away. That led to the study of linkage disequilibrium, which identified blocks of variants that were often as far as a million letters of DNA away from each other," Eric Lander explained in a talk. And, by the 1980s, molecular biology was a crackling field, and so much of everything seemed traceable to our genes; indeed, a brand new field of "population genetics" was emerging based on principles such as "population bottleneck," the sudden restriction or sorting of a gene pool into a far more limited tranche of genes.[297] In a bottleneck, the frequencies of genes that Mendel would call "recessive" may increase significantly. In effect, it's a sampling error. A bottleneck is one mechanism that can enable genetic drift, or change in allele frequency. Genetic variation is largely healthy, and reduction in variation is the reason that inbred groups, kissing cousins, proscribed peoples and self-sequestered colonies can have high rates of rare diseases – cystic fibrosis and Tay–Sachs are precipitously higher among the Ashkenazim Jews and Pennsylvania Dutch. And it is not for any reason but foolish chance. Carriers of *CFTR* mutants happened to get sorted and sequestered together in the happenstance of population movement. Autosomal dominant diseases such as Huntington's are rare, but they are highly visible, since inheriting just a single copy of the genetic variant will trigger the disease. Recessive diseases where two parents are carriers, and don't know they are carriers, are a harder problem for genetic counseling. "All of you," Lander told an audience, "carry a dozen disease genes." To eliminate human disease, it would take the impossible effort to use genetic screening on everyone, "not so likely to happen, not particularly realistic."

Barbara McClintock's "crossing over" mechanism, by which pairs of chromosomes tip their arms and shuffle copies of genes in a kind of gene swap, provided a means to study population genetics. Probabilistically, genes that are close neighbors on a chromosome are less likely to be broken apart by a chromosomal crossover than those which are far flung. However, all genes should be broken up through the course of time, measured in generations. Crossing over once per cell division takes many generations to recombine chromosomes, so genetic loci which had little variation were apt to be the ones undergoing drift. This is because the frequency of an allele is increasing in the population at a rate faster than chromosomal recombination. If chromosomal regions had been recombined at predictable rates, they were said to be in "equilibrium," but if not, they were said to be in "linkage disequilibrium." A genetic region that is in disequilibrium has a long stretch of DNA that is identical in many people in a population.[298] This could be a good or bad sign! If there was not much recombination at a genetic locus among members of a population, it might predict a recessive disease, which is the case of an inbred or sequestered population. But it also might signal the quick circulation of a beneficial gene and its flanking genetic region of "genetic hitchhikers" through a human population.

Consider that babies make lactase to break down their mother's milk. The default is to stop producing it in adolescence. Mutations in the gene that builds the enzyme enabled some people to continue to produce lactase into adulthood. The people with the mutated version on the gene began to take advantage of the calories of milk from herd animals. A selective group pressure to stick with the herd resulted in increased frequencies of the allele, which enabled lactase persistence into adulthood. Suddenly, everyone seemed to have that cool new version of the gene, which allowed us to drink milk into adulthood, as it swept into broad currency in a process called "selective sweep," a term which was instantiated and brought into common parlance by Harvard geneticist David Reich. Nick Patterson, one of Reich's collaborators, along with Alkes Price and Kevin Galinsky, later showed that that a few genetic variants were under significant selection in European Americans, including rs1229984, a coding single nucleotide polymorphism (SNP) of the alcohol-dehydrogenase gene (ADH1B) that has been shown to have a protective effect on alcoholism risk. ADH1B also swept independently through Asian populations, and many Asians are lactose and alcohol intolerant, rendering them especially incapable of enjoying White Russians. Mutations which are rapidly promulgated throughout a population of small breeding groups can result in a major competitive advantage.[299]

The influence of multiple genes on diseases and traits has been known since 1916.[300] In fact, hundreds or thousands of genetic and epigenetic variants can contribute to a complex disease or trait. "Broad-sense heritability" reflects the combination of additive, dominant and epistatic contributions to a trait or phenotype, referring to an observable characteristic in a tissue or organism. Additive means that the number of copies of an allele or copy number can affect the severity of the disease or the extent of the trait. Sometimes genes can undergo duplication events resulting in extra copies of that allele in a single chromosome, and the quantity or load of any single allele in a cell can actually exceed two copies, going up to three or four or more, a concept called "dosage." Dominant means that a single allele can control the trait; epistasis refers to interactions, meaning that the trait may only show up or magnify when a number of genetic variants interact and conspire together, confounding our abilities to make connections. Some interactions can even be negative, meaning one variant can neutralize the effect of another variant, a concept called "masking." Indeed, rare are the Mendelian diseases in which a single genetic variant can be connected to an observable trait. We began to study genetics through a "broad sense" of multiple sources of genetic variation contributing to a trait, whereby we simply consider the combined contribution of all the many additive, dominant and epistatic effects. Such a strategy turned out to be particularly important to selective animal breeding, human behavioral genetics or complex traits such as height. Heritability estimates vary from 0, indicating no genetic inheritance, to 1 for complete genetic determination. But importantly, heritability describes genetic contributions at a population level, and it is a distinct concept from inheritance, which refers to the transmission of a discrete gene from parent to child.

Heritability can lend itself to deception. Consider the following armchair thought experiment attributed to Professor Richard Bentall. "Imagine a world where everybody smokes 200 cigarettes a day. In this worrying scenario, the environmental factors are controlled (there is no environmental variance), therefore the only difference between whether a person gets lung cancer or not has to be due to individual differences in genes (it cannot be whether someone smokes or not since everyone's at it). As a result heritability is 100%... Hence the only explanation for differences between individuals is the genes." Now take away the smoking from people in this nicotine-obsessed environment. The number of people who get lung cancer drops to a negligible amount. The consequences of these considerations are not trivial since mental health issues are on the rise and arguably connected to economics and modern stressors. Heritability may be overestimated due to the contribution of a strong environmental stressor which is assumed to be neutral when it is ubiquitous in a population. More problematically, most of the identical twin studies, which are used to assess heritability in situations where twins maintaining similar genetics are separated by environment, rely on something called equal-environmental assumption. However, work by Jay Joseph and colleagues has suggested that environmental stressors are rarely if ever equal, and that this is a dangerous assumption to make. For instance, such twin studies have estimated the heritability of schizophrenia to be about 80 percent. By adjusting such studies for differential stressors, those scientists believe that the heritability of mental illness is not as pronounced."[301] Surveys suggest that social pressures exert a large effect on mental health.[302]

As Paul Thompson and colleagues wrote "heritability estimates measure the proportion of the trait variance explained by variations across the entire genome, it does not tell us anything about which specific genes contribute to it, how many genes are involved, or the impact of any one gene on the trait."[303] By comparison, the "narrow sense" of heritability has focused on single genetic variants or a small number of multiple genetic variants, which became the primary focus of most modern genetic investigations, since specificity is where drug-makers' interest primarily lies, through the identification of actionable targets. In fact, there are two main ways to localize a gene or a locus in a chromosomal region: *linkage* and *association*. Linkage disequilibrium, as mentioned, is based on a tendency for neighboring genetic variants to be inherited together on a single chromosome. Genetic loci get broken up during meiotic cell division. We know genetic variants run in those families which carry the disease, and so we can exploit inheritance patterns to test for "co-segregation" of the phenotypic trait and the genotype within the families. If a genetic locus is broken up then we can eliminate that part of the search, and if one is preserved and segregates with people in the family that have the disease, we can nominate it as a candidate for further study. Linkage varies across populations and such studies are limited to large families of related individuals and often at best narrows a search to a large genetic locus on the order of millions of bases. Linkage disequilibrium studies can be used to test rare variants that contribute to human disease, an intense area of research and elegant new methods.[304]

Association is based on statistical correlations which use an allele to predict a disease or trait. This is based on the "common disease common variant hypothesis," a basic belief that common disease shares a set of genetic variants or etiologies which must be, in a sense, also common to the disease. Such tests do not require large families of inter-related people, and are in fact sensitive to population ancestry, so you want to remove the effects of variants that tend to associate with people who live in specific localities. In 2005, the first successful genome-wide association study, or GWAS, was completed. These studies used thousands of subjects to allow us to identify single nucleotide polymorphisms which are common spelling mistakes. Such a polymorphism that occurs in more than 1% of a population is a common variant, while one that occurs less frequently than that is a "rare variant." An allele is a version of a gene which can be defined by single or multiple polymorphisms or spelling mistakes in our genetic code. An allele is therefore a means to typify a version of a gene by one or more mutations.

More often than not, we would observe variants in multiple different genes, but it turns out that complex diseases turned out to be more than a collection of Mendelian diseases. There are six or seven exceptions, including *NOD2* in Crohn's disease and *APOE4* in Alzheimer's disease, in which a handful of SNPs account for a significant risk on their own.[305] For instance, I worked on a GWAS study on Alzheimer's, and I have also published some results on the gene *BIN1*, which we think is neuroprotective and is clearly elevated in some cell types in Alzheimer's disease. *BIN1* includes something called a Clap domain, and participates in clathrin-mediated endocytosis, meaning that it has a role in ushering characteristic amyloid beta plaques into the cell for destruction. But while we know that it is upregulated in the disease, that doesn't mean that upregulating it further will provide any therapeutic effect. In most disease states, the body is already operating at its optimal performance for responding to the disease state. One of the mysteries of Alzheimer's is that drug companies have developed antibodies to clear amyloid beta plaques out of the brain but it has relatively little therapeutic effect.

William Klein at Northwestern University and others have proposed that its not the large plaques, but actually small species of amyloid beta which are soluble and diffusible, so-called "small oligomers," which cause all the problems in the disease by binding to insulin receptors and NMDA receptors which are important in the creation of long-term memories. The research shows that these small oligomers bind to receptors and cause a "gain-of-function" disorder, by which the receptors are constantly jarred open. This helps to explain why memantine (Namenda), the only drug with mild therapeutic effects, might work. Memantine is an inhibitor, and scientists have often wondered why an inhibitor would have a treatment benefit for Alzheimer's. It would if it was compensating for a gain-of-function disorder at the receptor level. Klein is now developing an antibody for small amyloid beta oligomers, which he says will work. In other work, Dennis Wright and Ben Bahr are developing a compound called PADK, which has been in the public domain since the 1970s and has an effect of "positive lysosomal regulation," meaning that it triggers the cell's lysosome, which works like a lasso, and catches tau deposits which build up inside the cells, to clean up more of its interior garbage. (The other garbage disposal unit a cell has is the proteasome, which works like a trash compactor, a tiny tube that proteins enter and are then chopped up.)

A few common hereditary diseases such as the blood disorder hemochromatosis are influenced by a handful of genes.[306] Perhaps hundreds of genetic variants with small effects can influence a highly heritable complex trait such as height.[307] Association studies become less tractable when we move to higher-order problems like predicting structure and function in the brain. As Thompson noted, "Most brain traits appear to be influenced by many common variants with relatively small effects and rare variants with larger effects."[308] Indeed, the common disease common variant hypothesis is credible, it's just not that useful when it involves hundreds or thousands of such variants. GWAS is a reasonably fast and powerful tool, and highly publishable, so scientists continue to turn to it for investigation, even when they know it will have little or no clinical impact. As Sherman Elias, a clinical geneticist, told me "when you have a hammer, everything looks like a nail."

In January 2016, a paper on schizophrenia was published in the journal *Nature*. An article in *The New York Times* about that journal article appeared the next day. "More than two million Americans have a diagnosis of schizophrenia, which is characterized by delusional thinking and hallucinations. The drugs available to treat it blunt some of its symptoms but do not touch the underlying cause," noted the newspaper.[309] "That risk, they found, is tied to a natural process called synaptic pruning, in which the brain sheds weak or redundant connections between neurons as it matures. During adolescence and early adulthood, this activity takes place primarily in the section of the brain where thinking and planning skills are centered, known as the prefrontal cortex. People who carry genes that accelerate or intensify that pruning are at higher risk of developing schizophrenia than those who do not, the new study suggests... People with schizophrenia have a gene variant that apparently facilitates aggressive 'tagging' of connections for pruning, in effect accelerating the process."

In fact, the researchers identified a genetic variant in a classic immune system gene called *C4*, which also localizes to "neuronal synapses, dendrites, axons, and cell bodies" and tags synaptic connections for pruning, which "continues from adolescence into the third decade of life."[310] *C4* was yet another example of a gene that has multiple functions. Steven McCarroll, an associate professor of genetics at Harvard, and Beth Stevens, an assistant professor of neurology at Boston Children's Hospital and Harvard, led the study through the Stanley Center for Psychiatric Research at the Broad Institute, which involved the analysis of more than 100,000 DNA samples and found the strongest single nucleotide polymorphisms were "embedded in an immune system gene called the major histocompatibility complex (MHC) locus on chromosome 6 which includes 18 human leukocyte antigen (*HLA*) genes that encode 'antigen-presenting molecules' which are the molecules that display fragments of microbes and viruses to immune cells in the body to flag them to initiate an immune system response. The *C4* gene resides in this locus, and comes in alleles or gene versions *C4A* and *C4B*." An allele is typically copied into as many as 8 to 12 versions of RNA, which undergo a process called assortative splicing and thus have sections called "introns" spliced out leaving only combinations of "exons" that differ in length and function.[311] In fact, each of these C4 alleles comes in long and short versions "as distinguished by the presence or absence" in one of its introns of a human endogenous retroviral (HERV) insertion, meaning a retrovirus that wormed its way into the human genome eons ago, went dormant and became part of its permanent record. The retrovirus also includes a long terminal repeat which serves as an "enhancer," meaning that it enhances the expression of a gene it is embedded in. In fact, the expression of the long form of the *C4A* allele is a predictor of schizophrenia.[312]

In *The New York Times*, McCarroll was quoted as estimating the variant would "increase a person's risk by about 25 percent over the 1 percent base rate of schizophrenia – that is, to 1.25 percent. That is not nearly enough to justify testing in the general population, even if further

research confirms the new findings and clarifies the roles of other associated genes... The finding... will not lead to new treatments soon,
experts said, nor to widely available testing for individual risk."[313] On
January 30, 2016, The *Economist* noted: "They were looking for regions
of the human genome that might be harbouring variants that increase
the risk for schizophrenia. What they found implicated more than a
hundred genes and provided a strong pointer towards a portion of the
genome associated with infectious diseases. Many of these genes did not
operate independently of each other." Eric Lander further noted that
10000 signals identified in the study combined to increase risk to 10%
for schizophrenia. You could correct those variants, but the major problem is that genes are often multi-functional; they have more than one
function. As Lander declared, in a moment of anticlimax, we don't want
to "mess with 10,000 things in the genome."

Schizophrenia is multi-factorial, meaning it locates some of its risk
in factors outside the genome. In her 2015 book, *Infectious Madness*,
Harriet Washington reported that 10 to 20 percent of neuropsychiatric
illnesses, including autism, are partly caused by pathogens. Book
reviewer Meghan O'Rourke explained the growing body of evidence that
has sought to explain a longstanding anomaly. "Schizophrenics are
about 5 to 8 percent more likely to be born in winter and early spring –
not a huge upward tick, but one that is consistent across multiple
studies in different countries. Schizophrenics also have elevated white
blood cell counts, suggesting they may be fighting an infection..."
E. Fuller Torrey, a psychiatrist, and Jaroslav Flegr, a Czech scientist,
each became convinced that *Toxoplasma gondii*, a parasite that cats
transmit to humans, was a driver for schizophrenia. Another doctor,
Hervé Perron, "has identified a virus, HERV-W, that he believes is
involved in schizophrenia; it turns out that "49 percent – nearly half –
of people with schizophrenia harbor HERV-W, while only 4 percent of
people without schizophrenia do," Washington writes. "One theory is
that viruses like the flu or infections like toxoplasmosis cause the body
to 'release' HERV-W viruses, overwhelming the immune system and
causing inflammation in some people," O'Rourke writes.[314]

One lesson here is that human genetics may not be the deciding
influence on mental health, but is one small contribution amid a raft
of contributors, including many environmental stressors. It may sound
critical to dismiss the work of geneticists, but the burden of proof is on

them, and while human genetics may influence the disruptions in neural networks, these connectivity disorders – and they are almost certainly that – have multi-factorial etiologies that may even emerge independently of our genetics. The allure of isolating a cause for schizophrenia or depression in a gene or infection is that we can avoid talking about economic inequalities, social pressures, and the effects of chronic stress and grief, which I think are real. There are a few reasons that I think it's unlikely that genetics will every lead to a clinical treatment for mental health disorders. The major problem is that our genes simply cannot predict the higher-order complexity of brain connectivity. Geneticists, and particularly those who use high-powered GWAS studies, engage in a misreading of mental health disorders, primarily by studying a highly diverse set of etiologies, as a single disease, when there is undoubtedly a spectrum of disorders. Thousands of genetic variants contribute to neural anatomy and function, and most probably have epistatic and pleiotropic effects, meaning their function is highly sensitive to their specific context or genetic background. In my estimation, genetics can contribute to the distribution and migration of cell types in the brain, including neurons and glia cells, and highly influences, but does not determine, the wiring or synaptic structure that is the "connectome," and to diseases that are "connectopathies," or aberrations of how neurons are communicating. There are some genes such as synaptotagmin 7, or *syt7*, a calcium sensor that dynamically increases neurotransmitter release, which may have a global contribution to connectivity, but we are hard pressed to locate genes which can determine or govern the structure and topography of those connections, and the connections seem highly dynamic. If genetics are complicated, then protein-to-protein interactions are even more so, given that there are perhaps a hundred thousand proteins which interact in complex and unpredictable ways. In one recent and unnerving study, scientists found that they could only replicate about 25 percent of protein-to-protein interactions, meaning that their findings of how proteins interact in an organism are speculative at best, highly sensitive to conditions.[315]

The "connectome" is driven in large part by the release and reception of neurotransmitters, which supply the signals that transmit from the axon of one neuron to the dendrite of another neuron. Both alcohol and benzodiazepines bind to receptors called GABA, which are ubiquitous in the brain and provide a mechanism to quiet or calm overactive anxiety centers in the brain. But these are highly dynamic systems, which ultimately undergo changes for reasons that are not hardcoded in the genes. The alcohol in a Budweiser or anti-anxiety drugs may bind to GABA (alcohol may also bind to an excitatory glutamate receptor called NMDA) and calm an overactive firing, but the result is the more we rely on those drugs, the fewer of those receptors the neurons produce, compensating to return to their baseline, as the English neuroscientist C. Heather Ashton wrote, suggesting a need for "tapering" off our medications. "People become tolerant to benzodiazepines probably because their nerve cells respond by producing fewer receptors for GABA/benzodiazepines. This phenomenon, known as 'down regulation', means that the number of 'high affinity' GABA receptors decreases in response to the enhancement of GABA caused by the drug. Such homeostatic responses, which tend to reinstate the status quo despite the continued presence of drug, happen with many of the drugs that people take regularly, including alcohol, opiates and even beta blockers, which are widely prescribed for heart disease. The adaptation of behaviour to overcome the actions of the drugs probably also contributes to tolerance.... Whatever the mechanism, the development of tolerance sets the scene for withdrawal effects. At this stage, the removal of benzodiazepines, or even a reduction in dosage, exposes the altered state of the brain, with fewer 'higher affinity' receptors for GABA to act upon... The body responds to the continued presence of the drug with a series of adjustments that tend to overcome the drug effects. In the case of benzodiazepines, compensatory changes occur in the GABA and benzodiazepine receptors which become less responsive, so that the inhibitory actions of GABA and benzodiazepines are decreased."[316]

There are a number of critical events that occur at the onset of adulthood in the prefrontal cortex, including engagement of "fast-spiking interneurons" which are GABAergic, meaning they produce GABA, and are therefore critical for determining the timing and spatial selectivity of pyramidal cell firing, the kinds of cells that release glutamate, an important excitatory neurotransmitter. Dopamine activates these interneurons through D1 and D2 receptors, but this mechanism only becomes activated in late adolescence, an important time to avoid drinking, drugs and undo stress.

Finally, and this is just my own gut instinct, it strikes me that people with mental health issues are, in a way, more open to experience, more honest and may often have experiences that are more genuine and closer to reality. That any of us can be killed in a car accident on any given day and sent into oblivion – the overwhelming sense of oblivion – is closer to reality than the hope that we can control and secure our lives through mechanisms such as genetics or biochemistry. That any of us has a cohesive sense of reality is the exception and wonder, not the default, holding together a sense of stability is a privilege, not a right. It's almost certainly a temporary situation. In many ways, mental health issues may derive from not less, but *more* exposure to reality. In *Crazy Like Us*, Ethan Watters wrote about how people with mental health issues who live in cultures with a high level of "expressed emotion" over their condition do worse than in those with low levels of concern, basically people in cultures who see a dark night of the soul as something transitory we can pass through. Genius, like madness, was also believed to be originally appreciated as transitory. As Joshua Shenk wrote, "Historically speaking, locating genius within individuals is a recent enterprise. Before the 16th century, one did not speak of people being geniuses but *having* geniuses. 'Genius,' the Harvard scholar Marjorie Garber has explained, meant 'a tutelary god or spirit given to every person at birth.' Any value that emerged from within a person depended on a potent, unseen force coming from beyond that person."[317] If genius and madness are indeed linked, it is probably largely driven by the function of stress and internal turmoil, and it's by no means hard to find families that include a mix of both. Jim Watson has a son who is schizophrenic. Four out of five of Ludwig Wittgenstein's brothers committed suicide. Kurt Cobain may have been bipolar.

The most compelling and realistic theory in the literature is that endophenotypes which contribute to a risk for mental illness, in short, manifesting themselves as subclinical traits, which we often characterize as schizotypal or psychoticism traits, enable people to perform better on measures of creativity. However, if these tendencies become overly pronounced in the cases of severe mental illness, the aptitude for productivity and creativity plummet – a concept broadly referred to as the "inverted U."[318,319] In effect, mild amounts of stress and disorientation can contribute to outside-the-box thinking, but a full spiral into a psychotic episode results in a rapid decline in insight and creative potential.

The connectome is a dymanic range of interactions in neurotransmitters and highly regulated by stress hormones such as catecholemines. That's why the idea of low-expressed emotion is so important to the treatment of mental illness; because it recognizes that the status is not entirely genetically determined, but along the continuum of a dynamic range, an "inverted U." To be sure, we're all someplace on this U, including me.

The irony is that most of the creativity and actually useful contributions to science and the arts come out of deep uncertainty, disorientation and self questioning as to the nature of reality and to systems and to our work. Importantly, mental health does not exist in a one-to-one relationship between druggable genetic variants or biological targets, but exists in a dynamic range, along an inverted U, and within its drama, its failing, emerges its ability to shift and gain new powers, sources of inspiration and life, to renew. Dynamism is why the connectome is the most appropriate level to interpret and study mental health.

Thompson and colleagues wrote, "The term 'connectome' refers to the totality of neural connections within a brain. It is currently not possible to assess all neuronal connections in a living organism, but using modern neuroimaging and specially designed analytic strategies, we can map the connectome at the macroscopic scale, in living individuals."[320] A few tools for imaging include resting state fMRI, which captures the movement of blood as a default state, which is a baseline while sleeping or awake, and accounts for "functional" connectivity, and diffusion tensor imaging, which captures the directional movement of water in the brain, so-called anatomical or "structural" connectivity. The imaging techniques account for quantitative traits and we can use genetics loci, known as quantitative trait loci or QTL, to predict those traits. In fact, you can use genetics to try to predict any type of biological trait, such as the expression of a gene, or a quantitative trait that is gathered from a brain imaging technique. "The primary goal of imaging genetics is to identify and characterize genes that are associated with brain measures derived from images, including connectomic maps." Researchers also use algorithms to create multi-dimensional maps or graphs. "The human brain connectome can be represented as a matrix, or a graph, containing regions of interest as nodes and connections or correlations between them as edges."[321]

Risk aversion, mirroring or empathic traits, or anatomical traits can account for an endophenotype, "a heritable trait that is genetically correlated with an illness and has much greater power to localize genetic loci than affection status alone."[322] The activity of the amygdala, a region that has a role in negative emotions, has been implicated with major depression or bipolar disorder, and hyperactive connectivity patterns have been observed in persons with schizophrenia and unaffected relatives, leading to an interest in identifying a genetic loci which can predict activity of that endophenotype.[323,324] Some of those endopheno-types may also provide competitive advantages, raising interesting evolutionary questions about whether we'd want to rid ourselves of their genetics, or counter them. Technologies will enable us to further test associations between genes and endophenotypes. The Allen Brain atlas includes data on genetically altered mice which allows researchers to observe the effects on anatomical structure of brain regions and also "relates connection maps to gene expression patterns compiled from multiple sources."[325] The Stanford neuroscientist Karl Deisseroth developed a system called fiber photometry, which uses light particles to track activity of neurons, and used it to observe that neurons express-ing D2 receptors in the nucleus accumbens (part of the striatum) influ-enced whether or not rats would make risky decisions. The signal from those cells spiked in rats who gambled and lost out on a food source, but in other rats who were chronic risk takers the signal was dampened. If the D2 receptors did not signal, the rat did not take a loss too seriously and just tried again. Deisseroth also helped to develop optogenetics, a system that uses light to trigger the firing of neurons and showed he could stimulate this subset of neurons and cause rats to learn from a loss, not to take a risk again.[326] The best our genetics will probably ever truly model is an endophenotype. One such subclinical trait to model is called "white matter integrity," which is assessed through the diffusion or one-way movement of water through the microstructure of the brain; in other words, movement that is anisotropic rather than isotropic (not sensitive to direction). Thompson and colleagues wrote, to some degree these measures "may reflect axonal packing, coherence and even the extent of myelination." Early work in the field showed the microstruc-ture of cerebral white matter was under strong genetic control, meaning high heritability, and also that it correlated with intellectual perform-ance on some tests in twin studies.[327] In a large family study, linkage analysis identified genetic loci at chromosomes 15q25 and 3q27 which co-segregated with depression and obsessive-compulsive disorder, phenotypes which had also been predicted by atypical white matter.[328] Time and again, the impulse is to move from genetics to endophenotype, and then to the phenotype. But since heritability of traits comes in the broad sense, "a highly heritable trait does not necessarily mean that a GWAS will produce significant results."[329]

There are a few notable exceptions, but these genes promote non-specific connectivity through the robust growth of neurons. Growth factors, or neurotrophins, influence brain growth and the guidance and migration of axons during development. In fact, the brain-derived neurotrophic factor (*BDNF*) gene modulates hippocampal neurogenesis, synaptic transmission and activity-induced long-term potentiation. The hippocampus is where "place cells" fire, and provides an internal map. A single nucleotide polymorphism in *BDNF* led to poorer episodic memory and hippocampal activation, and another study associated that variant to alterations in white matter microstructure.[330,331] Variants in the *NTRK1* gene, which encodes for a neurotrophin, could predict microstructure and a risk for schizophrenia.[332] The *HFE* gene, which is involved in iron metabolism, contains variants which are critical to neural development.[333] The *COMT* gene encodes for the catechol-O-methyltransferase enzyme involved in degradation of dopamine in the prefrontal and temporal cortex.[334,335] People with two copies of a mutation have a fourfold increase in *COMT* activity and decreased connectivity in the prefrontal cortex, implicating the ability of the gene to modulate resting-state connectivity through the modulation of dopamine.[336,337] A genetic variant in *CNTNAP2*, an autism risk gene, was one of the first to be used to link connectivity measures to a common genetic variant.[338] These common variants all sound very interesting, but they add up to effects that are shockingly small. Five genetic variants in genes *COMT*, *NTRK1*, *ErbB4*, *CLU* and *HFE* combined about 6% of the variance in white matter integrity in the corpus callosum, a conductor between brain hemispheres.[339]

Steven Pinker relayed some "naturalistic psychology" in his *The New York Time Magazine* story "My Genome, My Self," which revealed he and George Church would have their whole genome sequences made public. "Dopamine is the molecular currency in several brain circuits associated with wanting, getting satisfaction and paying attention. The gene for one kind of dopamine receptor, *DRD4*, comes in several versions. Some of the variants (like the one I have) have been associated with 'approach related' personality traits like novelty seeking, sensation seeking and extraversion. A gene for another kind of receptor, *DRD2*, comes in a version that makes its dopamine system function less effectively. It has been associated with impulsivity, obesity and substance abuse. Still another gene, *COMT*, produces an enzyme that breaks down dopamine in the prefrontal cortex, the home of higher cognitive functions like reasoning and planning. If your version of the gene produces less *COMT*, you may have better concentration but might also be more neurotic and jittery... Behavioral geneticists have also trained their sights on serotonin, which is found in brain circuits that affect many moods and drives, including those affected by Prozac and similar drugs. *SERT*, the serotonin transporter, is a molecule that scoops up stray serotonin for recycling, reducing the amount available to act in the brain. The switch for the gene that makes *SERT* comes in long and short versions, and the short version has been linked to depression and anxiety. A 2003 study made headlines because it suggested that the gene may affect a person's resilience to life's stressors rather than giving them a tendency to be depressed or content across the board. People who had two short versions of the gene (one from each parent) were likely to have a major depressive episode only if they had undergone traumatic experiences; those who had a more placid history were fine. In contrast, people who had two long versions of the gene typically failed to report depression regardless of their life histories. In other words, the effects of the gene are sensitive to a person's environment. Psychologists have long known that some people are resilient to life's slings and arrows and others are more fragile, but they had never seen this interaction played out in the effects of individual genes."

There are other genes like the serotonin receptor *5-HTT*, which has a famously complicated history on predicting resilience. Different alleles or versions of the gene produce receptors of different lengths, which have been associated with how resilient a person is to tragedy. Despite their etiologies, and they are complicated, I cotton on to the argument that schizophrenic, autistic and depressive types are not so much abnormal as they are *personality models* that come with advantages and disadvantages. In his classic reflection, *The Noonday Demon*, Andrew Solomon suggested one view of people with major depression is they hold a *more* realistic view of life. In his 2015 work *NeuroTribes*, Steve Silberman argued against "framing autism as a contemporary aberration," instead suggesting it had roots in "very old genes that are shared widely in the general population while being concentrated more in certain families than in others. Whatever autism is, it is not a unique product of modern civilization. It is a strange gift from our deep past, passed down through millions of years of evolution... Neurodiversity advocates propose that instead of viewing this gift as an error of nature – a puzzle to be solved and eliminated with techniques like prenatal testing and selective abortion – society should regard it as a valuable part of humanity's genetic legacy." In 2005, in *Development and Psychopathology*, Bruce J. Ellis of the University of Arizona and W. Thomas Boyce of the University of California published a paper "Biological Sensitivity to Context," which examined how sensitive children were to their family environment, suggesting the term *orkidebarn*, which means "orchid child," in contrast to *maskrosbarn*, or "dandelion child," who as the name suggests, are more psychologically resilient and able to thrive in any context. As Herbert Wray wrote in *Scientific American Mind*, "Orchid children, in contrast, are highly sensitive to their environment, especially to the quality of parenting they receive. If neglected, orchid children promptly wither – but if they are nurtured, they not only survive but flourish." In the authors' poetic language, an orchid child becomes "a flower of unusual delicacy and beauty."[340] The geneticist Danielle M. Dick of Virginia Commonwealth University and colleagues identified *CHRM2*, a gene which codes chemical receptors involved in learning and memory. Dick's team took DNA samples from 400 boys and girls who were part of a longitudinal behavioral study, and found that genetic variants in the *CHRM2* gene interact with parental negligence to result in aggression and delinquency, but also with attentive parenting to produce incredible teenage outcomes. As Wray wrote, "If *CHRM2* does turn out to be an orchid child gene, some earlier findings might now begin to make sense... the gene has also been linked to serious depression in some studies and to cognitive ability in others."

Genetics and the cult of neurobiology had fed into the very modern impulse to embrace a binary view of psychiatric disorders. In fact, the psychiatrist Emil Kraepelin is credited with the "categorical" position of psychosis, distinguishing between states of insanity and non-psychotic states, legitimate and illegitimate, and indeed, modern psychiatry and its manuals including the DSM are aligned with this view. In contrast, the psychiatrist Eugen Bleuler did not believe in a separation between sanity and madness, and instead believed that we are all on a continuum, most of us capable of entering into episodes of depression or psychosis. My instinct is that Bleuler is probably right. Life is much more devastating and unstable than most of us are willing to admit – indeed, half of us will have some type of mental health disorder at some point in our lives. In fact, psychologists put personality traits on a continuous scale, not a categorical one. Each personality is a dynamic and idiosyncratic model which exceeds in some places and fails in other lots in life. It is an enduring truism that artistic people are more open to trauma, but that may also be an advantage that works to their end.

Steven Pinker told me "there are several possible explanations of why the trait of openness to experience could be an individual adaptation. As with any trait that varies among individuals, there is the challenge of explaining why it does not take a single, optimal value in all members of the species. Among the possibilities are that it's the result of mutations that have not been weeded out yet; that different values are adaptive in different kinds of environments; and that it's frequency-dependent: it's only adaptive when it's not too common."

In his essay *A Supposedly Fun Thing I'll Never Do Again*, David Foster Wallace, amid a torrent of "hysterical realism" on a cruise ship, had a moment of stillness. It nearly undid him, "especially at night, when all the ship's structured fun and reassurances and gaiety-noise ceased – I felt despair, but it's a serious word, and I'm using it seriously." He goes on: the "marrow-level dread of the oceanic" and the "intuition of the sea as primordial nada, bottomless, depths inhabited by cackling tooth-studded things rising toward you at the rate a feather falls." At the least, there is a note of sincerity here, an instinct to move beyond the ironic and detached, to cope with an enduring situation. Wallace's own depression only adds to the reputation of writers as troubled and their troubled characters as autobiographical. In Herman Melville's *Moby-Dick*, Ishmael introduces himself as having "a damp, drizzly November in my soul." And author Olivia Laing reports that not much has changed between Melville and Wallace. In *The Trip to Echo Spring: On Writers and Drinking*, she documents the life of six literary figures, all alcoholic, teetering on the verge of psychic breakdown: Ernest Hemingway, F. Scott Fitzgerald, John Berryman, Raymond Carver, John Cheever and Tennessee Williams. Hemingway was wracked by insomnia, paranoia and depression, and drank himself into a catastrophic failure. As a teenager on the boulevards of Paris, Williams began abruptly to feel afraid of what he called "the process of thought" and came within "a hairsbreadth of going quite mad," describing his experiences as "the most dreadful, the most nearly psychotic, crisis that occurred in my early life." Wait, there's more: Faulkner, Poe, Woolf, Plath. Thom Jones's father died in a mental institution. Robert Stone's mother was schizophrenic and institutionalized. Andre Dubus II won MacArthur and Guggenheim fellowships, but his life was sad beyond words. In the winter of 2016 I read the obituaries of Pat Conroy, who wrote *The Prince of Tides* and Jim Harrison who wrote *Legends of the Fall* and was not at all surprised to read they each suffered from a lot of mental turmoil. Conroy was berated by a militant father, Harrison was slashed with a broken bottle in the eye and decided to go live in the woods as a child before suffering a lifetime of deep depression. In 1995, Arnold Ludwig showed a 77 percent rate of psychiatric disorders in eminent fiction writers. Researcher Jonathan Gottschall piles on more evidence for the instability of writers, noting that writers are 10 times, and poets 40 times, more likely to be bipolar than the general population.[341] Junot Diaz explained absences between his novels to the local bi-monthly events guide *Scout Cambridge*, saying simply he'd spent much of his life "nice and depressed and dysfunctional."

We didn't evolve to write books. Literary talent often does not emerge until the 30s and 40s because so much of it is based on endless draftsmanship. I suspect more fiction writers set out to write as a means to solve problems and rehash conflicts and sort out dysfunction in their lives, than there are fiction writers that write to put well-adapted talent on display. The production of literature, like music, is not even an adaptation, but may be a by-product of adaptation, sometimes called a "spandrel." "Certainly a cultural invention like writing, to say nothing of the even more recent invention of the novel, could not be an evolutionary adaptation," Steven Pinker told me. "There is a romantic cultural stereotype that authors themselves like to cling to – painful process, requiring a solitary cabin, you have to hate book tours. I doubt it's true for most authors."[342] Lorin Stein, a senior editor at the *Paris Review*, seemed to embrace the dysfunction of his writers. "You have to be inside the scene – the tactile world of tables and chairs and sunlight – attending to your characters, people who exist for you in nonvirtual reality. This takes weird brain chemistry. A surprising number of novelists hear voices, and not metaphorically. They hear voices in their heads. It also takes years of reading – solitary reading."

"My intelligence – whatever I call my intelligence – was assembled by that kid I was between the ages of 26 and 36 who just did not stop reading," Junot Diaz told *Scout Magazine*. "That kid build the edifice which I currently claim as my own." All serious writers begin as serious readers who have an almost crushing sense of their own deficits. As Diaz said on community television, "Every reader knows that they don't understand half of what they read; it's true, that's not a joke – because that's how real life is really like. People you love say shit and you have no idea what they mean." Serious reading begins with a stance that embraces antagonism, and incompleteness, and is sunken in process. David Foster Wallace had an almost punishing sense of curiosity and he was bothered most by the simplest things ("What is a number?"). The French philosopher Catherine Malabou called it "plastic reading," or beginning with a sense of understanding only partially what she read, bearing some interpretive power, and drawing on context to understand what she read. In *The Space of Literature*, philosopher Maurice Blanchot wrote: "What threatens reading is this: the reader's reality, his personality, his immodesty, his stubborn resistance upon remaining himself in the face of what he reads – a man who knows in general how to read."

Two hundred years ago, Hegel proposed a basis for narration in a concept he called "tarrying the negative," which contemplates what philosophers call alterity, or otherness, drawing perspective through conflict and opposing opinion. The Romantic poet John Keats codified an idea that sounds strikingly similar, which he called "negative capability," which implies suspension of judgement and thinking outside of context. If intelligence locates itself anywhere, it grows through the process and coping with its deficits, by collapsing and breaking into new reality. Psychologists have long noted that "creative people are *obsessed* with a lack of order in nature, and with the development of their own ethical code."[343] In *Wittgenstein's Mistress*, his stunning experimental writing on the condition of confronting nature in its stark realities, echoing a profound sense of loneliness and isolation, David Markson writes of a woman who is coming to terms with being the last person on Earth. She never gives us her name, but only reveals a deep despair that she is the only measure of her own life, as she wanders the globe on her own. "In the beginning, I left messages in the street."

In *The Mosquito Coast*, the novelist Paul Theroux imagined a Yankee inventor who becomes disenchanted with the superficial impulses and dwindling intellectual rigor of middle-class American life. He invents an ice machine that operates on fire rather than electricity and relocates his family to Honduras to live among savages and to forge a better life, bootstrapping his family into a purer existence. Fer Allie Fox, the main character's genius, and also his downfall, is a kind of self-punishing questioning and open-mindedness that rests not on past accomplishments, demonstrated facts and established status quo, the stability that comes from a few intellectual achievements which establish a person in the social mix, but rather on a blinding perseverance into unknown territory, a sense of rollicking insecurity and instability, and a sense of surging will.[344] Allie Fox is pretty much a man destined (doomed) to surpass himself. Theroux explains his character like this: "What he liked best was taking things apart, even books, even the Bible. He said the Bible was like an owner's guide, a repair manual to an unfinished invention. He also said the Bible was a wilderness. It was one of Father's theories that there were parts of the Bible that no one had ever read, just as there were parts of the world where no one had ever set foot." Allie Fox responds to this assessment of his character: "You think that's bad? It's anything but. It's the empty spaces that will save us."

We tend to think of intelligence in terms of the techno-scientific, quantifiable and monetized, while neglecting the value of approach. In *Ecco Homo*, Nietzsche talks about "amor fati," or the love of fate. "Not merely bear what is necessary, still less conceal it – all idealism is mendacity in the face of what is necessary – but *love* it." Jonah spent a dark night of the soul in the belly of the whale. Dante struggled through layers of existence. Intelligence springs from our genes, but at least part of it springs from continual questioning, its journey, as novelists say, its Bildungsroman. In fact, the "analytic rumination hypothesis" suggests an evolutionary basis for mild depression, such that it may have a functional purpose and occur based on social defeats or impasse, which can send the mind into withdrawal and circular thinking to rehash a conflict. Case studies abound: Superman, yes even he, retreated into hiatus at the Fortress of Solitude. In literature, the ghost is sometimes used as an expression of a real person stuck in rumination. In his typical counterintuitive analysis, Slavov Zizek suggested the important thing is not so much that ghosts startle real people, but that real people startle ghosts into returning to their senses.[345]

Zizek represents a radical social constructivism that is an extension of Michel Foucault and Jacques Lacan by which we find the roots of our psychology in the social order, but it is an oversimplification. Chomsky and the cognitivists have superseded this with a more realistic and mature vision of human nature in which identity and intelligence emerges through the order in our neurobiological wellsprings. The psychiatrist George Makari commented on his inability to fully embrace social constructivism. "I was a medical resident in psychiatry when I first studied Foucault's arguments, and I got the distinct impression that his 'madness' was often just a metaphor with which to challenge authority, not much related to the shaking, hallucinating teenager that I would soon return to on the wards."[346]

Foucault developed the influential notions of "biopower" and "bio-politics" which passed the "threshold of modernity" in order to give "power its access even to the body." In the words of Foucault, biopolitics is "the endeavor, begun in the eighteen century, to rationalize problems presented to governmental practice by the phenomenon of a group of living human beings constitute as a population: health, sanitation, birth rate, longevity, race." But even Foucault had yet to conceive of the deep biological history, a history of the body, to the extent that genetics could be harnessed for leverage. The relationship of biology to social pressures has become an active new frontier, for instance, through the auspices of epigenetic effects that are acquired through stress and diet, and which regulate our gene expression. As the Stanford neuroscientist Robert Sapolsky has noted, stress is distributed unequally across the social spectrum – and the poorer you are, the more stress you get. Hierarchies of wealth and power have institutionalized forms of stress.[347] And because chronic stress is debilitating, this trend has had the effect of fixing social hierarchies in body chemistry through social imprinting. "A canonical body of knowledge shows how stress in early life, particularly in the prenatal period can have predominantly adverse neurobiological consequences reaching long into adulthood."

"These effects can have an extraordinarily long reach, changing the trajectory of brain again, and even having multi-generational effects, through the non-genetic transmission of behavior and physiological traits. The mediation mechanism for these long-term effects has increasingly been shown to be epigenetic, a current focus of intense amounts of work."[348] Sapolsky spent decades studying hierarchies and status of baboons in Kenya and the effects of those relationships on stress. In 2003, Sapolsky and Gary K. Steinberg, also a doctor at

Stanford, began work on a "stress vaccine," which was a kind of prophylactic gene therapy.

Glucocorticoid is a stress-related protein that exerts a range of harmful effects when it is chronically elevated. Sapolsky and Steinberg developed a series of elegant experiments in which they spliced a gene that builds a receptor for glucocorticoid together with a gene for an estrogen receptor. They installed the construct into a herpes virus, which can infect neurons, using it as an injectable vaccine in rats. The scientists observed that an elevated glucocorticoid stress signal was transduced into a gentle estrogen signal.[349] Next, the two scientists took on stroke. Consider that most of the damage in heart attack or stroke actually happens during "reperfusion" when blood returns to the region. The reason is energy production in the process of oxidative phosphorylation is stopped dead in its tracks during a stroke, and when the mitochondria lurch forward back to work, they bobble electrons which cause "free radicals," molecules with unstable electron configurations that cause cell damage. Sapolsky and Steinberg spliced a genetic sequence for low-oxygen response elements to genes for neuroprotective factors that would protect against free radicals and stop cell death. In short, those protective genes would turn on as soon as a stroke event occurred, improving the survival of brain cells by 50 percent.[350] But there are a couple of reasons that these strategies might not work in the clinic for humans; in the case of stress, it is sometimes useful for a brain; in the case of stroke, a low-oxygen environment already induces a number of neuroprotective genes to begin to fire. Steinberg told me when I wrote to him, asking for an update on his progress, that he and Sapolsky "haven't pursued the gene therapy strategies for neuroprotection beyond the experimental, preclinical stage."

In an article in *Nautilus*, the journalist Taylor Beck wrote how a stress mechanism is gaining traction as a trigger for changing neural architecture, and is explaining mental disorders better than simple appeals to dopamine and serotonin which don't always correlate well with disorders. In fact, people who are falling in love can even have *lower* serotonin levels. As a result, some researchers are proposing the iconoclastic idea of using ketamine, otherwise going by its street drug name "Special K," as a kind of "depression vaccine" since it may preserve synaptic structure during stressful events. Beck wrote that "the correspondence between these chemicals (like serotonin) and depression is relatively weak. An emerging competitive theory, inspired in part by ketamine's effectiveness, has it that psychiatric disease is less about chemical imbalance than structural changes in the brain – and that a main cause of these changes is psychological stress." Gerard Sanacora, a psychiatry professor running a ketamine trial at Yale, was quoted as saying, "I really do think stress is to mental illness as cigarettes are to heart disease." The neuroplasticity "theory describes stress grinding down individual neurons gradually, as storms do roof shingles. This, in turn, changes the nature of their connections to one another and the structure of the brain. Ketamine, along with some similar molecules, acts to strengthen the neuron against that damage, affecting not just the chemistry of the brain but also its structure."[351]

Stress is often healthy and during spikes in cortisol, a stress hormone, "neurons are born and expand in the hippocampus, the seahorse-shaped finger of tissue responsible for forming new memories and understanding three-dimensional space, and rodents learn better. The student who gets stressed while studying is more alert and remembers more... the problem comes when stress is either too intense at one moment, as in a rape or violent attack, or too sustained, as in long-term poverty, neglect, or abuse... We usually think of our brains' adaptability as a good thing. Just as neurons grow during development, the wiring in the adult brain can change. After strokes or other brain injuries, neural signals re-route themselves around damage, allowing even very old people to re-learn lost skills... But the neuroplasticity hypothesis of mental disorder highlights the drawback of such neural liberalism: The human brain's flexibility allows regeneration, but also renders it vulnerable to being altered by stress."[352] Intriguingly, glucocorticoids, or stress signals, can decrease synaptic plasticity in the hippocampus and frontal cortex, but actually increase plasticity in the amygdala, the almond-shaped region related to fear. In Sapolsky's words, "evidence of plasticity in the adult nervous system" is demonstrated as "the excitability of synapses change, dendritic spines come and go within minutes, dendritic processes expand or retract, and circuitry remaps. And then there is, of course, the revolution of adult neurogenesis. Little in the brain, it turns out, is set in stone."

"Stress hormones' most important effect is to flood parts of the brain with glutamate, the brain's 'go' signal. Used by 80 percent of neurons in the cortex, this key neurotransmitter drives mental processes from memory to mood. Glutamate triggers neurons to generate sudden bursts of electricity that release more glutamate, which can in turn trigger electrical bursts in nearby neurons. This cellular signaling is called excitation and is fundamental to how information is processed in the brain... Other neurotransmitters, like serotonin, are called 'modulatory,' because they change the sensitivity of neurons that secrete glutamate (among others). Less than 1 percent of neurons in the cortex signal with these modulators...

"Glutamate moves like a ship between neurons. The sea it sails is called the synapse, the shore it departs from is the presynaptic neuron, and the destination, on the synapse's far side, is the postsynaptic neuron. Another component, called a glial cell, works to remove glutamate ships from the synapse and recycle them. The glutamate system is affected at each of these points by stress hormones: They push the first neuron to send more ships, interfere with the glial cell's recycling, and block the docks on the distant shore... Indeed, depressed people's brains, or at least animal models of depression, show all three of these problems, leading to long-lasting excesses of glutamate in key portions of the brain... This superabundance of glutamate makes a neuron fire sooner than it should and triggers a cascade of signals inside the cell, damaging its structure... Each neuron has tree-like branches, called dendrites, which are used to communicate with other neurons. When overdosed in glutamate, this canopy of branches shrinks, like a plant doused with herbicide. First the 'twigs,' called spines, disappear. After prolonged stress, whole branches recede... The mood drugs in wide use now focus on modulatory neurotransmitters like serotonin. Ketamine, however, works directly on glutamate signaling... directly on mature neurons, fertilizing them to grow branches more robustly, or protecting them against damage."

One reason we might find few strong genetic signals to predict neuropsychiatric disorders is due to the influential role that stress plays in shaping the structure and density of synaptic connections. The handful of genetic variants we have found to predict schizophrenia and depression seem to bear out these assumptions. As Sapolksy wrote, "A good example of this is seen with the immunophilin *FKBP5*, which, as a glucocorticoid receptor co-factor, is highly pertinent to stress neuroendocrinology; variants of the *FKBP5* gene are associated with altered risk of depression, anxiety and PSTD. As another example, consider the *DISC-1* gene (Disrupted in Schizrenia-1) whose cytoskeleton protein product interacts extensively with the signal transduction pathways of stress signals;

despite the specificity implied by *DISC-1's* name, abnormalities in the structure or regulation of the protein have been implicated not just in schizophrenia, but in depression and bipolar disorder."[353]

It is almost certainly the case that genes predispose us to psychological resilience or mental disorders, but the academic track record for such findings results in very weak associations, and seems to suggest that our neuroplasticity plays a role in our intelligence and resilience. Biology is often talked about in terms of balance and settings, which can be thrown out of whack. For instance, the journalist Kate Murphy wrote in her article "Do Your Friends Actually Like You?" in *The New York Times* about the health effects of broken relationships. "Not only do the resulting feelings of loneliness and isolation increase the risk of death as much as smoking, alcoholism and obesity; you may also lose tone, or function, in the so-called smart vagus nerve, which brain researchers think allows us to be in intimate, supportive and reciprocal relationships in the first place." Sandeep Jauhar took that concept of getting "thrown out of whack" a step further in the same newspaper, describing an alternative theory to homeostasis, which is called "allostasis" and extends our typical thinking about calibrating the body's internal conditions in terms of homeostasis to extend to external conditions and social circumstances.

"Hypertension disproportionately affects blacks, especially in poor communities," Jauhar wrote. "This may in part be because of genetics, but it is doubtful that this is a major factor; American blacks have hypertension at much higher rates than West Africans. Moreover, hypertension is also common in other segments of society in which poverty and social ills are rampant. Peter Sterling, a neurobiologist and a proponent of allostasis, has written that hypertension in these communities is a normal response to chronic arousal ... which prompts release of 'stress' hormones such as adrenaline and cortisol which tighten blood vessels and cause retention of salt. These in turn lead to long-term changes, like arterial wall thickening, that increase the blood pressure set point. The body adapts to this higher pressure and works to maintain it." The body is not out of whack from its normal set points, but rather the set points are recalibrating to fit the circumstances, since, "in the allostatic formulation nothing is 'broken'."

Scientists seek to isolate variants they can replicate and monetize, and, in doing so, avoid the harder problem of balance and homeostasis – or, if you prefer, allostasis. That's why the common plea that *if we only had more expensive data, we'd have the answers to most of our problems,* falls short. It's precisely because the belief in data often ignores context, and it especially ignores how we operate in space. That's the basis of my argument for why I think that science can obscure our sense of reality, and why the space of literature and arts often provides a more trustworthy sense of reality, which we should at times yield more authority than data-driven science. There is nothing that boggles my mind more, or is more obnoxious or even hurtful to me, than the modern maxim that all the answers are in the data. Noam Chomsky, our most important citizen, wrote in *New Horizons in Language and Mind* that "Plainly, a naturalistic approach does not exclude other ways of trying to comprehend the world. Someone committed to it can consistently believe (I do) that we learn much more of human interest about how people think and feel and act by reading novels or studying history or the activities of ordinary life than from all of naturalistic psychology, and perhaps always will." Steven Pinker hung his hat on naturalistic psychology when he wrote me an email: "There is a vast amount of work establishing the heritability of intelligence, and the reliability of measuring it. We know the genes are in there, but because each one accounts for such a small proportion of the variance, they are hard to pinpoint."

In 2014, the first genome-wide association study on childhood intelligence with children age 6 to 18 was reported on 17,989 individuals. No "individual single-nucleotide polymorphisms (SNPs) were detected with genome-wide significance." However, the authors show that "aggregate effects of common SNPs explain 22–46% of phenotypic variation in childhood intelligence." And the variants in one gene, FNBP1L, combined to be significantly associated with childhood intelligence. The authors report that "these genetic prediction results are consistent with expectations if the genetic architecture of childhood intelligence is like that of body mass index or height, suggesting the "heritability and polygenic nature of childhood intelligence,"[354] but also betraying our inability to tease out the complex interactions between genetic variants, suggesting intelligence is partially inherited through a combination of genetic code which would be nearly impossible to recreate or reconstitute synthetically. In 2016, the psychologist James J. Lee at the University of Minnesota followed that up by publishing a study in *Nature* on 329,000 young people which identified 74 SNPs which combined to predict 20 percent of the variance in the years of education completed in school. However, speaking to the Lee paper, Pinker wrote me an email saying, "I doubt that we'll see parents using Crispr to implant any of them in their kids, for a number of practical reasons – there are too many genes, the effect of each one is small, we don't know which ones have negative pleiotropic effects (meaning they may contribute to a weaker effect when combined with different genetic backgrounds in different people) and the safety impediments to allowing the procedure are almost certainly too steep."

In *The Washington Post*, Pinker explained the problem of trying to use genetic engineering to change a multitude of weak genetic variants: "Most of the 'Gene for X' claims of the 1990s turned out to be false positives that resulted from snooping around genomes in paltry samples. The discrepancy between the robust results from classic family research and the failures of the gene-hunters is called the Mystery of the Missing Heritability. But new studies looking for small effects of thousands of genes in large samples have pinpointed a few genetic loci that each accounts for a fraction of an IQ point. More studies are in the pipeline and will link those genes to brain development, showing that they are not statistical curiosities. The emerging picture is that most behavioral traits are affected by many, many genes, each accounting for a tiny percentage of the variance. Biologists are solving a related mystery: What is the additional factor shaping us that cannot be identified with our genes or families? The answer may be luck. We've long known that the genome can't wire the brain down to the last synapse, so there is tremendous room for unpredictable zigzags in development. Random accidents also shape the genome itself. Each of us inherits about 60 new mutations, and as we live our lives, our neurons fill up with still more mutations, which can affect how our brains work. We are all mutants, so our genes may have an even bigger role in shaping us and our children than we thought: not just the ones we inherited from our ancestors but the ones that we mangled ourselves."[355]

Intelligence is difficult (for me) to accept as a construct since it's not simply an input–output system, but explicated as an ability to hold two or more opposing thoughts in your head at the same time – or two opposing opinions and to oscillate between them, essentially an ability to deal with multiple realities. Some of what we call intelligence is certainly "ergodic," meaning that no matter what path we take in life we couldn't shake some inevitable aspect of who we are, a concept concisely stated in the title of David Lipsky's book on a road trip with David Foster Wallace, *Although of Course You End Up Becoming Yourself*. But there is also something quite arbitrary about life, which happens concomitantly, which is called "path dependency," meaning that developmental patterns and identity are contingent on accidental events, which ushers in an eerie, if existential, feeling that things could have always been otherwise ("Could I have been a parking lot attendant?")

In fact, much of the complexity of biology seems to lie in the interactions within the "edges and nodes" of the immune system or brain networks, whereas a node is a real object such as a cellular receptor, or protein, or cell, and an edge is the connection between those objects. Genes build the nodes, or objects, but don't necessarily determine all the edges, or connections. The idea that the wiring is genetic suggests that the nodes are genetically determined, which they're probably not. Genes influence cellular migration and cell type distribution, and anatomical structure, but not necessarily the connections.

Indeed, that there are elaborate rules involved in how cells are connected or work together, or how psychological traits, or even commonplace use of language is formed, is an idea that has been under increasing attack. Take language acquisition and use. In the 1980s, Chomsky took a "principles and parameters" approach to positing rules that govern a "faculty of language," which was well established to be innate, which has commonly been compared to web spinning in spiders or echolocation in bats. These grammar rules were first contrived to solve what Chomsky called "Plato's problem," in other words, how to account for descriptive adequacy to explain the incredible variation in languages throughout the world, while maintaining explanatory adequacy of a simplistic enough model of grammar that could be formulaic. The tack he took was by establishing a "deep structure" of grammar that could be permuted at a surface structure as a transformational grammar. But, by the 1990s, Chomsky had ditched deep structure and most of his highly theoretical principles and parameters in favor of a much more simplistic mechanistic approach which he called the "minimalist program." Through this program, he and others suggested that only the sparsest of functions exist, namely "merge," which built noun phrases and verb phases from the bottom up, and "move," which is basically move anything anywhere in a sentence. The only other mechanism he held onto was the principle of recursion, which is the idea that not only can we build a countless variety of phrases, but our sentences are extensible since we can embed components of sentences inside other larger sentences. He argued that language may have even emerged for reasons other than social communication; "the phonological component of private speech might help serialize private cognition, focus attention on one train of thought, and increase the capacity of short-term memory."[356] By comparison, Pinker and Ray Jackendoff argued that recursion exists in other biological domains, such as vision, and suggested that language evolved piecemeal and was most certainly derived as a social adaptation.[357,358] What I find so intriguing about Chomsky and the neurobiological revolution he helped to sweep in, is that his fascination with the language faculty was not only in its limitless combinational power, but also in its ubiquity – his rhetoric is dry, his sensibility is that cognitive powers are in no way unique to a single person, but rather that that intelligence is ordinary, broadly distributed and co-extensive. What I dislike about how neurobiology is interpreted as a rationalization for special privileges, and to make exceptions. The fascinating thing about the language faculty is that it seems to be undergoing a shift to radical simplicity. The rules that govern grammar are simply not that complicated, and as such, human intelligence is probably far less complicated and stratified than we think it is. And if the edges of the connectome largely emerge through associative learning, that means there is little hope to fix psychiatric disorders or improve intelligence through alterations to our genes.

Jon Gordon expressed his great doubts we will ever use gene engineering to improve intelligence. "A useful way to appreciate the daunting task of manipulating intelligence through gene transfer is by considering the fact that a single cerebellar Purkinje cell may possess more synapses than the total number of genes in the human genome. There are tens of millions of Purkinje cells in the cerebellum, and these cells are involved in only one aspect of brain function: motor coordination. The genome only provides a blueprint for formation of the brain; the finer details of assembly and intellectual development are beyond direct genetic control and must perforce be subject to innumerable stochastic and environmental influences."[359] But the willingness to explore alterations to our brains is evident, which anyone can discover with a simple PubMed search. In 1999, Joe Tsien and his colleagues at Princeton University shocked the world when they reported genetically engineering mice with better memories. They achieved the effect by popping an extra copy of the NR2B gene into their genomes. This gene encodes the NMDA receptor, which is used in memory formation and can affect a trait that neuroscientists call "long-term potentiation." The press dubbed the super smart mouse pups "Doogie mice," after the popular television show Doogie Hauser MD (then in syndication). At the time, Tsien said, if it worked in humans, everyone would want to use it, since "everyone wants to be smart." It's worth mentioning that, by the end of the series, Doogie Hauser becomes jaded with modern medicine and quits to become a writer.

Daniel Keyes anticipated Tsien's experiment decades before in his 1966 book *Flowers for Algernon*. The book unfolds though progress reports written by Charlie Gordon, a 32-year-old bakery worker with an IQ of 70 who grew up in the Warren State Home and Training School. Using misspelled words and broken sentences, Charlie explains to readers that scientists have told him they've found a means to rapidly increase his intelligence. In fact, they say, they have already engineered a mouse named Algernon to become super smart. Charlie's IQ eventually soars to 186. He struggles with relationships as his intellectual development outpaces his emotional development. People at his bakery job start to resent him. During his courtship with a love interest, Alice, he starts to get close to her, but senses that "Old Charlie" is near. He becomes too self-conscious to be close to her, and she claims all he wants to talk about is "cultural variants, and neo-Boulean mathematics, and post-symbolic logic." Thus, his character is divided into antithetical halves, as he struggles to reconcile his capacity for slicing insight with lagging emotional development. Charlie decides: "Intelligence is one of the greatest human gifts. But all too often a search for knowledge drives out the search for love. This is something else I've discovered for myself very recently. I present it to you as a hypothesis: Intelligence without the ability to give and receive affection leads to mental and moral breakdown, to neurosis, and possibly even psychosis." *Flowers for Algernon* is based on an old story, and it is virtually the same story as *Frankenstein*, each written in epistolary form, an exegesis of the old Promethean myth.

In Aeschylus' telling of the original mythology in the sixth century BCE, Prometheus is a titan who has a penetrating ability to see into the future and uses his keen foresight to raid the workshop of Hephaistos and Athena on Mt. Olympus. He steals fire from the Gods and bestows it to mankind by

hiding it in the embers of fennel stalk. The "fire bringer," is often associated with Lucifer, or "light bearer," who pilfered light from the heavens
and brought it down to Earth. Thus, the "fall of man" implies an age when
mortals are illuminated with knowledge.

Prometheus bestowed not only fire, but also the entire Catalogue of
Arts, including technology, arts, sciences and medicine, to mankind. It
angered the Olympians, who chained him to a rock on Mt. Caucasus
while an eagle, "the dark-winged hound of Zeus, pecked out his liver
each day under the blazing sun, only to have it re-grow each night – thus
he functions as a proto-Christ figure, one who takes on exceeding responsibility and pain – and like Christ, he suffers, fixed to a mantle. Such as it
is, in the tragic version of literature, a character must take a hit, and
suffer dire consequences for their transgression or misdeed, which he
does for the love of mankind. That we would someday tap into the raw
forces of nature – electricity, fire, genetics, atomic energy – is not right
or wrong, but confers unspeakable new forms of power, privilege, risk
and harm. The tether suggests an unbreakable responsibility for his own
life and deeds. "Your kindness to the human race has earned you this,"
the Olympians tell Prometheus, who as the proto-Christ figure is
tethered to the rock. "Power newly won is harsh." Once Prometheus
expropriates his fire, he can no longer curse the heavens, rather left to
his own devices, the things he creates return to petition and haunt him.

The eagle has an identical function as the fiend in Frankenstein, or the
escaped dinosaurs in Jurassic Park. Each is a piece of technology or a
natural force that is called upon that exceeds our capacity to handle it,
coming with a steep learning curve and takes a while to master – what we
are really trying to do is to master our own minds. Psychologists tell us
that we search for an "external locus of control," an external agent to pin
responsibility. The emergence of a hero or titan who can appropriate
natural forces indicates dissolution of the separation between the heavens
and the Earth. If not a metaphysical God, then we locate His incarnation
in technology. Everyone understands the allusions: we summoned something more powerful than us and it got out of control. The plot is that
technology is merely an extension of ourselves, and as the drama wears on,
the masterful technology we and our characters create has an eerie,
haunting effect, gradually revealing that we alone are the source of our
own suffering. And that's why it is so proto-Christ. The anti-climax is that
the authority and responsibility of God is revealed to be embodied in man.

Today the myth is unfolding anew, in the sense of personal genomics, which disposes us to omniscient forecasting by using prognostic genetic mutations to read or "see" into a future disease condition. The tethers are real in the sense that we are tied to our genes, and if we expropriate the natural power to change our genes, then we are tethered or bound to whichever variants we create. The allure is powerful. In one stage of the myth, the Olympians send Pandora down to Earth to trick the Titans, but Prometheus, who has the gift of forethought, recognizes the dangers at hand. He warns his dim-witted brother, Epimetheus, who only has the gift of afterthought, but Epimetheus falls for the ploy anyway, opening the jar she gives as a gift, and scattering "burdensome toil and sickness that brings death to men." Thus, an element of the myth is containment, in the literal sense, such as a rogue genetically engineered species, such as in *The Andromeda Strain, The Stand* or *Jurassic Park*. This aspect of the myth is also expressed not only in the creation of rogue species, but in the protocol of using Cripsr-Cas9 as a medical tool, and in the unleashing of this cheap, easy-to-use technology that it will be virtually impossible to legislate, regulate or contain. Once Prometheus steals fire, he is bound to the rock, but it's prophesized that in 13 generations he will be freed by one of his descendants, a hero, Hercules; as the Gods bound him, they prodded, "How are your mortals going to cut this knot for you?," suggesting not only the burden of foresight, but also that gene edits will stay with us for generations. That we are bound to whatever genetic engineering we engender in agriculture, aquaculture, mosquitos and especially genetic variants we create in people is a literal meaning. To retread the words of Robert Sinsheimer from the 1970s, "What we are doing is almost certainly irreversible."

George Church disagrees. He suggested to *The New Yorker* in an interview that: "It strikes me as a fake argument to say that something is irreversible. There are tons of technologies that are irreversible. But genetics is not one of them. In my lab, we make mutations all the time and then we change them back. Eleven generations from now, if we alter something and it doesn't work properly we will simply fix it."[360] Easier said than done, in a human with a trillion cells, or genetically engineered seeds, crops or aquaculture which leak into the wild. And if some countries are restrictive of germline engineering in people, but others, such as China are more lenient, best of luck in using the borders of a country to contain those engineered hominids.

In some kinder, gentler versions of myth, near the end of the story, Prometheus reconciles with Zeus and the ascending Olympian gods in a cosmological struggle which results in conquering the old order of Kronos and other gods. The reconciliation between Prometheus and Zeus signifies a new establishment of hierarchy and law. Therefore, while technology may signify a break with existing standards and practices, and test the boundaries of legal authority, resulting in a synthesis, a new version of order that re-emerges as genetic engineering becomes a fluid part of modern life which is regulated.

The Greek playwright Aeschylus wrote *Prometheus Bound*, one of the first standard versions of the story, and also introduced us to the idea of *"deus ex machina,"* a device in which an unresolvable problem is suddenly and abruptly resolved by some unforeseen circumstance. In the Greek tragedy, a machine such as a crane (mechane) was used to bring actors playing gods onto stage or a riser used to bring actors up through a trapdoor. Aeschylus often used the machines to get his characters out of trouble; and Christ's disappearance from the tomb was a deux ex machina, a trap door for an impossible situation. Tellingly, people who came to see Aeschylus' plays reportedly found the *deus ex machina* unsatisfying and not particularly realistic.

Immanuel Kant was the first to modernize the term, when he nicknamed his pal, Benjamin Franklin, "the Prometheus of modern times" for his nifty work with kites to disarm thunder of its light. In the 1980s, the Harvard scientist Richard Mulligan took genetic code and wrapped it up in a virus, returning it to mankind as a tool; it was not unlike Prometheus' theft of embers from the gods as he wrapped them in a fennel stalk returning it to man. Leon Kass, an ethicist and advisor on biotechnology to George W. Bush, warned that "human control of genetic makeup represents a Promethean seizure of God's power." The story seems to re-cycle through every generation, with a perpetual reoccurance. But, it was Mary Shelley, who better than any other, captured its essence.

"The year without a summer," as it was known, 1816 was bleak, if not strangely gothic. Mount Tamboro in Indonesia had erupted the year before, pitching volcanic ash into the atmosphere and obscuring the sun. Torrential rains pressed deep into the year, resulting in global crop failures. The birds quieted down by midday, as darkness descended, and for days at a time, a group of writers huddled by candlelight in a rented mansion on Lake Geneva. The dashing 23-year-old poet Percy Shelley and his 18-year-old companion, Mary, who had already taken to calling herself "Mrs. Shelley," traveled to the lake to spend the summer with the poet Lord Byron. Also in company were the physician John William Polidori, and Mary's stepsister Claire Clairmont, pregnant due to an affair with Byron, who was now in the grips of writing a poem, simply called *Darkness*. Mary had already given birth to two children by Percy, one of whom was dead, and the other, soon to be dead, while Percy's actual wife, Harriet, at the brink of exhaustion, drowned herself in the River Westbourne by the end of the year.

This was a brief moment of refuge. Byron had rented the Villa Diodati, where the group convened during the "incessant rain," which held out for days at a time, discussing their literary projects late into the night. Polidori, the physician, offered a counterbalance of reason and evidence as Percy and Byron speculated on "the principal of life," while exchanging German ghost stories. Then on the night of June 15, 1816, they all read ghost stories aloud. And then Byron suggested they each try their hand to *write* one.

Mary would write her stunning exegesis *Frankenstein, or The Modern Prometheus* in just under 11 months. She set forth to write a penny dreadful, but wrote a stinging commentary on the times that came to her in a flash, a waking dream. A collision of forces discharged in her writing, and she produced something more than a ghost story, but a "book of ideas." This was the height of the Industrial Revolution. Many in her generation, including Percy, sought to break with traditional values such as the monarchy, military, marriage and social class, opting instead for the reason of scientific inquiry, free love and atheism; but this shift to impersonal rationalism also triggered recoil. Mary's mother, Mary Wollstoncraft (yes, also dead; childbirth), author of Vindication of the Rights of Women, "attacked the hierarchical system that required underpaid mechanics to support the rich and idle aristocracy and deprived women of any chance to realize their human potential. She demanded equal political rights for all English persons deprived of the vote – which meant, at the time, most members of the middle class, all workers, and all women regardless of class," wrote the New York University literary scholar Walter James Miller in his circa 2000 foreword to Shelley's novel. Her father, William Goodwin, author of Enquiry into the Principals of Political Justice "believed, like Voltaire, in the power of pure reason to solve all social, political, and personal problems. And like Rousseau, Goodwin felt that humans are by nature benevolent and become evil only when abused by society. Government, he preached, and other institutions like marriage and the family, impose evil restraints on citizens and must be abolished" urging "well-educated citizens working toward a better world by repressing emotions and reasoning person-to-person." In his August 2016 article in *The New Yorker*, "Down with Elites!," Pankaj Mishra explained how Jean-Jacques Rousseau, a child of the Enlightenment, had, in fact, been at odds with Voltaire, as the new era of scientific inquiry resulted not in a doing away with social stratification, but the reemergence of new classes of artistic and scientific elites, anointed by Voltaire, and antagonized by a counterrevolution of populism as articulated through the writings of Rousseau. After contemplating an essay competition entitled "Has the progress of the sciences and arts done more to corrupt morals or improve them?," in 1750 Rousseau wrote "A Discourse on the Moral Effects of the Arts and Sciences," in which he ironically expressed his discontent with the age of the "light of reason" or, at least, how it was rationalized, applied and used to justify the dominance of power. Rousseau believed the secret workings of financial systems were a means of "putting freedom and the public good on the auction block." The "obstacle" existed in "the insatiable craving to secure recognition," which led "each individual to make more of himself than of any other" and would lead people to subordinate others. In Mishra's words, "even the lucky few at the top of the hierarchy would remain insecure, exposed to the envy and malice of those below, albeit hidden behind a show of deference and civility. This pathological inner life was a devastating 'contradiction' at the heart of modern society." Insomuch as Mary's father, William Goodwin, raised her in this new era of "free inquiry," it was still a world in contradiction, one in which men would use their advances to suppress their competition, to justify their abandonment of basic social responsibilities and duty. Mary's father was not affectionate, her mother, dead, and she grew up an intellectual heiress to a newly liberated world – with few close companions.

Mary "would brood all her life on the plight of a person brought up without a real mother: notice how many characters in Frankenstein struggle with the problems of the orphan or of the broken family," Miller notes. Her father, William Goodwin, did extend his love of books to Mary, and "trained his daughter in the stimulating practice of reading several books concurrently. And he allowed her to sit in on social evenings he'd staged for other literary giants like William Wordsworth, Charles Lamb and Samuel Taylor Coleridge. One awesome evening she actually heard Coleridge read aloud his *Ancient Mariner*. Her impressions of the sailor supernaturally punished for his violation of Nature would clearly influence her conception of her scientist Frankenstein." In 1814, she returned from a voyage to Scotland to find a handsome, visionary poet Percy Shelley, "a frequent visitor at her father's house." Just entering his early twenties, Percy had published numerous stories, nine verse cantos, seventeen prose notes, and several inflammatory pamphlets, one of which had gotten him expelled from Oxford. He was, very much, an extension of the anti-establishment impulses that Mary's parents had promulgated in their writings. "Having thus ransacked the ideas of Godwin and Wollstonecraft, Shelley now took their daughter as well," Miller notes. Percy was already married and a father, but he absconded to be with Mary, as they eloped to Europe. They began collaborating on writing (after Percy's first wife died of a suicide at the end of the year, Mary became Mary Wollstonecraft Shelley).

Percy and Mary read, and they read; they read John Locke's *Essay on Human Understanding* and Humphrey Davy's books on chemistry and scientific progress, which praised "modern masters" who "penetrate into the recesses of nature." Percy was busily drawing on science writing to instruct his writing, having written poems including "two that would loom important in her thinking about Frankenstein: 'Mount Blanc,' which helped her with her settings, and Alastor, a long poem about a young man who, obsessed with seeking Ideal Truth, unwittingly loses all the benefits of human companionship."

By June 1816, reaching the respite of Lake Geneva, Mary was struggling to bring competing ideas into a "symbolic synthesis," which, as Miller notes, included "her anguish as the neglected child of a genius" and "her dread of her father's impersonal rationalism and her husband's unconditional love of science." The trick she pulled on the men in her life was to let them win to the full extent – the name of the main character in her novel, "Victor," is ironic. "I have described myself as always having been imbued with a fervent longing to penetrate the secrets of nature," the scientist tells us. Frankenstein sets out to create a perfect human. So shall it be. The figure that he creates has a penetrating intelligence, and a ferocious love of life. He is eight feet tall and bolts through the Swiss Alps with stag-like swiftness, and has translucent, yellowish skin. He is, in a sense, engineered as the perfect machine.

But no one loves him. He is alone, and his loneliness and existential grief drive him mad. As Miller notes, Mary Shelley "wanted to show that he, according to Rousseau's teaching that she was following, was born virtuous and gentle and that only society's mistreatment of him could turn him violent and malevolent. She was also testing out John Locke's psychology. He'd taught that each human is born a tabula rasa, a blank slate, and that society, writing indelibly on that slate, determines much of an individual's character." The irony is that even in the instance of the scientific mastery, when all scientific hurdles were cleared, the miseries of psychology may persist.

Shelley's novel begins at the end, in epistolary form, based on letters between Captain Robert Walton Saville and his sister on the mainland, as the captain explains he has rescued Victor Frankenstein from an ice flow, bringing him back up upon the deck of his ship, which is on expedition in the North Pacific. Frankenstein tells him the strange tale of how he created an eight-foot superhuman and how it all backfired. In fact, the fiend started out good. He saves a young girl who falls into a slipstream, but a mountaineer calls it out for malicious intent, shooting him through the shoulder with a shotgun. In Miller's words, "Shelley actually tells how the well-meaning monster saves the girl from drowning. Then he is shot by somebody too terrified by the looks of an eight-foot creature to grasp the situation." The fiend proceeds to seek friends. He stares through windows. He has incredible intelligence and ability, but he cannot connect. This perfect figure is everything science could hope to dream about, but he is a neglected orphan. He soon demands companionship. Frankenstein tries to explain to him that the fiend must go since he is under his own control. But the fiend will not go. Victor learns he is bound to the figure he creates, which results in a haunting effect. While hiking in the Swiss Alps, Frankenstein encounters the monster, once again, and tells him that he must go. But the fiend asserts his own sanctity in defiance. "Life, although it may only be an accumulation of anguish, is dear to me, and I will defend it," he says. Deeply distraught by his loneliness, the fiend stalks members of Frankenstein's family, killing William, then, his adopted daughter Elizabeth.

In fact, Frankenstein has repressed many of the details of the story until this moment. He had a breakdown that occurred early on in the story, when his younger brother William was murdered. He now comes to terms with the reality that the fiend, which he created, killed most of the members of his family. All of this is crashing to the forefront of Victor Frankenstein's consciousness, as he is rescued onto the deck of the ship.

In Miller's words, "Victor found he could not confide the truth about what had caused his breakdown." When news from Geneva originally came that Victor's young brother William had been strangled and their servant Justine charged with the murder, Victor suspected he knew who the real murderer was. Hiking in the Swiss Alps, Victor comes to encounter the fiend, who is dislocated and wandering, in a state that the existentialists called "unanchoring;" by now, "embittered by this and other rejections," he had set out to seek revenge on Frankenstein's species. In a famous passage, delivered during their confrontation, the monster explains, "I was benevolent and good; misery made me a fiend." Miller notes the "misery-made-me-a-fiend speech" and its passages "constitute one of the strongest attacks on the patriarchal 'work ethic' we have in Western literature."

As Harold Bloom noted in a 1965 afterward to the novel, the "greatest paradox, and most astonishing achievement, of Mary Shelley's novel is that the monster is more human than his creator." Indeed, most critics, he notes, accept that "the monster and his creator are the antithetical halves of a single being." It would be overly simplistic to say that intellect and intuition was the split, but rather, as Miller explains, "the monster is an extension of certain of Frankenstein's powers that he is unwilling to take responsibility for. This would include intellectual forces and savage, instinctive forces he is afraid to recognize in himself." When the fiend murders William, he plants evidence that leads to the conviction of a servant, Justine, which Frankenstein buys into. "Certainly, we have to consider Frankenstein as the ultimate cause of the monster's misdeeds. Moreover, starting with the murder of William, Frankenstein was morally obliged to reveal his secret. His refusal to do so, with rationalizations convincing only to himself, makes him an accomplice. What he can only dream of doing – killing Elizabeth – he in effect allows the monster to do." Shelley's awakening is demonstrated by her insistence on "recognizing and coming to terms with the role of the irrational in human affairs – this, mind you, long after Shakespeare's emphasis on it had been down-graded by the Age of Reason and long before Freud, Jung, and Lacan would upgrade it again in modernist times."

Shelley showed how an age of evidence that demotes the life of experience and represses our intuition makes us less responsible and more at risk. "To show how deeply this self-destructive trait is ingrained in the Western male, Shelley first has the scientist condemn it, as above, and then relapse into it. In Frankenstein's dying hours – in one of Shelley's most bitter scenes – he tries to shame Walton's crew into pursuing their goal against hopeless odds, even using the patriarchal tactic of accusing them of not being real men," Miller wrote. The reconciliation between the two scientists is important, since Captain Walton is presumably worth saving from this blindsided scientific ambition. The Captain also has strong ambitions in science, but oscillates between his scientific voyage and thoughts of his family. In Miller's words, "Walton's polar expedition provides a dramatic, enhancing framework for Frankenstein's confessions. It also supplies a foil and a parallel for Frankenstein's own exploits. The explorer's work, like the scientist's, is bold and risky. But at least Walton is the Baconian scientist, whose work is public and offered for the general benefit of humanity. Frankenstein represents the Faustian scientist, working in dark secrecy, ostensibly for public good but largely for personal power (as master of a super race), and concealing all responsibility for his action. Walton's struggles are more objective, external; Frankenstein's deeply subjective, internal. Finally, Walton's expedition makes is easier for Shelley to drive home one of her main points, and with a magnificent twist of irony. Early in his stay on board, Frankenstein told his rescuer how he regretted having neglected family, friends, and fiancée to finish his years-long project: If only the study to which you apply yourself has a tendency to weaken your affections and to destroy your taste for those simple pleasures in which no alloy can possibly mix, then that study is certainly unlawful, that is to say, not befitting the human mind."

When I set out to write my book *Modern Prometheus*, I knew that I had found clear parallels with Shelley, who invented science fiction, and whose novel offered a plot device for so many modern tales, including *Flowers for Algernon* and *Jurassic Park*. After all, Crispr-Cas9 is a powerful new genome editing tool that may allow us to engineer new species, awaken some form of extinct ones and to engender new "transhumans," which are engineered as the perfect machines of parentless children. As Miller points out, "Frankenstein invents the ultimate technique for siring heirs without having to love a woman;" in fact, some of us express the subconscious desire to do that today. Just about a month before the bicentennial of the famous literary night of June 15, 1816, which upon Lake Geneva, launched Shelley into her year-long odyssey of writing *Frankenstein, or The Modern Prometheus*, it sunk in how Shelley's vision had anticipated a reality of our times.

In May 2016, nearly 150 scientists, lawyers and ethicists converged at a "secret" invitation-only meeting at Harvard Medical School to discuss fabrication of an entire human genome from scratch. George Church, Jef Boeke, a systems biologist at NYU Langone Medical Center, and Andrew Hessel, a "self-described futurist" and employee at software company Autodesk, and who first proposed such a project in 2012, organized the meeting. The project introduced was first called "HGP2: The Human Genome Synthesis Project," but later changed to "HGP-Write: Testing Large Synthetic Genomes in Cells."[361] An invitation stated the primary goal "would be to synthesize a complete human genome in a cell line within a period of 10 years." Nancy J. Kelley, a legal expert, had planned to engage the public and policy makers; in fact, the meeting was originally planned to be streamed over the internet. However, organizers had submitted a paper to a journal, and when the publication was delayed in the review process, the authors agreed to a code of silence in discussing details of the meeting until the paper was published—a common practice known as embargo. "Scientists are now contemplating the fabrication of a human genome, meaning they would use chemicals to manufacture all the DNA contained in human chromosomes," wrote the journalist Andrew Pollack, who cobbled together a story based on interviews with organizers and available information. "The prospect is spurring both intrigue and concern in the life sciences community because it might be possible, such as through cloning, to use a synthetic genome to create human beings without biological parents."[362]

If the quest to sequence the human genome amounted to a revolution in "reading" the genome, we were now at the beginning of a new revolution in "writing" genomes. In 2009, Church and colleagues at the Wyss Institute created MAGE, "a machine that harnesses the natural principles of evolution to do all the heavy lifting of genome design and automates these steps to dramatically shorten the time scale.[363]

Billions of different mutant genomes can now be generated per day. Mutants of interest are kept, and mutants that do not have the desired properties are discarded." The MAGE machine works by introducing "oligos," or small molecules of nucleotides, which can incorporate into the genomes of a cell, engendering billions of variants every three hours. It's high-speed evolution. "The speed and ease with which MAGE can alter genomes will transform how we approach the manufacturing and production optimization of industrially significant compounds in the bioenergy, pharmaceutical, agricultural, and chemical industries." In 2013, J. Craig Venter said he had built a prototype of the "digital biological converter," which worked as a fax machine, and which would allow operators to input code, and to print out DNA at the other end of the call. Venter suggested that his machine may have uses in space travel, but may also be a common household appliance of the future.

As Jeff Benson, a chemistry student at Harvard wrote in a blog, "the process of making artificial DNA is similar to letterpress printing – each character is painstakingly assembled in the correct order. The result is chemically identical to naturally-occurring DNA."[364] The global market for synthetic DNA was estimated at $1 billion annually, as we were witnessing the emergence of the "gene as a commodity." Biotech companies were rapidly sprouting up to sell lengths of genetic material as if they were rolls of fabric. In fact, it was more than genes, but fully operating genomes. In 2010, at a cost of $40 million, J. Craig Venter chemically synthesized a complete bacterial genome, *Mycoplasma mycoides* (JCVI-sny1.0) at a size of around 1 million bases – the synthetic genome which was inserted into the cell took control and began to run the cell.[365] In effect, Venter had created life from mere molecules. In 2014, Boeke synthesized a chromosome of yeast, a microorganism that is a eukaryote cell with software that is considered more complex. In March 2016, Venter and colleagues followed up with a stunning feat of synthesizing the minimal components required for a bacterial life form to function, with "retention of quasi-essential genes" to synthesize a 532 kilobase genome – half the size of the first attempt – with a mere 473 genes which was called JCVI-syn.3.0.[366] Notably, the authors declared "its genome is smaller than that of any autonomously replicating cell found in nature" – a minimal scrap of code that could provide instructions for a fully operational life-form.[367]

But the human genome has long been the *locus classicus* in the codex of life by which to test reading or writing. And, the quest to synthesize a fully operational human genome was, for geneticists, like putting a man on the moon. By 2016, improvements in technology had reduced the cost of writing "building blocks of life," in little more than a decade from four dollars to just three cents per individual letter or "base pair" of DNA. The cost to synthesize a human genome was estimated at $90 million, and confronts limitations in manufacturing capacity and speed, which is why a major conference had been organized – to try to consolidate private and public funding around such a "grand challenge." But questions quickly arose, pertaining to whose genome would be synthesized. Pieces of Einstein's brain were available, and The Leonardo Project, had been engaged to locate the whereabouts of Leonardo da Vinci's grave. "For example, would it be OK to sequence and then synthesize Einstein's genome? If so how many Einstein genomes would it be OK to make and install in cells, and who would get to make and control these cells?" asked Drew Endy, a bioengineer at Stanford, and Laurie Zoloth, a bioethicist at Northwestern University, in a statement of criticism they threw it up online at MIT. Endy and Church are co-founders of DNA construction company Gen9, Inc., while Church was an organizer of the meeting, Endy was a chief critic, speaking to deep rifts on issues of human code.

Endy and Zoloth's statement pleaded caution, such that "while we strongly agree that sustained improvements in DNA construction tools are essential for advancing basic biological science and improving public health we are skeptical that synthesizing a human genome is an appropriate demand driver. We recall how controversies associated with many of the earliest genome synthesis projects produced unintended consequences. For example, a project that made polio virus from scratch in 2002 led to cancelled public funding for DNA synthesis research, unwittingly hindering research across diverse and unrelated fields, as policy makers struggled to imagine how such a technology could ever be controlled. From a simple technical perspective, we argue that synthesis of less-controversial and more-immediately useful genomes and also greatly improved sub-genomic synthesis capacities (e.g., real-time plasmid printing) should be pursued; alternatives that would deliver broad and diverse benefits. Other topics on today's agenda included changing the human genome itself. For example, could scientists synthesize a modified human genome that is resistant to all natural viruses? They likely could, for purely beneficial purposes, but what if others then sought to synthesize modified viruses that overcame such resistance? Might doing so start a genome engineering arms race?" The authors asked for deeper public discussion on "whether and under what circumstances it is morally right to proceed" and suggested the "first actors at the table mostly have a significant material interest in proceeding" and as such, the project "risks out-of-control competition between public and private interests, ethical conflicts of interest, and temptations to manipulate human subject consent." A number of questions arise.

"In a world where human reproduction has already become a competitive marketplace, with eggs, sperm and embryos carrying a price, it is straightforward to brainstorm various uses of human genome synthesis capacities." The "primary question," the authors said, emerges when we move from "just because something becomes possible" to "how should we determine if it is ethical to proceed?"[368]

Shelley's novel is visionary to all of this. She anticipates the recoil to genetic engineering and technological accelerationism, not in being anti-technology, but through her insistence that technology does not remove us from the situation of life. But she also achieves a subtle message. The murder that is pervasive in Shelley's novel is reflective of a solipsistic logic which achieves its authority in science and eliminates any contention. The orphans that are left in it – and Shelley is obsessed with the orphan – exemplify an existential grief and loneliness that continues to permeate life, even in the case of scientific mastery. In fact, she shows us, an over-reliance on science and technology can cause us to ignore the basic contemplations of our situation and its gravity.

Indeed, such a naïve view on the insistence on genetic science as a wellspring of meaning in every aspect of our lives, and the spotlight for an illuminated reality on everything from schizophrenia to cancer, is at odds with the changing and often context-dependent nature of genetics and biology, and the dark forces of nature that promise us that whatever laws we know and trust may someday be overturned, if not sooner than we think. That data functions as we expect it in some conditions, and not in other conditions, genetic backgrounds and biochemical and neurochemical conditions, is a more literal message here. We think if we only had better data – we'd have complete control. But Shelley shows that putting too much emphasis on evidence we are losing our grip on the depth of our situation, its gravity, and losing our sense of contemplation. Data has illuminated everything, so much so that we can no longer imagine a deeper reality, or a counter reality as expressed in a "year without a summer."

The modern impulse that a full reality is in the data ignores activity of data framing and the partiality of data. The subconscious – and this is important – does not provide access to a complete self, but only other partial information. This is why we can have a human nature as Steven Pinker and the cognitivists have elucidated it, smashing the theory of the blank slate, and still remain in a state of turmoil and conflict. Many people will say the age of experience has been eclipsed by an age of evidence, and I asked myself many times whether reading a 200-year-old book is just a pleasant diversion or a rigorous exercise, and I have to say I think it still fights to be serious and relevant. As Robert Pogue Harrison observed "timeless truths do not exist," but there exist "books so pregnant with meaning that they never finish saying what they have to say." Shelley showed that an age of evidence can never fully eclipse an age of experience. What remains bothersome to us today is her enforcement of a plot in which science fails to confine reality or to be a final purveyor of truth, one in which scientists are not free of eclipse.

Shelley evoked the irrational, applying it as "necessary counterpoise" against accelerationism of science and progress which exceeds itself. In the case of germline genetic engineering, the principles of Shelley's novella have clear parallels. Clones would be parentless children, a "product of science," while germline engineering would engender a quality of "otherness." The "industrialization of the human genome" likewise conceals the plot, in a real sense, as the myth appears to us in its full reification, irresistible enough to try, nearly plausible. The only certainty is that any genetically modified organisms attain sanctity in their own right, and a will to survive, which may exceed or conflict with our own intentions. If technology does not provide a route to utopia or salvation, it opens a potential for dystopia, as it simply shifts the terrain into new balances of power. Those genetically modified organisms, including people, perhaps our own children, achieve their haunting effect through a capacity to run counter to our ambitions, to petition and haunt, and to demand more. That there is no complete or unifying technology, but that the enduring condition of life is to remain incomplete or partial, drives us into an accelerated progress with no refuge, but more acceleration. Shelley was alive to this status of the human condition, and for her, the answer was not to neglect the available network and resources we have, our ability for progress unending, our time fleeting. When I set out to write my own book, I wanted to break with the tradition of recent popular science writing, which is didactic and instructive, and to write in the spirit of Shelley, Keats and Nietzsche, for whom the form of drama and tragedy is to show that something is at stake that is *more* real than our science, or our writing.

"After Frankenstein appeared," Miller reminds us, "Mary's life was a mixture of new tragedy and muted triumph. Her second daughter, Clara Evelina, and her son William, were dead by 1819, the same year that Percy Florence was born. Mary's fifth pregnancy miscarried in 1822. She was saved from bleeding to death by her science-minded husband: he sat her down in an ice bath until the doctor arrived. Three weeks later he was heading home from his skiff Areil, sailing off the coast of Viareggio and – as Mary tells us in her brilliant and sensitive notes to his poems – he was 'wrapped from sight' by a thunderstorm and when the 'cloud of the tempest past away, no sight remained of where' he had been. Ten days later his body washed ashore and was cremated."

6   Biopolitics

Societies have the authority to regulate science, and scientists have a responsibility to obey the law.

–The Hixton Group[369]

"Prosecutors in South Korea have seized documents from a biotechnology company linked to a controversial sect which claims to have created the world's first cloned baby," reported a correspondent from the BBC in typical breathless fashion. After smashing through windows and grabbing documents in a raid on the offices of BioFusion Tech Inc. in the southern city of Daegu, officials had questioned staff members to see if they had participated in the cloning project on an American woman said to have led to the birth of a daughter, Eve (b. 26 December 2002). The technique was not illegal, except in the case the group had been conducting medical research without a license. The Raëlian cult had chartered its own corporation to engage in human cloning. The leader of the cult, who calls himself Raël (formerly Claude Vorilhorn, the editor of a French motor sport magazine), believes all humans were created in the laboratories of the planet Elohim. He says the Elohims have instructed Raël and his followers to develop cloning on Earth to provide earthlings with a type of immortality. Raël claims in 1973 he found a spacecraft shaped like a flattened bell in a volcano. Inside the craft, a 25000-year-old human-like extraterrestrial told him a story of "those who came from the sky," and gave him his marching orders. The church was operating without issue, despite some fairly liberal views on sexuality, and an honest effort to construct a $20 million "embassy" for extraterrestrials in Israël with a landing pad for spaceships to dock. The money for the embassy was partially raised, but the Israëlis balked when they learned that the aliens, just by chance, used a swastika as their symbol. But it was the sect's overt plans for human cloning that starting ringing alarm bells in the scientific community. Raël was called to testify before Congress, and he actually showed up, dressed in a futuristic white jumpsuit.

"No one knew how serious to take them," recalls Marcy Darnovsky, director of the Center for Genetics and Society. "One thing they had were plenty of beautiful young women who would do anything they asked, and they would certainly act as surrogate carriers." The same year, Italian fertility doctor Severino Antinori, working with physiologist Panos Zavos, having no extraterrestrial authority, but indeed having some scientific chops, claimed he had the first cloned baby. But despite the claims, no darling little cloned babies were ever produced as evidence. Human cloning was not yet a reality, but it was *almost* real – and that's why the stories launched an international dialog and became such a potent piece of science fiction. As the *New York Times* writer David Itzkoff has noted, sci-fi writers must adhere to "the pact." To put together a truly compelling piece of sci-fi, a writer must honor the "unspoken understanding that exists between readers and writers of speculative fiction: the reader will suspend disbelief as long as the writer starts with basic scientific fact before weaving his science fiction." The Raëlians had the attention of Congress and the world because their story was based on a scenario of human cloning that was plausible. "Somatic cell nuclear transfer" involved plucking a nucleus from a skin cell and dotting it into an enucleated embryonic stem cell, and as everyone knew, that had already been done in 1996 in a sheep, Dolly, a curious incident in the history of recent science.

The other facet that made the Raëlian's story compelling was their tapping into the endemic lust for the cinematic events of space opera. "One of the mysteries of cinema history is the sudden eclipse of the Western in the mid-1950s," wrote social critic Slavov Zizek. "Part of the answer is the fact that, at the same moment, space opera emerged as a genre – so one can venture the hypothesis that space opera took the place of the Western in the late 1950s. The dialectical point here is that the Western and space opera are not two subspecies of the genre 'adventure.' Rather, we should shift the perspective and start *only* with the Western – in the course of its development, the Western then encounters a deadlock and, in order to survive, has to 'reinvent' itself as space opera." If nothing else, Raël knew how to spin a good yarn, win female attention by centering those young ladies at the heart of an intergalactic space drama – one which must have seemed even more credible when their leader was asked to address Congress. And perhaps unintentionally, what he did that was most important, was to cast a narrative arch for the debate on human cloning that was needed within the social and Congressional spheres. These were issues that needed sorting. And fast.

Congress asked Antinori, and then Raël, to testify, at least for the sake of understanding the drive for human cloning and heritable modifications to the genome. The primary argument in favor of human cloning, to create an identical duplicate copy of a person, a double, a true Doppelganger, was libertarian in spirit. The cult leader Raël wished to spookily make many copies of his tribe, a form of immortality, like a paper angel opening into a chain of angels, everywhere mirror images of his clones in white jumpsuits. Severino Antinori posed a less fantastic argument for his clients' "right to have a genetically-related child."

And yet, the uncontestable truth is that reproduction comes with the implicit hope that we will have "better" children, offspring with a brighter future. Building mere duplicates dashes that hope. As the novelist Douglas Coupland quipped, "Cloning is great. If God made the original, then making copies should be fine." Or take it as the technologist Nathan Myhrvold did: "Suppose that every prospective parent in the world stopped having children naturally, and instead produced clones of themselves. What would the world be like in another 20 or 30 years? The answer is: much like today. Cloning would only copy the genetic aspects of people who are already here." Human cloning, while technically impressive, seemed to contradict our most sentimental of impulses, that for an extended, *better* future. In contrast to human cloning, more emphasis, at least in academic circles, was placed on the implications of heritable alterations to cells. If history was any guide, genetic modifications passed on to future generations (providing an enhancement) could translate to complicated new stratifications in the social sphere, which had been muddled by rifts in ethnicity, class and wealth. How exactly people would harness this technology, nobody knew. As the philosopher-physician Leon Kass, head of George W. Bush's bioethics council from 2001 to 2005, put it in the context of genetic engineering: "though well-equipped, we know not who we are or where we are going."

To an informed citizen, or a member of Congress, what the Raëlians purported to be doing was not all that inconceivable. The physicians Patrick Steptow and Robert Edwards had helped to conceive the first "test tube baby" by *in vitro* fertilization to form an embryo in a laboratory. On July 25, 1978 in Oldman General Hospital in England the wonderful outcome of Louise Brown was born. In many ways, it evidenced "positive eugenics," using technology to promote and advance life, and alter population demographics. Louise Brown appeared under a newspaper headline that read "SUPERBABE" on the front page of the *Evening News*. Doctors were becoming capable of handling a clump of living cells in a lab, and if they could do that, it meant that they could inspect and interrogate those cells at a "preimplantation" stage for telltale signs of disease. "Preimplantation genetic diagnosis" was a kind of diagnostic "check-up" on an embryo *in vitro* before it was ever implanted as an attempted pregnancy. In 1990, the first birth from the technology demonstrated doctors' abilities to detect a disorder in a laboratory before the embryo ever became a baby. If scientists could carefully handle an embryo before implantation, then they might add a nucleus from a skin cell into an egg cell to conduct human cloning, or using genetic engineering techniques, begin to alter our heritable code.

Importantly, scientists wanted to use their *in vitro* techniques to isolate an embryonic stem cell from an embryo, which could be used to repair tissues or nerve cells. In 1994, a federal panel on human embryo research instructed the government to permit the usage of embryonic stem cells for research to treat human disease. Congress changed course a couple of months later and attached language to the National Institutes of Health budget that made it illegal to create embryos with federal funding. James Thompson, a developmental biologist in Wisconsin, in 1998 continuing with *private* funding, reported he had isolated the first human embryonic stem cell line, "master cells" that give rise to all other cells in the body. Embryonic stem cells can be culled from those embryos at the eight-cell growth stage, and be coaxed into progenitor cell lines that might repair spinal cords or damaged heart tissue, and did require the destruction of human embryos.

Humans were on an inevitable march to engineer their own DNA. Once again, Hollywood captured the concept just ahead of the zeitgeist. The 1997 cult film "Gattaca," set in the "not-so-distant future," explored issues of desired traits being selected in a scheme of eugenics. Traits were selected from a clump of cells *in vitro* at the preimplantation stage, before attempting a pregnancy, and some figures in the film were selected for genetically "superior" traits. "They used to say a child conceived in love has a greater chance of happiness. They don't say that anymore," lamented Ethan Hawke, who was cast as Vincent Morrow, a hero of sorts. He was a "normal" child born in the backseat of a Buick. He was diagnosed with a host of genetic maladies, including a heart problem predicted to end his life by age 30. His younger brother, by comparison, was conceived in the labs of the Eighth Day Genetic Center, and named Anton, a boy "worthy of his father's name." A councilor made changes to Anton's genome to eradicate genes for "prejudicial conditions" such as premature baldness, myopia, alcoholism, addiction, violence and obesity. "You want to give your child the best possible start," the councilor said. "Keep in mind, this child is still you, simply the best of you. You could conceive naturally a thousand times and never get such a result." And yet, in the film, "non-engineered" people are shunned as "de-gene-erates" or "invalids." Indeed, Gattaca explored the naturalistic fallacy that genes are all wrapped up with values. The plot proceeds as Vincent assumes a false identity of an engineered human to enter the clandestine world of the Gattaca Aerospace Corporation. His love interest, played by Uma Thurman, becomes wrapped up with genetics. Herself a "normal" person, she believes her "inferior" genetics make her unworthy of love and fails to see the possibility of a relationship with Vincent. "You are the authority on what is not possible, aren't you Irene?" Vincent said, defying her to have some faith. "They've got you looking for any flaw, that after a while that's all you see. For what it's worth, I'm here to tell you that it is possible. It is possible."

If the first gene splice in 1971 served as the first axis in genetic engineering, then circa-2001 served as the second axis in the field. What resulted was a barrage of arguments and debates relating to the ethics of genetic engineering in the human germline. From the outset, Annas had emphasized the issues relating to perceptions of values, such that "the new 'ideal' human, the genetically-engineered 'superior' human, would almost certainly come to represent 'the other.' If history is a guide, either the normal humans will view the 'better' humans as 'the other,' and seek to control or destroy them, or vice-versa." University of New Mexico academic David Correia suggested the wealthy might use genetic engineering to translate power from the social sphere into the enduring code of the genome, effectively as "legacy" genetics, establishing "permanent capitalist social relations."

In 2001, in the East Wing of the White House, the first draft of the human genome had been announced. The press conference headed by President Bill Clinton brought together NIH head Francis Collins and Celera head Craig Ventor who had raced to bring the first draft to completion. Not everyone was convinced of the benefits of sequencing the genome, due to its enormous cost, and due to the inability to do much at all therapeutically to any genetic targets we might find. The ethicist George Annas cautioned on the dangers of decoding the genome, likening the initiative to sequence the genome to Precolumbian cartographers who "drew their maps to the extent of their knowledge, and then wrote in the margins, 'Beyond this point there are dragons.'" The public was taken aback by the surge of incredible science. George W. Bush appeared on national television in his first term in summer, August, 2001 and stem cell science was at the forefront of the national agenda. Conservative Republicans had stonewalled a ban on modifications to cells used in "reproductive" science when a proposal failed to also include cells that were used in "research" projects. As a result, policy guiding the science of genetic engineering was never properly shaped. Bush's response to the impasse was to forge a compromise: the NIH could give grant money to scientists who did research on cell lines derived from human embryos, while accepting a determination by Clinton-era lawyers that stated research on cells was allowable under law, though it was not permitted to destroy embryos in the process. In effect, the compromise had the weight of removing a funding stream from embryonic stem cell research, while theoretically allowing it to go forward. But no one seemed happy. Michael J. Fox was apoplectic that stem cell science was being thwarted by removing its funding. Bioethicists thought the compromise failed to achieve necessary guidance on human engineering since people could still legally clone themselves and industrialize the human genome. Raël continued to fundraise to build his embassy. The policy was half-shaped, but momentum of the moment died, because then 911 happened and everything changed.

The biologist Lee M. Silver took a favorable view of germline modification, while posing a cynical stance that laws would essentially be feckless and ineffectual to stop it. In the words of Annas, Silver staked the position that "these technologies, while not necessarily desirable, are unstoppable because the market combined with parental desire will drive scientists and physicians to offer these services to demanding couples. Similarly to the way parents now seek early education enrichment for their children, he believes that parents of the future will seek early genetic enhancement to achieve for them a competitive advantage in life." Silver went so far to argue that it has the potential to lead to the creation of two separate human subspecies, the "GenRich" and "the naturals." In his 1998 book, *Remaking Eden: How Genetic Engineering and Cloning Will Transform the American Family*, Silver advanced a positive view on human cloning and designer babies, suggesting the advance of gene engineering technology was inevitable, and that parents had the authority to use it. By comparison, George Annas adopted a cynical stance of biotech marketers and has argued that public policy and regulation is needed for gene engineering. He has written that heritable modifications would set divisions between our children, muddling our children's right to an "open future," summoning Vaclav Havel's concept of "species consciousness," to argue against the industrialization of the human genome.[370] "The challenge is to get beyond the literary archetypes, the stereotypes, and the clichés, and to work together to develop a coherent set of goals against which to judge scientific priorities and actions," Annas wrote.

In 2002, Annas, Lori Andrews and Rosario Isasi felt the issue was urgent enough to write a policy paper called "Protecting the Endangered Human: Toward an International Treaty Prohibiting Cloning and Inheritable Alterations," a document that categorically opposed all cloning and/or heritable modifications to the human genome. Around the same time, Francis Fukuyama thusly called transhumanism "the world's most dangerous idea." In his book *Our Posthuman Future* he qualified his original "end of history" thesis, suggesting that human genetic engineering might allow humans to control their own evolution, putting liberal democracy at risk. Fukuyama's "end of history" hypothesis had locked on the fall of the imperial nation state, and singular history, and suggested the emergence of a democratic arena where history would be dialectic and subject to redraft. Fukuyama's idea wasn't new, it was Hegel's. But Fukuyama envisioned that genetic engineering now put liberalism at risk. His use of the word "future" in the title of his book, signifies a machine-like future, one which rather than being open, is characterized by the capacity of technologists to control it for us – a new "singularity," which was characterized by an increasing dependence of biology on electronics, psychoactive drugs, gene dosing and the like. If there was one imperial power left on the world stage, Fukuyama argued, it was biotech. "What should we do in response to biotechnology that in the future will mix great potential benefits with threats that are either physical and overt or spiritual and subtle?" he asked in *Our Posthuman Future*. The answer "is obvious. *We should use the power of the state to regulate it.*"

The battle lines were being drawn. "Bioconservatives" wanted regulation and little or no tinkering in human genomes, while "transhumanists" believe that alteration of our genetic code with technology is precisely the thing that separates us from other species and makes us human. In the tradition of Paul Ramsey, Annas, neoconservatives like Fukuyama, Leon Kass, and aligning in a strange coalition with leftist activists such as Jeremy Rifkin and Bill McKibben (who has written books including *Enough* as a warning against the advance of biotechnology), pushed a pro-regulation agenda that sought to ban the modifications outright. On the other hand, in the tradition of Joseph Fletcher, the Oxford ethicist Julian Savulescu and others were arguing that it was not only a right but a duty to manipulate our genetic code.

"Reprogenetics" suggests that genetic manipulation be taken up in the process of reproduction. In the words of Jonathan Moreno, "reprogeneticsts see themselves as advocates of market and reproductive freedom. They also cite the fact that class and economic privileges notwithstanding, parents are permitted to finance 'improvements' in their children's competitive position with SAT tutors and tennis lessons." Lee M. Silver seemed to think that government couldn't stop genetic engineering in humans, even if it wanted to. By the early 2000s, right smack at the time two highly publicized deaths were widely reported in the genetic engineering field, these policy issues hit a peak of recognition in the public sphere. The two camps had staked their claims and were divided along very clear lines: either align with the pro-biotech wing, with those who want to allow genetic modification in humans because they think it's our natural right or because they think states cannot thwart the progress, or encamp with a pro-regulation people who read faith into the democratic process and insist that humanity is an "endangered species" and that we must ban operations on genetic engineering.

Dartmouth ethicist Ronald M. Green stepped forward in 2007 and released a forceful and compelling book *Babies by Design: The Ethics of Genetic Choice*, in which he argued for a qualified form of "parental libertarianism," reading nuance into the debate. Green argued, essentially, that it is up to the parents, not the governments, to make the decisions on heritable alterations to the genomes of their families. As long as it didn't compromise the health of the child, then, fair game. He advanced a family-centered, favorable view on genetic engineering in step with Silver. Green thought that state regulation did have a role in providing guidelines or rules to families, while granting parents a status of limited or qualified authority. Green interjected into the debate by countering the move to categorical obstruction from the conservatives.

"I, too, am a bioethicist, but I disagree profoundly with this conservative direction... In this period of retreat, I want to draw attention to the impending revolution in genetic technology that will allow us to select or modify our children's genetic inheritance. I believe that the issue of gene selection will dominate bioethics in the decades to come and emerge as a major focus of debate, dividing those opposed to biomedical advances from those committed to them. Gene modification will encompass the first hesitant steps to *improve* the genetic endowment of our children so they can flourish in new ways." Green wrote four guidelines, which concisely define his libertarian stance. First, genetic interventions should be "aimed at what is reasonably in the child's best interests," citing the Christian ethicist Sondra Wheeler, "any proposed intervention must pass the tests of being undertaken directly and primarily for the sake of the child rather than the parents or other parties." Green goes further: "The word 'reasonably' here is important. It both constrains the parents and empowers them. It constrains them because it implies a larger standard of judgment than mere parental wishes or beliefs. It is not enough for parents to think that something is in their child's best interests; their judgments must accord with that of most other informed members of society." Secondly, genetic interventions put into play should be almost as safe as natural reproduction. Thirdly, Green argues we should avoid and discourage interventions that confer only "positional advantage," in other words, stronger memories for rich kids, and muscle doping for athletes. He cited Garrett Hardin's "tragedy of the commons," as a case where a limit to resources causes some to lose out, and dynamics of doping such that "one competitor's use of drugs puts pressure on everyone to do the same." Fourth, he says genetic interventions should not "reinforce or increase unjust inequality and discrimination, economic inequality or racism," while softening that claim, channeling the ethicist Arthur Caplan who observes "it is possible – in fact, probable – that if nothing were done to ensure access to brain-enhancing technologies, inequities would arise," but adds that the best solution "is to provide fair access... not do away with the idea of improvement."

Shoukhrat Mitalipov had completed his PhD in Moscow and set up a lab at Oregon Health & Science University. Actually, he set up two labs. One of his labs was set for research funded by the National Institutes of Health, and one was set for research experiments that were exempt from federal funding, but which were not illegal: human cloning and genetic engineering in embryonic stem cells. Masahito Tachibana was a visiting researcher from Sendai, Japan, and in 2013 he added the capstone to a five-year stint of research in Mitalipov's lab with an article in the journal *Nature*. It proved the strategy for modifications to germline cells that could be transferred to future generations. In effect, it would allow for the birth of the first transhumans. The group then put on stunning display an optimized technique of "somatic cell nuclear transfer," plucking the nucleus from a skin cell and inserting it into an embryonic stem cell. They could clone a human, they said. Did the public want scientists intervening in the code that gets transferred to future generations, in effect, inserting themselves into human evolution? The questions scattered into plain sight when Tachibana kicked the hornet's nest. Paul Knoepfler, a University of California stem cell scientist, rattled out a blog post that cloned babies could be a reality in five years. "Some crazy person will try to clone humans."

Mitalipov and Tachibana had published a strategy for engineering humans based on the method of plucking a cell nucleus from an embryonic stem cell, and inserting the nucleus into an enucleated embryonic stem cell from another woman. This second donor cell included all the working machinery, including mitochondrial DNA, but no nucleus. If a woman knew she had a mitochondrial disorder that ran in her family, it essentially put a death cast on all future generations. The Oregon researchers' argument, and a powerful one, was that if the FDA would allow them to simply swap the nuclear DNA into the context of a donor cell that carried good copies of mitochondrial DNA, they'd stop the disease in its tracks. Our cells contain hundreds of mitochondria, technically organelles or tiny organs, which contain their own circular copies of DNA. Mitochondria only get transferred through maternal lines, and thus it's true, there is something only a mother can impart upon us. In fact, they're as vital as our very breath. Mitochondria create a chemical fuel called ATP (a widely used currency of energy, the US dollar of the body) in a process called oxidative phosphorylation. It's done by stealing electrons from oxygen molecules each time we breathe. Sometimes in the process, those electrons get misplaced, resulting in "free radicals," oxidative species, just to get a smidge technical, that now have an unpaired electron and a "dangling" covalent bond. The result is a molecule that is unstable and prone to interacting with other molecules in damaging ways. It's the reason that foods are promoted as "antioxidants," because in a real sense, they reduce free radicals.

Lynn Margulus rocked biology in her 1967 paper "On the Origin of Mitosing Cells," advancing her "endosymbiotic theory." She argued for a position that mitochondria began as microbes! All of our human cells are eukaryote type, while bacteria are prokaryote type. Margulus' hypothesis suggested that, once upon a time, a eukaryote ancestor cell engulfed a prokayote, probably of the type *Rickettsiales* (an invasive microbe that can be found in streams and causes Rocky Mountain Spotted Fever), but this time the cell got the best of the conflict, trapping the microbe within its confines and syphoning off its energy production. In fact, the cell held it forever as its captive.

Marcy Darnovsky, a director at the Center for Genetics and Society, wrote a scorching position letter in the journal *Nature* titled "A Slippery Slope to Human Germline Modification," in which she derided the UK for moves to back germline therapy. "Germline modification is the hydrogen bomb of this whole field," Darnovsky told me. She argued that in the case of familial mitochondrial diseases, the technique did not actually count as therapy, since it did nothing for living generations. "It's not therapy," she said. "That's the distinction that we are making." Instead, it allowed mothers to create new children who were disease-free. Darnovsky also questioned whether the technique, which worked in monkeys, would translate effectively to humans. The work involves snapping together cells "like Lego," she said, where two cells are "smushed together," but it's not entirely known how "disruptive this will be to interactions between nucleus and mitochondria" organelles which are engaging in "cross talk," and how well a hybrid cell will "resume intercellular conversation," she told me.

Ethicists were largely aligning in a consensus, that if genome editing could be proven safe, it could be used to edit disease-causing mutations that were strongly evidenced in the scientific literature, especially if the diseases were very serious without alternative pharmacological treatment courses. But questions were emerging if insurers and taxpayers should pay for engineering techniques such as mitochondrial therapies or germline editing therapies prior to a child even being born, since as Darnovsky notes, it's not therapy.

Nuanced questions were emerging as to who would pay for "stress or stroke vaccines," such "prophylactic" gene therapies. A group of researchers led by David Pepin at Harvard Medical School showed that they could install a modified version of a gene that builds a protein called Müllerian inhibiting substance, by using the adeno-associated virus to deliver the gene into the cell, and suppress the growth of "chemotherapy-resistant" ovarian tumors in mice. It was one of many trials ongoing that were ushering us into the age of the "cancer vaccine."

By 2013, Crispr-Cas9 was in broad use, and ethicists were beginning to debate whether to edit our gene variants such as *APOE4* that serve as a genetic "risk factor" for Alzheimer's. In some cases, insurers may someday want to pay for gene editing. Crispr-Cas9 might be used to end blindness caused by dominant forms of retinitis pigmentosa, prevent myocardial infarctions that kill patients with homozygous familial hypercholesterolemia, or edit liver cells to restore a functional copy of the gene encoding low-density lipoprotein receptors. A one-time gene edit may within decades be cheaper than a lifetime of cholesterol drugs. But if we started intervening with Crispr-Cas9 as a "prophylactic" or "preventative" therapy, it would lead to an almost endless mining and alterations of our genomes. It would be no big surprise to learn that almost all of us have variants that predict a disease to varying degree. Geneticists call this penetrance. In dire cases, it's people who have the repeats of the motif CAG in a single gene who are almost certain to get Huntington's disease, or those with mutations in the *PDK* gene family, which are highly likely to cause polycystic kidney disease. It's the actress Angelina Jolie, who in the film *Tomb Raider* fought off a six-armed guardian statue, armed mercenaries and a robot named SIMON. But it was a typo in a molecule that put her at the greatest danger.

Carrying mutations in *BRCA1* put a woman's risk at up to 60% for developing breast cancer. These were not simple thought experiments. By the end of 2015, Jennifer Doudna was reporting she was having sleepless nights, while receiving hundreds of emails from people asking if Crispr could be deployed as a preventative tactic. In one email, "a 26-year-old woman told how she had discovered that she carried the *BRCA1* mutation, which gave her a roughly 60% chance of developing breast cancer by the time she was 70. She was considering having her breasts and ovaries removed, and wanted to know whether the approaches made possible by Crispr–Cas9 meant that she should hold off."[371]

Insurers might not be so quick to cotton on to preventative gene editing. Consider the 1994 case Katskee vs. Blue Cross Blue Shield of Nebraska. Sidnie Katskee had her ovaries removed as a precaution against cancer. Her mother and aunt died of ovarian cancer with diagnoses at 47 and 48 years. The insurer refused to pay, saying it was not "medically necessary." A trial judge ruled for the insurer, saying Katskee did not have a "bodily illness or disease," but the Supreme Court of Nebraska reversed the decision and ruled in Katskee's favor.

Marcy Darnovsky, director at the Center for Genetics and Society in California, raised skepticism for the high price tags with treatments running into the millions. Gene therapies, she said, are "risky and the costs of this medical technology are jaw dropping." The whole field posed issues of "distributive justice," she said. Annas wrote that "the new genetics" will likely blur the distinction between prevention and treatment, since spotting a mutation that causes a disease is close to spotting the disease. But he cautioned that treatments based on a predisposition might be cost prohibitive, after all, "we will all die of something."

In many cases, genetic risk factors are "balanced polymorphisms," meaning they have a bad effect coupled with an unrelated good effect. A mutation in the *TP53* gene protects mice against cancer, but causes premature aging. Many genetic variants have only weak contributions to a disease, and others may appear to be false signals. A controversy over "personal genomics" tests was mounting over the reliability of such tests. In 2013, Harvard professor Robert Green had held a talk announcing that the American College of Medical Genetics had a new policy. Anyone who had their genome sequenced would now be required to be screened for 56 genetic markers that could predict conditions such as breast cancer, heart disease and other known diseases. Like it or not, the patients would have to be subjected to their genetic predispositions. But the decision was not embraced by everyone. And Green was preparing to conduct a personal genomics project as a form of newborn screening called "Baby-Seq." As The New York Times science writer Nicholas Wade once quipped "when genomes can be decoded for $1,000, a baby may arrive home like a new computer, with its complete genetic operating instructions on a DVD." Wade's predictions had now become a reality. Once again, the progressive edge of genome science found a town crier in George Annas, and his close ally Sherman Elias, a clinical geneticist. "We were kind of taken aback," Elias told me. "The rationale was that if someone carries a genetic mutation that is 'actionable,' meaning that doctors can do something about it, then the patients and doctors must be informed." Elias and Annas believed the College was over-reaching, smug about the abilities of therapeutics to correct many conditions, and unduly subjecting patients, children in some cases, to information that might only contribute to stress. Genetics was moving fast, with sexy new tools like whole genome sequencing, which could pinpoint mutations that were highly predictive of some diseases. But those mutations, or predictive markers, are often only "associated" with a certain disease. But as Elias has pointed out, many of the mutations in breast cancer genes *BRCA1* and *BRCA2*, for instance, have been identified through studies of high-risk families, which conceal a conundrum of multifactorial origins of disease. In other words, families share a lot of genetics in common, and so their study is prone to identifying signals that are nested in complex genetic relationships (sometimes called epistasis, interactions that happen "above" the genomic template) and a variant may not cause the disease in people outside that family. "Most of the probabilities have been determined from studies of high risk families, genes have many functions; there are parts of the genome, which we don't understand. What are the probabilities? We don't know."[372]

But, we are starting to know. In August of 2015, Manolis Kellis and colleagues published a study in the *New England Journal of Medicine* on obesity, which described a new circuit in cells that controls metabolism by causing adipocytes, or fat cells, to store fat or burn it. The strongest association to obesity had been variants in a gene called *FTO*, the focus of many obesity studies for the past decade, and suggested a link with brain circuits controlling appetite and the initiative to exercise. But the study showed that cell circuits can contribute to obesity in a brain-independent way. In at-risk individuals, a change to a single nucleotide referred to as marker rs1421085, which involved the change of a thymine (T) to a cytosine (C) nucleobase, disrupted a regulatory brake on a cellular circuit and enabled the rampant expression of genes, which have a role in thermogenesis, whereby the adipocytes, or fat cells, dissipate energy as heat, instead of storing it as fat. In fact, these two genes regulate or put brakes on other genes. Thus, if they are turned up, it results in less dissipation of heat and more fat storage. Kellis and colleagues edited a single nucleotide position using Crispr-Cas9 and showed they could switch between lean and obese gene signatures in human cells. "Knowing the causal variant underlying the obesity association may allow... somatic genome editing as a therapeutic avenue," Kellis said.[373] But not everything that works in a mouse may work in a human. As David Altshuler once quipped, "It turns out the best model for a human ... is a human."

Obesity might best be corrected in the germline, since then it would ensure that all cells have this correction. The same is true for the genetic variant that causes Huntington's disease, which might be best edited at an eight-cell embryo, which turns into all the different cells of the body, including neurons, so that a fully grown adult would have a brain with billions of neurons that each contains the correct fix. If you tried to make the edits to their billions of neurons as an adult, it would be impossible to successfully correct all of them; many neurons would remain with the defective genetic variant.

"Some human genetic diseases can really only be effectively attacked by germline gene therapy, providing gene correction in fertilized eggs or very early embryos," Dana Carroll added. "This raises serious ethical issues, of course." Marcy Darnovsky argued that even if the tools were safe and effective, she wanted to prevent an opening to germline modification where anything goes in the genome. "We'd be introducing brand new types of inequality into the world," she said. "The gene therapy field has historically been linked to a lot of hyperbole." And yet, modifying the germline and human cloning were two techniques where "we must draw the line." "It will take public policy," Darnovsky said. "Without it, there's a slippery slope to a Gattaca type future – that's where we're headed." In his office, Phil Sharp echoed to me that while there is "not much sensitivity in this country on somatic tissues, for instance, using gene therapy to treat defects in bone marrow and liver, there is great sensitivity in the debate on alterations in the germline. If you try something like higher-order intelligence, and you achieve this, would these people be treated like real people? Should man start engineering man? I see a lot of sensitivity in that issue. From the humanistic side, I don't think we should do it."

A raft of opinions were flooding into the marketplace of ideas. Oxford bioethicist professor Julian Savulescu was arguing that it is not only possible, but our *moral obligation,* to dose ourselves with genes for cognitive enhancers like serotonin, whereby we could turn those genes on and off like switches with pills. Savulescu was arguing for genetic germline engineering that is transferred to future generations, which he called "procreative beneficence." Questions were emerging on who will receive genetic benefits, to become something we can call "gene rich." If a child was not given a new gene that could help them, was it some type of moral slight? A few ethicists, including Savulescu, were extending the concept of "parental neglect" into a new term called "genetic neglect." But these opinions were not without staunch opposition.

"We need a halt on anything that approaches germline editing in human embryos," warned Ed Lanphier, chief executive of Sangamo BioSciences. "Such research could be exploited for non-therapeutic modifications. We are concerned that a public outcry about such an ethical breach could hinder a promising area of therapeutic development."[374] With much contention in the space of discussion, and confusion as to just who had the authority to make these decisions, ethicists and policy groups were in a scramble to throw up blogs and letters with suggested guidelines. In 2015, the Hixton Group, an international consortium on stem cells, ethics and law, released a statement with guidelines to suggest a halt to using germline editing on human cells, but to continue going forward with embryos from fertility clinics that could provide fertile ground for research. Hixton suggested a pressing need to shape policy "to inform the plausibility of developing safe human reproductive applications. These distinctions are important to make clear that, even if one opposes human genome editing for clinical reproductive purposes, there is important research to be done that does not serve that end. That said, we appreciate that there are even categories of basic research involving this technology that some may find morally troubling. Nevertheless, it is our conviction that concerns about human genome editing for clinical reproductive purposes should not halt or hamper application to scientifically defensible basic research." Hixton cites a concern of mosaicism, in other words, if an eight-cell embryo is edited, what happens if only five of the cells are successfully edited, and three are not. Thus, they suggest unexplored problems in engineering humans that are "mosaics" of multiple variants of cells. "Of note, most supernumerary IVF embryos available for research will have progressed beyond the one-cell stage, such that the use of genome editing techniques will likely lead to mosaicism."

Hixton released recommendations: "Decisions about research and clinical uses of genome editing technologies should be made through inclusive, deliberative processes that will make engagement with the public and policymakers substantive, and should aim to strike the best possible balance between free scientific inquiry and social values. Further, best methods for integrating the outputs of public engagement into the policymaking process should be identified and utilized." However, the group noted that "any constraint of scientific inquiry should be derived from reasonable concerns" and "policymakers should refrain from constraining scientific inquiry unless there is substantial justification for doing so that reaches beyond disagreements based solely on divergent moral convictions. In the case of human genome editing, as with all science, it is important to target restrictive policy... proportionate to the magnitude of what is morally at stake."

In fact, at least 29 countries have laws or guidelines that ban the practice of genome editing, according to a 2014 review by Tetsuya Ishii, a bioethicist at Hokkaido University in Sapporo, Japan. However, whether or not it is entirely restricted in the United States is a provocative question. If it is treated as a drug, then it certainly comes under the restrictions and full force of compliance with the FDA, but many *in vitro* fertility clinics in the United States already offer preimplantation genetic diagnosis, and so it tempting to conceive of genome editing as a kind of service that allows for modifications to an embryo before implantation. In the US there were murky questions on whether genome editing at fertility clinics is or is not really grounded in law, whether or not IVF clinics are restricted from doing this. And worldwide, clinics may have questionable standards and practices. As Ishii noted, "there are already a lot of dodgy fertility clinics around the world."[375]

Just who was in charge, the thought leader and the authoritative body, was not entirely clear, not as clear as I had expected. The National Academy of Sciences set up a meeting for the fall of 2015 in Washington to vet just these issues. Eric Lander had just dashed out an opinion piece in the *New England Journal of Medicine*, laying out the stakes and calling for caution, and suggesting that scientists should draw the line at germline editing to create "designer babies" and "genetically engineered humans."

"The discussions that will begin in the fall may solidify a broad international consensus that germline editing should be banned – with the possible exception of correcting severe monogenic disease genes, in the few cases in which there is no alternative. For my own part, I see much wisdom in such a position, at least for the foreseeable future. A ban could always be reversed if we become technically proficient, scientifically knowledgeable, and morally wise enough and if we can make a compelling case. But authorizing scientists to make permanent changes to the DNA of our species is a decision that should require broad societal understanding and consent. It has been only about a decade since we first read the human genome. We should exercise great caution before we begin to rewrite it."[376]

7   Life in a Bubble

I hope it doesn't deter him, because I want grandchildren. Maybe science will be even better by then.

– Jennifer Golliday, mother to Jamey, who was born with a heritable X-SCID immune disorder

By July, the swelter of summer was upon us, I was feeling locked into the crucible of Boston and I headed west by highway. The roads were lined with milkweed and purple violet; the breeze was cool. I drove with the windows rolled down, past a sprawling wind turbine farm on I-55. The sky opened up big, with rainclouds coasting in the distance. The horizon in the Midwest is longer. I forgot that. It lends an expanse, and I felt as if I was driving into a chasm. But then, I was there.

I met Jamey Golliday, a blue-eyed boy, age 2, on a small patch of lawn in Bloomington, Illinois at his grandfather's house. Jamey's grandfather, Warren, lives on a circular street, in a subdivision with spacious lawns, hardwoods and river birch. He has silver hair, shiny skin and was wearing shorts and a short-sleeved shirt. The early afternoon was hazy. The neighbors were burning lawn debris, and the air contained a light hint of combustion, of burning, of calcium carbonite, oxides and potash, and fly ash was swirling in the sky, big fluffy flakes, falling lightly all around us.

Jamey's older brother, Shawn, age 5, showed up with a black *Star Wars* T-shirt, and two plastic light sabers, and promptly flipped one to Warren, as in, "you better catch this if you think you're going to defend yourself." And within seconds, Shawn was on the advance, hacking his way through to his grandfather, who was fending off the angular blows and there was a steady bat-bot-bat-bop of batting plastic. The fly ash continued to fall from the controlled brush fire in the neighbor's yard, lending the effect of a cosmic rain as the saber fight continued through the yard, and the situation was quickly turning galactic.

Jamey was wearing a white shirt with stripes, shorts and Crocs. His mom, Jennifer, 31, was cradling him in her arms, and they retreated to a quieter spot in the acre-sized yard, near some box gardens and trees which receded into darker woods. Jennifer hung him back down to the ground, and he was helping her to pick up sticks and put them into a wheelbarrow. "It's super sad," Jennifer told me. "He sees kids off in the distance and points at them. I know he wants to interact."

Jamey can interact with his family, but for his entire life, he has been without friends. That's because he has a rare disease called X-SCID, or Bubble Boy disease, which means he was born without a working immune system. In effect, Jamey has a defective copy of the *IL2*-gamma receptor gene on the X chromosome, which was transferred to him from his mother. Since women have two copies of the X chromosome, they serve as carriers of the disease, while they are protected by a second functioning copy of the *IL-2* gamma receptor. And that's why there is a Bubble Boy disease, but no Bubble Girl disease. Jennifer was a carrier, but she didn't have the disease, and her father Warren did not have it. That means it might be traceable through Jennifer's mother's side of the family. The other possibility is that it is a *de novo* mutation, meaning that it emerged in this generation.

For much of his short life, Jamey was "bubbled" or kept in a sequestered environment to prevent him from catching his death of cold. But the previous year he had a gene therapy treatment at Cincinnati Children's Hospital, in which doctors added a working copy of the *IL-2* gamma receptor. Now he was on the rebound. A rudimentary immune system began to take up arms in his body. He was still not allowed to interact with other children, or people outside his family. Jennifer allowed him to go barefoot in the backyard, jaunting among sprinklers, picking up sticks, rocks and clumps of grass. "He loves to be outside. He loves to run around and scream, and laugh for a long time. He cries when he has to go back inside."

He was just a baby when his mother discovered a bump on his left hip. It was a sore that didn't go away; in fact, it was becoming a deep infection. A pediatric surgeon at Saint Francis Medical Center in Peoria, Illinois said he thought it might be a tumor. The clinic excised the bump, drained it, and a doctor returned, telling Jennifer he had cancer. "It was a very scary week," Jennifer remembers. The doctors said her baby boy had diffuse B-cell lymphoma. But it was such a rare disease for a baby to have. Jamey also had PCP pneumonia, a rare situation, and he had a small cold – which he was fighting for about a year. He was signed into the emergency room, and his breathingwas fluttering at about 100 breaths per minute. Doctors now thought they had his breathing under control. "They told me it was fine," Jennifer said. A machine was recording his breathing down around 40 breaths per minute, but Jennifer disagreed. "Come over here, and count his breaths," she told the nurses. Soon doctors began to question the cancer diagnosis. Then there was an entire reversal of circumstance. Further tests would show that Jamey had X-SCID. That's why he had a persistent pneumonia, and why his body couldn't patch up his hip. B-cells had been clumping near his infection, to try to fight it, but B-cells must work in co-ordination with T-cells, and since Jamey had no mature T-cells in his system, the B-cells were feckless and ineffectual, just clumping and convening there. His sore just wouldn't heal up. And the clumping of those useless B-cells, imitated a cancer, a situation that doctors call "phenocopy."

An accurate diagnosis was now in hand, Jamey was flown in a medical jet to Cincinnati Children's Hospital. For two months, doctors exhausted options for a bone marrow transplant, the traditional method of treatment. "I did do a lot of researching. In fact, that was nearly all I did," Jennifer said. Her baby had been diagnosed with cancer and pneumonia, but those two symptoms were now revealed to be a single immune deficiency, changing the state of play. "I didn't go outside for the first two months we were there for fear of bringing germs back to him. Back to the original point, they first mentioned it to me in Cincinnati. The relief from being down to one potential life threatening problem from two was immeasurable."

To contemplate matters, the trips back and forth to hospitals were especially tough on Jamey's brother Shawn, who was so often left out of the loop and in the absence of his mother as she waited in hospital halls, pondering the gravity of having a baby boy with no immune system. Shawn had become opposition-defiant and starting a light saber fight was only a milder act of aggression. For Jamey, a bone marrow transplant was considered to introduce some functioning cells into his body, to patch the communication of his immune system. In fact, doctors make the determination of a bone marrow match based on a profile of human leukocyte antigens, or HLA, which are molecular badges that the immune system uses to tell the difference between self and foreign cells. But even with a close match, sometimes a terrible side-effect occurs, called graft-versus-host disease. X-SCID kids face even worse odds. David Vetter, born in 1971, was perhaps the most famous Bubble Boy. As a baby he lived in a sterilized cocoon bed. When he was older he lived in a bubble, using only items sterilized with 140-degree ethylene oxide gas. He often wore a yellow C-3PO T-shirt, and attended a special showing of *Return of the Jedi* at a local theatre, which he traveled to in a transport chamber. NASA built him a spacesuit. But it was to no avail. As he grew older, he became increasingly unstable due to a lack of normal interactions, and he was wracked with nightmares about the "King of Germs." In 1984, at age 12, a bone marrow transplant was tried from his sister, Katherine. But an Epstein–Barr virus was sleeping in that marrow, putting the slip on researchers. David Vetter died 15 days later of Burkitt's lymphoma, a cancer triggered by the virus, which is normally suppressed by our immune systems.

Jennifer knew the risks of a bone marrow transplant. By comparison, gene therapy was not without its dangers. A decade earlier, trials using the retrovirus to treat X-SCID resulted in five patients coming down with leukemia-like conditions. One of those patients died. But scientists now thought they had a handle on it. They had made some alterations to the virus used to deliver a new gene, deleting some of its dangerous elements. They said the procedure was safer. Jennifer read about some young patients in England who were having gene therapy treatments for X-SCID using "safer" retrovirus tools. None of those young patients had so far developed a cancer.

In the US, scattered gene therapy procedures were being tried at Boston, Cincinnati and UCLA. But the FDA had not yet approved a gene therapy drug in the United States, and a wide body of scientists remained deeply circumspect. "They told me they'd call me at the first sign that something went wrong," Jennifer said. "It was scary in some aspects. I was willing to risk it."

One of Richard Mulligan's students had been David A. Williams, now chief of hematology at Boston Children's Hospital. In the early 1980s, Mulligan had engineered retrovirus into a cloning system, so that it could install a new gene into a cell *ex vivo*, meaning outside the body. The first cells to be engineered with gene therapy were hematopoietic cells, the class of cells which emerge in the bone marrow and give rise to red blood cells and the immune system's white blood cells. Hematopoietic cells circulate and can be easily removed from the body, giving rise to an interest in treating them with gene therapy for sickle cell disease, thalassemia and severe combined immune disorders. Williams had been one of the post-docs in Mulligan's lab who was interested in using gene therapy to engineer immune cells. But in the first trials in Europe in the late 1990s by an alternative group of researchers, something when awry. Retrovirus randomly inserts into the human genome, and in some cases it landed next to an important developmental gene called *LMO2*. This threw those T-cells into a non-stop growth cycle, causing a leukemia-like condition in many X-SCID patients treated with the gene therapy. A patient died in 2003.

Williams continued to work on retrovirus technology. Years later, while conducting research at Cincinnati Children's Hospital with colleague Christopher Baum, he decided to try to delete enhancers and promoters, elements in the retrovirus which are strong switches that could slam on cell growth and cause cancer. Consider that the human genome is literally a graveyard of viruses. When the genome was first published in 2001, it was found that more than 10 percent of it was comprised of long terminal repeats, or LTRs, traces of retroviruses that had at one time integrated into the genome, and had since gone dormant. LTRs include regions called a promoter and an enhancer. In fact, proteins called transcription factors dock at the promoter and begin sliding down the gene, expressing the gene, as the wheels of the genome's publishing house begin to turn. It turns out that retrovirus has strong versions of these promoter regions which turn on gene expression, and so if a virus integrates next to a gene in a human cell, it could also turn on the expression of the gene next door. And so, if the gene that it installed next to was involved in cell division, the virus could kick on runaway cell division, leading to a cancer. Williams and colleagues replaced those elements of the virus with elements of genetic code from a woodchuck and a promoter region found in a gene called *EFS*, which is a gentler initiator of gene expression.

This time, if the virus randomly installed near a proto-oncogene, its expression would be calmer. It might not slam up the volume on a gene that drives the cell cycle, and initiate non-stop cell growth. In fact, a storm of technical improvements had contributed to make gene therapy game-ready, and investment was flooding back into the field as a consensus was emerging that the tools were safe enough to be applied to a spectrum of different rare diseases. Bluebird Bio, Inc. of Cambridge, MA was developing a lentivirus as a tool, as opposed to a retrovirus. Mitch

Finer, chief scientific officer, and a one-time student of Mulligan, squiggled schematics of viruses on a white board in a conference room with colorful markers, when I visited him in his office that same summer. He drew boxes for promoter regions and triangles for deleted elements of sequence. Whether retrovirus or lentivirus was the better tool for inserting genes into humans "has been a topic of contention for years," Finer told me. "And the guy who brought this to the forefront was Christopher Baum." Baum had been Williams' collaborator at Cincinnati, where they figured out how to build a safer retrovirus to treat X-SCID. But he also then applied a test to compare the safety of retrovirus and lentivirus. When a virus added to cells in a lab triggers a cancer, those cells continue to grow non-stop, achieving something called "immortality." He found that lentivirus triggered immortality less often than retrovirus. Baum wanted to know why. He used a new method, which was developed by another German colleague, Crist of von Kalle, also on Williams' faculty at Cincinnati, to determine the sites where the viruses were installing. The scientists saw that retrovirus had a preference for installing in gene-dense regions, and even more interesting, preferred to jump into regions related to cell cycles, where it can turn up the volume on cell division. Lentivirus did not have this preference for installing in gene dense regions. It was safer to use, they started to believe.

By now, retooled versions of retrovirus and lentivirus were at the rough-and-ready stage to use as delivery vehicles to treat a raft of rare diseases. Finer explained that researchers could now install promoters along with new transgenes that would only turn genes "on" in specific cell lines. Genes could be installed in stem cells, but wired up to only turn "on" in blood cells. He continued to scribble with marker on the white board, detailing a complex schematic of a newly engineered lentivirus, one which he said, was a safer "next generation" gene therapy. If the drawing Mulligan scrawled for me on a scrap of paper was the Model T of gene therapy, a "Tin Lizzie," then the carriage Finer drew for me was a Model A, still rickety, but profoundly safer.

The company gutted the lentivirus and installed a gene called *ABCD1*. Its first use would be treatment of adrenoleukodystrophy, a downright awful disease that results in long chain fatty acids building up in cells throughout the body. Cells have small packaging rooms called organelles, and one of those is a recycling room where boxes get broken down called a peroxisome. The *ABCD1* gene builds a tiny door called an ATP-binding cassette transporter, and when that door is broken and doesn't work right, the fatty acids never get moved into the recycling room. They don't get broken down. And they can't be taken out with the trash, because the trash man says they must be recycled. Among the tragic consequences is demylenation, or removal of tiny sheaths that protect neurons, resulting in children rapidly deteriorating into a vegetative state. Patrick Aubourg at San Raffaele-Telethon Institute for Gene Therapy in Milan, Italy led a trial in 2009. In just a handful of those patients, the treatment had stopped disease in its tracks. Bluebird was betting high stakes on its first major trial. If gene therapy could cure inborn childhood diseases, and it looked like Aubourg had provided "proof-of-principle," then thousands of rare diseases provided a market for its drugs.

"Early on, there were some hiccups in the field," Richard Smith, a Bluebird executive at the time, told me. "The science has moved ahead, and we can predict the safest elements of the lentivirus to use, and which must be deleted." These were diseases that laid children to waste. A month after I visited their offices, Bluebird's collaborators in Italy reported the results of a study on three children with metachromatic leukodystrophy, an unrelated disease, which results from mutations in a gene that builds enzyme arylsulfatase A. The disease results from a trash disposal room in the cell called a lysosome. This enzyme resides in that room, and its malfunction means the lysosome fails to take care of the trash. The trash builds up, resulting in accumulation of molecules called sulfatides, which also, once again, degrade the tiny sheaths that protect neurons. There is no current treatment and children usually die within a few years. Luigi Naldini, who headed the gene therapy study and is widely considered the "Father" of lentivirus, reported to the press that "at this stage, the patients normally have brain damage or are dead. Instead they are alive and thriving."

Bluebird obtained orphan drug status for its drug from the FDA, a fast-track approval that would allow the company to use its drug on a small cohort of patients. The company tapped Williams to supervise a trial of its gene therapy drug on adrenoleukodystrophy, starting in late 2013 at Children's Hospital Boston. If things went well with that trial, the company would be just a step away from bringing the first gene therapy drug to market in the United States. Much had been accomplished. Williams and colleagues had stripped the viruses of the elements that were likely to cause a cancer, believing that they had solved a key problem in the gene therapy field, and further shifted research from retrovirus to lentivirus as a backbone. A decade after the deaths that rocked the field, gene therapy had come roaring back. Trials were in the works throughout the US. Gene therapy had come full circle. And Williams would apply retrovirus, once more, to treat X-SCID, or Bubble Boy patients.

June 29, 2012 was storming in Cincinnati. Nurses carried a cooler full of Jamey's cells across the parking lot toward the hospital. Jennifer Golliday watched from a window. "Nerve-wracking," she said. The wind was gusting. "I kept thinking the cooler was going to blow away." A cluster of nurses' heads and cameras were visible in the hallway window. A head nurse injected a vial of Jamey's cells, which had been edited to now contain the *IL-2* gamma receptor gene, into a central line that fed into his blood stream near his lungs. He was gently napping when the procedure began, which took two minutes. His father Rob cradled him in his arms. His dad was wearing a St. Louis Cardinals jersey. The reintroduced cells had been kept icy cold in a cooler. When they re-entered his body, Jamey's head snapped to attention with sudden curiosity. "The cold startled him awake," Jennifer said.

Five days before, bone marrow had been harvested from Jamey's hip, and enriched in a culture so that a greater proportion of stem cells remained. In fact, these were hematopoietic stem cells, which give rise to blood and immune system cells. Scientists used viruses as tiny pilots to travel to the genome of the stem cells, and install new cargo: the *IL2*-gamma receptor gene, which receives a signal from a protein called interleukin 2, a type of signaling molecule called a cytokine. When microbes and viruses enter the body, they show badges, called antigens, to T-cells. All the adult cells in our bodies are issued correct badges by the body's surveillance community, but pathogenic cells don't have the right badges, they don't have authorization to enter the system. When T-cells pick up on an intruder without the correct credentials, they release *IL2* which stimulates the development of mature T-cells, which in turn, interact with B-cells and mount a system-wide defense. It happens that some of those mature T-cells have memories, keeping track of past intruders and "prime" the immune system. In the event of a future

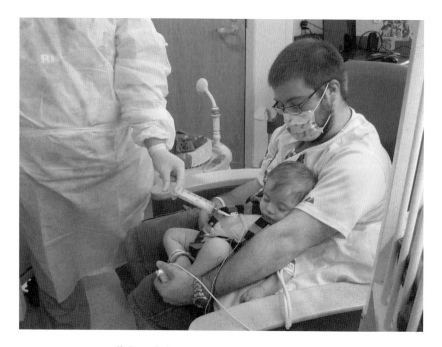

FIGURE 5 Jamey Golliday's father, Rob, held him during a gene therapy procedure. Jameson was born with no immune system, commonly called Bubble Boy disease. Image courtesy of the Golliday family.

invasion, the response is swift. Jamey now had a shiny, new *IL2*-gamma receptor gene. That night, Jennifer slept with him, curled up in his crib. For the first night in a while they fell fast asleep.

Doctors began taking blood samples from Jamey in the weeks that followed to see if they could detect any mature T-cells. But the first few times, they found none. Then a month passed, then another. Finally, a test showed a fledgling count of 13 mature helper T-cells per microliter. Jennifer cheered. Shortly thereafter, the stuffy nose and cold which Jamey had been nursing for a year suddenly disappeared. "It was our first victory," she said. Jennifer felt alone. Other parents had dangerously sick children, but none were treated with gene therapy. "All the other parents had each other. My child was in gene therapy. No one understood what that was." Jamey stayed at the Ronald McDonald House for nine months during his treatment. His mother transported him to the hospital in a "bubble stroller" that she improvised from a baby stroller and a rain tarp.

Tests kept coming back. Jennifer was charting the rise of helper T-cells in Jamey's blood. A year later, in the summer of 2013, his

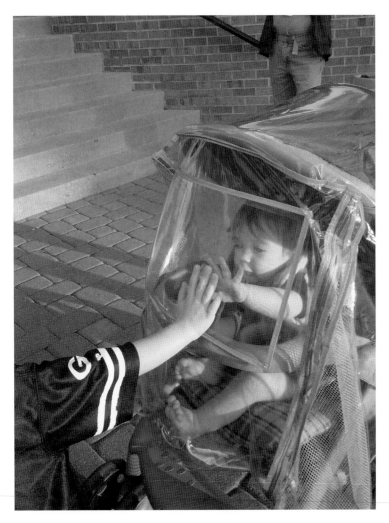

FIGURE 6 Jamey Golliday, then age 2, in an improvised "Bubble stroller," making contact with his older brother Shawn. Image courtesy of the Golliday family.

T-cell count was up to 133 per microliter (healthy adults can have a count of up to 1000, while adult HIV patients go on retrovirals when their count dips below 500, a threshold considered pausing). Jennifer allowed Jamey to remove the mask that he had been wearing, and to play outside in the grass. Yet he wasn't yet allowed to interact with other children, or to use high-contact playground equipment at the park. Williams and colleagues had by now treated two young X-SCID patients from South America at Children's Hospital Boston. An X-SCID child was treated with the new tool at UCLA. Jamey was running free in his backyard, a year after his treatment at Cincinnati Children's. It had been two years since the first applications of the "safer" tool on patients. No leukemia was seen in any of the new X-SCID patients. But in prior trials, leukemia wasn't spotted until the three-year mark.

Jamey had taken to drawing with crayons on the walls inside his house. Jennifer had a degree in psychology, and she pondered what type of career she might want to have in the future. But for now she stayed home. She went for walks and did work in the yard. She picked up crayons. She sanitized counters and washed laundry. And she was waiting for any sign that his immune system was going to restore. She was still waiting, a stay-at-home-family, when I showed up at their front door step in the summer on a hazy afternoon with brush burning in the neighbor's yard.

By mid-afternoon, fly ash continued to fall. It was swirling in the sky, large white fluffy flakes. The saber-fight proceeded through the ashen storm. It was a pitched and pivotal battle, son versus grandfather. The Resistance (Shawn), at last, was confident about its position in the light saber fight against the Dark Side (his grandfather, Warren). Shawn chucked his sword into a tree, and sat down on a swinging chair in the front yard. Just then, Ms. Baird, a preschool teacher who had won his trust, swung by on a walk. Shawn had been oppositional, but now his mother was back from Cincinnati, giving him attention, and he learned Ms. Baird lived nearby. "We didn't even know she lived in the neighborhood," Warren said. Shawn would begin kindergarten in the next month, with Ms. Baird, he said. But "No," his grandfather said, it would be with a new teacher. He sat quietly, now on the bench, thinking about school, and thinking about that. "I'm excited," Shawn said.

"Once we brought the family back together, everything has been OK," Jennifer said, of the situation with Shawn. By the summer 2013, Jennifer had put away the bubble stroller, and let Jamey take off his mask while he was playing in the backyard. He still was not allowed to play with other children, and he couldn't go near playground equipment or high-contact surfaces. Jamey hid his eyes from Ms. Baird when she approached. Jennifer's theory is that he associates most women, except his mom, with nurses, and expects that they will poke him with a needle. He still has a port in his chest, which is used to inject mature IgG antibodies into his system, every few weeks, until his immune system is robust enough to mature them on its own. He hates his port, and he pulled up his Polo shirt and showed me its location, a tiny bump under his collarbone, which takes needle sticks of monoclonal antibodies. Jamey could not yet have vaccines such as an MMR shot, for instance, since it would overwhelm his system. I asked Jennifer if she thought her son should have children, since if he has a daughter, and she has a son (his grandson), the baby would have a 50% change of having X-SCID. "I definitely hope he would have a child, and he can make up his own mind," she told me.

As a child, Jamey was quick to walk, but slow to talk. He liked to draw, and now he and his mom were scribbling on the driveway with hefty pieces of sidewalk chalk. Jamey's T-cell count was now up to 154 cells per microliter, and apparently on a steady rise. He might even start preschool on regular schedule, his father said. Earlier in the afternoon, Jamey had been delivering sticks, leaves and clumps of grass to me, while his mother had pushed the wheelbarrow around the yard, evidently, I suppose, confident that as a male, I wasn't going to stick him with a needle. I let him drop clasps of grass into my hand, but was careful not to touch him. He hadn't yet had any contact with anyone outside his family, even as his mom was feeling more courage as his immune system was restoring, she said. And then, he came back to me once more, and thrust his tiny arm, skyward. "What's he doing?" I asked his mom. "I think he wants to hold your hand," she said.

It was a very brave moment from a mother who had guarded her baby boy from contact with the outside world for more than a year. The gravity of gene therapy began to hit me, and driving out of Illinois, I knew that engineered viruses had enabled him to have contact with me, and that meant that in another year he might be interacting with school children his own age on the playground. Once I got back to Boston, I sent Jennifer a letter and a package which included the book, *Darth Vader and Son*, by Jeffrey Brown. Jennifer and I traded emails and letters over the course of the next three years, as I wanted to check in with her on the status of Jamey and her family. I wrote, again, in March, 2016, and opened up my email box to see her reply.

"He is in preschool now as you know. He is loving it but the transition was hard. He cried when I left him for the first few weeks. Now he is ready to go and excited on school days. He is not afraid of women specifically anymore but he is incredibly shy around adults. When someone talks to him he often will hide his head or move to hide behind my legs. He does improve as he spends more time with someone. And with other children he seems to do just fine. Shawn is in second grade cub scouts and Jamey frequently attends the meetings and runs around and plays with the boys talking and trying to make them laugh. It is great to see and it is hard to stop watching him. The feelings of amazement at how he is doing are pervasive and lead me to spend a lot of time enjoying just watching him be a kid. I'm so grateful that he is able to. He loves ocean animals and space and says he wants to be an astronaut when he grows up. We recently took him to the Science and Industry museum in Chicago and he was fascinated by the real space suit they had on display. I think he could have stayed in that part of the museum all day. We are completely out of isolation. The nurses and doctors no longer wear gloves, gowns, and masks. We are able to take him anywhere and do anything that we want. I never thought this day would come but am so happy that it did.

"Medically he is doing well at last check his CD3 were in the 300's. They have been very stable. So I am not expecting them to go up significantly. The function check shows them functioning well into the normal range. So though his quantity remains low they are of good quality. This winter he has been getting colds frequently, most likely from preschool. None have been very bad and he has not needed any medication or doctor visits to deal with them."

"In the spring, the plan is to go off of IVIG (intravenous immunoglobulin) and test his IGG levels monthly. If they remain stable we can take out his port and start vaccines. I'm crossing my fingers. This is the last medication he is on. It's been four years of slowly testing the waters and getting more comfortable with a new normal as we allowed him more and more freedoms. I am still happy that we chose to go with gene therapy. While his numbers aren't normal, he is still able to live a normal life. We haven't experienced any negative side effects and have had no real issues at all. I don't think I will ever be completely free of worry for him but I am definitely enjoying life with him out of the bubble!"

8   To Summon a Leviathan

> If men are (not) naturally in a state of war, why do they always carry
> arms and why do they have keys to lock their doors?
>
> –Thomas Hobbes, *Leviathan*

It was a rainy October morning. Quiet had fallen on the streets. Students shuffled through soggy, rusty leaves and carried umbrellas, hiking through the pitter-patter of rain. The Perelman School of Medicine at the University of Pennsylvania is the oldest medical school in the US with looming brick and iron gates. Inside the hospital is a tangle of hallways, old laminate tile floors, decades old. Bruce Levine was in his office, his desk plastered with papers. He earned his doctorate from Hopkins, and spent the better part of the 1990s as a postdoc and then a staff scientist with the Naval Medical Research Institute with Carl June. He has silver hair and a steely blue gaze.

Levine is now a collaborator with June, David Porter and Stephan Grupp, who together just a few short years ago emerged on the scene with a radical new strategy to fight cancer. It is exceedingly rare for an event in the cancer world to upend things, to be earth-shaking, to startle peers, to resemble anything that could be called a magic bullet. But June's group has now treated hundreds of patients with pernicious forms of leukemia that had repeatedly come back upon them and exhausted all standard treatment options.

The group was now enrolling patients to try the strategy, called "chimeric antigen receptor" T-cells, or CAR T-cells, on solid tumors of mesothelioma, breast, brain and pancreatic cancer.[377] These solid cancers are harder to treat because they can be wrapped in a sheath of connective tissue called stroma, and cancers of the organs tend to be detected late. Researchers had been deciphering the suite of tricks cancer cells had at their disposal. The immune system and cancer cells are engaged in an arms race, and cancer often wins by locking out the immune system or turning its dials down. CAR T-cells are special forces that can decipher the locks on cancer cells and focus the intensity of the immune system onto the cancer once again. "The past 26 months have been a tipping point," Levine told me. "We've published, others have published; interest has been white hot."

In the 1980s, researchers had learned to engineer viruses as tiny pilots to travel into the nucleus of a cell and install good copies of working genes. The tools had been engineered as synthetic composites of run-of-the-mill viruses, and each of the tiny crafts carried cargo of a human gene. Once it had entered the nucleus, viral-encoded genetic material could insert itself into a chromosome, and thereby install a new gene, popping it in like a cassette tape. Each of these carriages is an "expression cassette" and the cargo it delivers is a "transgene." These genes could be virtually anything. Replace a gene that was defective, or add new synthetic code to life's little instruction book, it was all possible.

But now, researchers at Penn were taking things a step farther. In effect, the team had engineered T-cells to fight cancer by adding a gene that did not exist in nature. It was a gene designed on a computer and then cobbled together, incorporating bits of genetic code from mice, cows and woodchucks and packaged in the delivery vehicle of a disabled HIV virus, which would pilot it into a human T-cell. If "chimera" signifies a new species, a hybrid that did not exist before in nature, in this case, it was a chimeric molecule of DNA. June noted the hodge-podge of code made it a "Rube Goldberg-like solution" and "truly a zoo."[378]

This synthetic gene provided the code to build a receptor on the surface of a T-cell that could guide the immune cell to a unique marker on a cancer cell. In effect, it was a new means to weaponize a patient's own immune cells into a precision-guided strike force. In short, genetically engineered T-cells focus the body's own immune system on a target, calling it to task like a leviathan to fight the cancer. But summoning the wrath of the immune system, and doing it swiftly, can result in a dark and powerful response. Doctors saw it wipe out 3.5 to 7.7 pounds of cancer in a matter of days among three different patients. The deployment of CAR T-cells can also stimulate a cascade of "adverse events" including "cytokine release syndrome," which is an effect of activating T-cells en masse, in effect, sending the immune system into overdrive with cascades upon cascades of cytokines being released, swirling up fevers, a collapse of blood pressure, very rarely, death. Not only that, but patients can be at risk for "tumor lysis syndrome," which is a constellation of metabolic disturbances that can occur when a glut of cancer cells are decimated all at once, spilling out all the breakdown products of dying cells, leading to skyrocketing potassium and phosphorous levels, and plummeting calcium levels, ions, or electrically charged molecules that maintain cellular homeostasis, and their disruption can lead to organ failure.

In 1999, Levine came to Penn, an expert in culturing T-cells on a plate of beads. It was a necessary first step to doing any genetic modification to these cells outside the body, *ex vivo* engineering, since scientists first had to develop protocols to grow a T-cell. Levine had conducted a T-cell trial a few years before, and CAR T-cell trials, which involved the addition of chimeric genes to T-cells to give them a trained targeting power to seek and destroy cancer cells, were tried in collaboration with Cell Genesis around that time. T-cell therapies were an advancing suite of new potential treatments for cancer, and Levine was eager to begin his own trials. But he arrived on campus at the most inauspicious time. The FDA had slammed down a hold on Penn's trials in 2000 due to the revealed dangers of immune reactions to gene therapy which killed one young patient at Penn. CAR T-cells would start appearing in trials, but it would take years for consensus to build around their safety. "The early trials were more hampered by lack of efficacy than anything else," Levine told me. The Dutch scientist C. H. J. Lamers had published the first cancer trials using the technology in 2006, demonstrating minimal efficacy. Levine would publish results by 2011. CAR T-cell therapy appeared to be safe enough to use in patients and gene therapy was on the rebound. Suddenly, things began to move fast.

CAR T-cells mark the emergence of a new breed of one of the oldest and most potent forms of medical treatment, known as "biologics," treatments such as blood transfusions, enzyme replacement, vaccines, antibodies and gene therapies, which make use of nature's spare parts. In fact, the study of antibodies goes back to the 1890s, when Paul Ehrlich hypothesized the existence of a breed of nearly magical proteins, made by human cells, which work as homing devices to search out molecular badges, or antigens, on microbes or viruses.[379] In 1894, Emil Fisher had offered the metaphor that an antibody and its target substrate, or antigen, functioned as a "lock and key." Instructive theory suggested the fusion of antibody to antigen enabled an interaction between an infectious agent and receptors on human immune cells; antibodies emerged formless, achieving their specificity by molding like clay around an antigen they contacted in their environment. This might explain why there was such a stunning suite of diversity of antibodies: simply, they obtained their structure by molding around their target, and then, through a mechanism called "mass action," would rapidly scale up large armies of a specific conformation to bind to the target antigen. If we could learn to manufacture quantities of these antibodies in the lab, scientists realized early on, they could be used to train the immune system on virtually any target. Scientists soon declared that antibodies would be a "magic bullet" to treat all that ails us (a reference to the German folk myth of Der Freischütz). In fact, antibodies turned out to be Y-shaped proteins that come in perhaps one billion forms. How they could be generated in such a stunning variety of epitopes was explained not by instructive theory, but instead by an awakening that cells had an innate knowledge to code for all of them, and in fact did so in small titers.[380] An encounter of a specific antibody with its infectious target led to its rapid, large-scale production. Thus, the differential response of the immune system became selected for and ramped up based on need. In the words of Rockefeller University scientist and Nobel laureate Gerald Edelman, "early explanations of the immune system were that antibodies were 'instructed' whereby an antibody, as it was formed, would fold around the shape of the injected foreign molecule (or antigen)... The idea was beguilingly simple, and it turned out to be wrong."[381] Geneticists would add the insight that antibodies are built by shuffling gene segments. Very powerful secrets lay in our genes.

In the early 1980s, Japanese scientist Susumu Tonegawa had been studying under Renato Dulbecco at the Basel Institute for Immunology. Up until this time, scientists were fascinated at how the human body could produce such a diverse suite of antibodies. B-cells mature in the bone marrow (hence the B) and tout antibodies, while T-cells mature in the thymus (hence the T) and each then circulates through the lymphatic system, hence they are both lymphocytes, one type of leukocyte or white blood cell. Tonegawa showed that regions of DNA can actually "shuffle" to create immune system diversity, for instance, leading to the generation of millions of antibodies. It would become known as V(D)J recombination, otherwise called "somatic recombination," a mechanism of genetic recombination that occurs in the early stages of immuno-globulin and T-cell receptor production. Tonegawa discovered four sets of "gene segments" including Variable, or V (44 kinds), Diverse, or D (27 kinds), Joining, or J (six kinds) and Constant, or C (one kind), which where shuffling or jumping about. In fact, he found that antibodies are composed of light and heavy chains of amino acids. The heavy chains are composed of random combinations of all four of the gene sets VDJC, while the light chains only include VJC. The shuffling of the genes along with a mix of reactions, and the subsequent joining of light and heavy chains, results in a suite of antibody or receptors, which may be on the order of a billion forms or "epitopes."[382]

Tonegawa's explanation of what was happening became one of those events of biology that was stranger than fiction. He suggested the enzymes that eukaryote cells use to carry out this recombination of antibodies were hijacked from microbes! In fact, somatic recombination might have its origins in the transposable elements or "jumping genes," molecules discovered by Barbara McClintock, which hop around chromosomes.[383] Antibody genes make use of an enzyme that is similar to the transposase enzyme that McClintock's mobile elements used to jump and hack into our genomes. Recombination-activating-genes *RAG1* and *RAG2* have a similar sequence to an enzyme called "trans-posase" which McClintock's mobile elements used to chop their way into genomes.[384,385] Once the RAG genes made a double-strand break into antibody gene segments, those segments were repaired back together by the mechanism of "non-homologous end joining," or NHEJ. Our cells repurposed reckless mobile elements, wiring them up with the mechanism of NHEJ, into a cut-and-paste system that could randomly generate a billion varieties of antibodies and receptors on the fly to sense and respond to any pathogen.

Due to the randomness in the shuffling of these gene segments, the immune system was able to diversely encode proteins to match a stun-ning array of antigens from bacteria, viruses, parasites, pollens and tumor cells. These recombined antibody sequences then go through a second step, it was later learned, whereby an enzyme called a deaminase built by a gene named *AICDA* carried out a process whereby it would create a kind of DNA damage on *purpose*, turning a cytosine base into a uracil, which triggered a DNA repair pathway called base excision repair to cause a break in one strand of the double-helix. Because this could happen on both opposing strands, and more bases could be removed through an enzymatic process commonly called "chew back," it could lead to a second double-strand break, and more refinement in the variable gene segment, refining the antibody's epitope, or changing the class of the antibody by switching its constant region in a feat called "class switching." The process was called "activated induced deaminase affinity maturation" or AID.

Researchers began manufacturing "monoclonal antibodies," which were mature forms of antibodies no longer undergoing somatic recombination or affinity maturation, for very specific medical tasks, ramping up their production on their own, in labs and factories. The first antibody was approved for sale by the FDA in 1986, and two decades later about 40 antibodies had been approved by the FDA for sale in the United States. Dartmouth scientist, Tillman Gerngross, started the company GlycoFi, Inc., where he would hijack yeast machinery to complete a delicate step called glycosylation to refine antibodies for use in humans, selling his technology for $400 million in cash to Merck. The mechanism of antibody action had been well clarified. Once arriving at the site of the antigen, antibodies would stick to an agent, tagging it to be disposed by scavenger cells; or else B-cells and other "antigen presenting cells" would lock on the target, and then present the antigen on their cell surface at a site called the "major histocompatibility complex." Helper T-cells would then notice the structure, or "epitope" of the antigen, lock onto the antigen, and then send signals to stimulate the B-cells to rapidly scale up this version of antibody, unleashing the powerful wrath of signaling molecules called cytokines to stir up the immune response. And furthermore, "killer" T-cells would uptake the antigen and carry out a lethal attack on microbes carrying the unauthorized badge. T-cells are white blood cells that orchestrate an immune response through a complex signaling system of hundreds of cytokines, which boost or temper aspects of an immune response. T-cells carry a powerful thwack, but without the precision targeting of the antibodies, they act as rugged storm troopers without much guidance.

Zelig Eshhar, an immunologist at the Weizmann Institute in Israel, came up with a plan to combine the precise targeting of antibodies with the rugged attack power of T-cells. By 1989 he had invented "chimeric antigen receptor T-cells," or CAR-Ts, first describing them as "T-bodies."[386] It was a scrambled virus carrying a brand new human gene. The first applications came as a means to dissect cell signaling. In other words, scientists add a gene to a cell and see how it affects the activity of a suite of other genes and molecular pathways, and also the activity of genes in other cells in the neighborhood. This has been the primary revelation of genetic engineering since the get-go: alter the function and activity of a gene and see what it does to the cellular landscape, and then you know the function of that gene, what it does. But, ideas for therapeutic applications soon emerged. A chimeric gene could be developed that would build a new receptor on T-cells that would mimic the targeting function of antibodies, and would guide those genetically engineered cells to lock on a target, an "antigen" marker on cancerous B-cells. June and Levine, and colleagues elsewhere, would improve CAR T-cells.[387,388] For instance, the initial versions Eshhar developed had been wimpy. They didn't grow up in the context of a biological system, a network of signals that biologists call "cross talk." June in 2003 heard St. Jude pediatric oncologist Dario Campana describe the use of a booster signal, called 4-1BB, which had been under investigation in June's laboratory projects on the nature of T-cell activation.[389] It turned out to be the right motherly voice to get the T-cells to mature.

"Carl and I knew of 4-1BB in the late 90s through our work on T-cell signal transduction (meaning signaling). Campana described the use of 4-1BB in a CAR in a murine (mouse) retroviral vector (retrovirus used to deliver the new gene). Carl June's lab put it in a lentiviral vector and we made it work in humans," Levine told me. June would use lentivirus to install a synthetic gene in T-cells, which would express a chimeric receptor on the surface of T-cells. That receptor would enable the T-cells to seek and destroy cancerous B-cells. Gene therapy was coming into its own, in part due to the "unwieldy, but critically important translational work of Carl June," Mulligan told me. Soon there was a "Patient Number One."

William Ludwig was a 64-year-old retired corrections officer living in Bridgetown, New Jersey in 2010, when he received a near-hopeless cancer prognosis. The Abramson Cancer Center at the University of Pennsylvania had run out of chemotherapeutic options, and Ludwig was disqualified from most clinical trials since he had leukemia, lymphoma and squamous cell skin cancer – three cancers at once. In a later interview, June described Ludwig's condition as most dire. "Almost dead," is how Dr. June described Ludwig.[390]

Alison Loren, an oncologist at Penn, had been taking care of Ludwig for five painful years as he fought cancer. If chemotherapy is not effective early on, each new round brings diminishing returns, and it becomes more and more toxic, she told me. In Ludwig's case, its toxic side-effects were outdoing any progress it was making in scaling back the battalions of cancer cells. By this point, the chemo was suppressing Ludwig's immune system, since it was his immune system's B-cells that were cancerous (technically, chronic lymphoblastic leukemia, or CLL, an uncontrolled expansion of white blood cells in the bone marrow), precisely the cells being targeted by the chemo treatments. An infection from an old chicken pox virus broke out in his right eye. And the cancer now appeared to be mobile, or more technically, what doctors call "motile," riddling far-flung sites in his body. Ludwig's skin cancer looked to Loren as if it had metastasized from his bones. It was about that time when Loren approached her patient to tell him about a new arrow that doctors at Penn had in their quiver. It was an ingenious strategy, and a radical and dangerous one. "William is the most lovely, humble human being," Loren said. "I don't think he realized how groundbreaking this would be at the time. He was almost casual about it. He looked at me, and shrugged, 'I'll give it a shot.'"

Scientists had a means to code a homing device into Ludwig's T-cells. In effect, the plan was to engineer a small population of his T-cells into a lethal security force, a sort of contract law enforcement added to aid the national security forces of his immune system. With the engineered cells added to the fight, scientists said his faltering immune system might be tactical enough to defeat the cancer. It would be a new type of high-tech cancer warfare, one far more mobile, responsive and lethal. The team hoped it would do so with great fury, while not causing extensive collateral damage to his healthy tissue. All of the pieces were in place.

Loren explained the procedure to Ludwig in detail. Blood would be drawn from one of his veins and run through a machine that would separate out from it a portion of T-cells. Those cells would then be edited by sending a virus into them that would travel into the cell nucleuses and install a synthetic gene at a random spot in his genome. That engineered gene would code a protein to build a receptor that would enable the T-cells to recognize certain chemical markers on Ludwig's cancerous B-cells, giving them a precision guidance system. The doctored cells would then be returned to his blood, and then, hopefully, they would go on the attack. There was a chance that his immune system would go into overdrive, and there was a chance that the edited T-cells wouldn't have the potency expected. The medical team just really couldn't be sure what would happen. And, Loren said, just one caveat: it had never been tried before. So it was that William Ludwig became known, for a time, as Patient Number One. He was checked into the hospital on July 31, 2010 as the very first patient to have the genome of his T-cells edited with a new chimeric gene. For a few days, nothing spectacular happened. He had a second infusion. But then, 10 days later, before the third and final infusion, things broke into all-out chaos. Ludwig's whole body shook. His heart rate shot up, his blood pressure collapsed. He had a fever. "I was put into intensive care. I wasn't supposed to survive," Ludwig recalled. The nurses didn't know it then, but his T-cells were killing the cancer. "A cytokine storm," Loren told me. "The engineered T-cells were 'engrafting' in the body, meeting up with target antigens, and unleashing a whirlwind of cytokines." Those signaling molecules were firing up the immune system, stirring fevers and opening up capillaries so immune cells could rush through the highways of the blood stream to reach the targets. If the immune system has been primed to a target by exposure to a similar type antigen earlier in life, then a storm can be especially intense. But, Loren said, "We now know from watching many patients that a strong immune response means the therapy is working." The storm that Ludwig was thrown into was counted in hours, but with intensity an order of magnitude beyond which most of us experience in our worst case of the flu. And just as quickly as it began, the storm was over.

Almost a month had passed, and clinicians came into Ludwig's hospital room on a Tuesday to ask for a bone marrow sample to test for cancer. "It's not very pleasant, and I'm a tough person to ask for a bone marrow sample," Ludwig told me. He reluctantly agreed. "Bill doesn't love them," Loren confessed, regarding the draw of bone marrow biopsy. Loren pierced his hip bone with a needle and drew a cord of bone marrow about 1 to 2 centimeters long, and resembling a coffee stirrer, also about a tablespoon of aspirate, a liquid that would demonstrate the composition of cells in circulation in the body, and then set forth to the lab. Bone marrow biopsies that are healthy include a balance of red blood cells, platelets and immune cells, hodgepodge cells that belong to the "hematopoietic" family of cells. The marrow is well balanced. By comparison, marrow that is cancerous is dominated by one cell type, "sheets and sheets" of lymphocytes, Loren said.

On August 31, Loren peered under the microscope. "It just didn't seem possible," she said. There were no sheets of cancer cells in the bone marrow. She had seen the striated layers of sheets under the same microscope, just a month ago. Two days later, the hospital people came back into Ludwig's room and asked him for a second bone marrow sample. On September 3, Loren was peering back under the microscope at that second sample. No sheets. "I couldn't believe it. This type of thing doesn't happen in medicine," Loren told me. She peeked into Ludwig's room the next week. "Can you believe it? The staff mixed up the samples and I had to repeat the bone marrow test," Ludwig complained, grumpily. "Not so," Loren chided. "The first draw wasn't a great sample. It was diluted with blood. We really didn't think the first test was correct," Loren said. "Honestly. We didn't know what to say. William, there is no more cancer in your body."

Loren remained circumspect. Months passed. "We kept waiting for the other shoe to drop," she told me. A year after his treatment, Ludwig leaned over to Loren, and prompted her. "Alison, why don't you ever say that I'm cured?" Loren explained to him that definitions for a cure, for say, treating cancer with a bone marrow transplant, are based on decades of research, hundreds of patients, mountains of data. "William," she told him. "You're the only one."[391]

A small population of mercenary cells appeared to have defeated the cancer. But that cell population might not last forever. I asked Ludwig what will happen when the small troop of cells finally die out. In other words, what will happen when the synthetic security forces pull out and leave only the national security forces to defend the body? Would it be a strong enough defense system. Or could the cancer return? "That was the first question we all asked," he said. "No one knows."

June estimated his genetically engineered T-cells had wiped out two pounds of cancer in Ludwig in less than a month. "Drugs don't do that," June told a reporter at the time. June's group had shown it could harness the immune system to the task of fighting cancer. The gambit worked in trials. Soon there was a Patient Number Two, and then, a Patient Number Three. Within a few years, hundreds of patients' saw their bodies cleared of cancers, in a stunning display of the tool. June's group at the University of Pennsylvania and colleagues at the Children's Hospital of Philadelphia were reporting jaw-dropping success in the use of CAR-Ts to treat acute lymphoblastic leukemia, a childhood cancer. Emily Whitehead, age 7, of Philadelphia and Avery Walker, 10, of Redmond, Oregon were splashed all over the pages of major newspapers. "Young cancer patient's good news: 'Total remission!'" trumpeted the *Philadelphia Inquirer*. "In Girl's Last Hope, Altered Immune Cells Beat Leukemia," declared *The New York Times*. Not all of the cancer patients had responded. And no one knew why gene therapy threw some patients, like Ludwig, into violent convulsions and tremors, and why some patients responded only with a slight fever. Emily Whitehead, then age 7, had the same procedure to treat childhood leukemia, and her body reacted so violently to the gene therapy treatment that it truly almost killed her. But days later, the fever was gone, and so was her cancer. Avery Walker, also had the treatment. "We were all waiting for the big storm," her father Aaron Walker, told the *Philadelphia Inquirer*.[392] But she only obtained a slight fever.

Loren was beguiled. June's group was developing the strategy to try on a number of solid tumors, cancers including mesothelioma, breast, brain and pancreatic cancer.[393] These new strategies were enabled by rapidly developing technology. For instance, all B-cells have the CD19 cell surface marker, so deploying a CAR T-cell to attack the cancerous B-cells meant that doctors would also target the healthy B-cells, wiping those out, too. CAR T-cells were now being tweaked so that their receptors had a stronger binding affinity to markers that were over-expressed, or more prevalent to cancer cells, so that those cancer cells could be preferentially targeted. In one study, scientists at Penn showed they could develop CAR T-cells with high affinities to cell surface targets ErbB2 and *EGFR*, which are "amplified," or highly expressed on cancer cells such as breast cancer, and "are also expressed, at lower levels by normal tissues." By "affinity tuning" the receptors, they could deploy the CAR T-cells to target the cells which are cancerous and have higher representation of these cell surface markers, and virtually ignore the healthy cells with lower levels of these ubiquitous markers. Emerging research sought to train CAR T-cells "cancer-specific" markers.

Gene therapy's transition from an obscure set of techniques to treat rare orphan diseases, into a tool that could be applied to cancer, meant that it was primed to draw big bucks investment. And yet, this ground-swell of investment contributed to new competitive pressures, lawsuits and ethical questions. In February 2014, Renier Brentjens at Memorial Sloan-Kettering Cancer Center reported 14 of 16 adults with relapsed ALL, or acute lymphoblastic leukemia, had responded to the treatment. At the National Cancer Institute, Daniel "Trey" Lee reported in October 2014 that 14 of 21 child patients who had relapsed for ALL were in complete remission. Novartis, Juno, Kite and Bluebird Bio were among the tech companies seeking to develop the therapies commercially. By the end of 2015, more than 250 people had been treated with the CAR T-cell approach. Novartis paid $12.25 million to Juno Therapeutics to resolve a tense three-year patent battle for the rights to commercialize technology related to CAR T-cells. Novartis had licensed CAR T-cell technology from Penn and Juno had licensed from St. Jude Children's Research Hospital. Since then, Juno has discontinued clinical trials.

Three years later, Ludwig was chatting-it-up at his neighbor's house when I telephoned him on a lark on a Sunday afternoon. I assumed he was doing fine, but was he? "I'm no spring chicken, but I think I'm doing well for someone my age," he said. He had an atypical skin growth, a chronic cough, a sinus infection, a puddle of fluid at the bottom of his lungs, a virus in his right eye and bad heart burn. He gobbled down six Prilosec a day, a drug used to treat acid reflux disorder. But something he didn't have was cancer. He just returned from an RV trip to New York City with his wife and two grandkids, and was bound for the Adirondacks. "Being Patient Number One is overwhelming to think about sometimes," Ludwig said. "I knew my days were numbered. I had nothing to lose." His wife stuck with him for more than a decade as he fought it, "a spectacular person," he told me. Not more than a week later, Ludwig and his wife were driving the RV to Cooperstown with another couple to watch baseball. The verdant summer was upon them, the windows rolled down, the couples in their shirt sleeves, coasting on the old highways of upstate New York, clear and starlit.

In January 2016, Vice-President Joe Biden swung by Penn and shook hands with Carl June and Bruce Levine, announcing that Penn would be a keystone site for launching a new "moonshot" initiative to cure cancer. "For Biden, the emotional undertones of his mission are difficult to avoid," *The Associated Press* reported. "After his 46-year-old son, Beau Biden, died from brain cancer in May, Biden entered a period of painfully public mourning, followed eventually by his decision not to enter the presidential race."

The moonshot was not launched without criticism. Public skepticism on cancer cures has run deep. Richard Nixon initiated the "War on Cancer," while introducing the National Cancer Act in 1971, which set national priorities, schedules and funding apparatus to focus on a cure for cancer, but scientists at the time had underestimated the diversity of genetic variants that cause cancer and how truly disparate the disease is in etiology and molecular tricks. By 2012, whispers of concern circulated through the halls of academia and industry when Amgen published its review of cancer studies in leading journals and found that results of only 6 out of 53 papers could actually be replicated.[394] The genetic drivers of cancer initiation and progression were emerging as disparate and context dependent. Most conservative estimates suggest that eight to ten key mutations must occur in a cell in order for a cancer to begin, but as cancer cells progress, they incur as many as 10000 mutations and all sorts of chromosomal rearrangements.[395] Most of these "passenger mutations" have nothing to do with the mechanisms of cancer and therefore confound research findings by masquerading as molecular underpinnings of a cancer.

In 1971, Alfred Knudson codified his idea, called the "two-hit hypothesis," which suggested the loss-of-function mutations in both copies of the same gene were required to initiate the start of at least one type of childhood cancer of the eye, called retinoblastoma. Knudson's study was developed based on the theory that some children inherited one of the mutations, and incurred the other in their development; other children incurred both mutations during development, as so-called *de novo* mutations. But basically, his idea was that if there was at least one functioning copy of a protective gene, the cancer wouldn't develop.[396] Robert Weinberg would later clarify the function of a gene called *RB* (which is shorthand for "mutated in retinoblastoma") as the first "tumor suppressor" gene, which accounted for lifting the breaks off a normally tightly regulated cell cycle. In his book, *The Biology of Cancer*, which is now the cancer bible which most students (including me) have been assigned, Weinberg also talks about discovering the first "oncogene" Ras, which participates in what we call mitogenic signalling, or promoting cell division. Whereas a tumor suppressor is a brake, an oncogene is a gas pedal.

Getting to the root of cancer has captured much of our recent focus, and the cancer "stem cell hypothesis" has suggested that a small population of slippery, amorphous stem cells actually give rise to the growth and spread of a cancer.[397] It has long been known that cancer cells undergo a program of dedifferentiation, and lose the specification of adult cells, becoming more innocent and naive, undergoing a process called EMT, or epithelial to mesenchymal transition. This transition is thought to bestow ability for enhanced migration and propagation, but it has also suggested that stem cells may already have the properties that make them closest to cancer cells. Weinberg and Eric Lander co-founded the company Verastem, Inc. to create a lead compound to target cancer stem cells, but by the spring of 2016, their compound failed and the public stock was worth about one dollar.

Cancer cells also rely on escape mechanisms, which we call "checkpoint blockade" mechanisms, which allow them to escape or avoid the immune surveillance of the body (more on that soon) and they alter their energy use. Our cells use two mechanisms to generate energy in a molecular form called ATP, one of which is oxidative phosphorylation, and the other anaerobic glycolysis, which makes use of glucose, or blood sugar, to create energy without oxygen. The German scientist Otto Warburg noticed that cancer cells undergo a shift to glycolysis even in the presence of oxygen, which became called the "Warburg effect," which is a predominant attribute of cancer cells. In fact, new emphasis has been placed on the genes, including one called *AKT*, which drives the effect of changes to energy production in cancer cells. "The protein created by AKT is part of a chain of signalling proteins that is mutated in up to 80 percent of all cancers," noted a recent newspaper article. Craig

Thompson, president and chief executive of Memorial Sloan Kettering Cancer Center, "discovered he could induce the 'full Warburg effect' simply by placing an activated AKT protein into a normal cell."[398] In 1997, Chi Van Dang, director of the Abramson Cancer Center at the University of Pennsylvania, showed that *MYC*, one of the most widely cited oncogenes, also "targets an enzyme that can turn on the Warburg effect."[399]

Agios Pharmaceuticals, a company co-founded by Thompson, is testing a drug that inhibits mutated versions of the metabolic enzyme IDH 2, which also has a role in altered energy metabolism in a cancer cell.[400] In December 2015, Bradley Bernstein of the Broad Institute published a paper in *Nature*, describing how brain tumors grow so fast.[401] Gliomas are the most common type of brain tumor, and the researchers showed that 80 percent of low- and moderate-grade gliomas have a mutation in the gene called *IDH*, for isocitrate dehydrogenase, which has a role in metabolism, or energy production. When the gene was mutated, it caused the cancer cells to take on a lot of epigenetic markers called methylation groups, which can weaken or even silence the expression of a gene. In effect, Bernstein found that the added methylation tags were, in turn, impairing a gene called *CTCF* that builds walls within a coiled DNA strand, which would be more than six feet long if unpacked from a cell and stretched out into its full length. Instead, the DNA is compact and scrunched together, and separated by the *CTCF* walls. But without the walls to segregate its parts, different genomic regions can come to interact with each other. For instance, this "unwalling" of the genome, resulted in a gene called *PGDFRA*, which makes cells grow and is seldom turned on, to come under control of other, adjacent genetic regions which keep it on in perpetuity. Thus, the brakes of this cell growth gene are removed, and the cancer cells grow like gangbusters. "What this tells me is that I know a lot less than I did before," Jeremy Rich, a brain expert at the Cleveland Clinic told *The New York Times*.[402]

In fact, research tells us that "calorie restriction" can do wonders for prognosis in the aftermath of cancer treatment. Restricting excess fats and sugars can not only starve cancer cells, but shift the body into a mode of ketosis, where it begins to fuel itself from old cellular debris, in effect living off old junk and storage. Crispr may be able to perturb many small genetic mutations, and allow scientists to learn more about the causes of cancer. It may also allow them to cause mutations in cancer cells on purpose to learn not only how a cancer starts, but how it can be weakened or defeated. But cancer cells are notoriously heterogeneous, meaning that their molecular and genetic alterations are often highly diverse, while multiple cancers may look highly similar at the level of biopsy. Levi Garraway at The Broad Institute is among those who are studying melanoma drug resistance. Melanoma cells with *BRAF* mutations which can be killed with a drug in treatment express genes in a pathway that contains the gene *MITF*, a master regulator of melanocytes, while other melanoma cells express a different program, under regulatory control of a gene called *AXL*. Anyone with cancer who has tried to enrol in an experimental trial knows that such trials are becoming increasingly selective, and that they almost always come with a prerequisite of screening for specific genetic variants. A drug in a trial may only work for selective forms of a cancer, those with a specific genetic mutation or alteration in a molecular pathway. About a decade ago, Garraway's work led to founding, along with Eric Lander and others, the company Foundation Medicine, Inc. which provides next generation sequencing of genomes from cancer patients to enable a more precise enrolment in trials and treatment strategies.

The use of "precision medicine" as a stepping stone to cancer treatment has been coming under increasing attack. Andrew Porterfield wrote in a blog for the Genetic Literacy Project, "Most people die because of cancer cells that break off from primary tumors, and settle in other parts of the body. This process of metastasis is responsible for 90 percent of cancer deaths. However, only 5 percent of European government cancer research funds, and 2 percent of U.S. cancer research funds, are earmarked for metastasis research." James Watson, whose description of the double helix in 1953 helped to usher in an age of molecular biology's gene-focused approach to cancer, told a newspaper reporter "that locating the genes that cause cancer has been 'remarkably unhelpful'– the belief that sequencing your DNA is going to extend your life 'a cruel illusion' suggesting that biochemistry was more important than genetics to interpreting cancer."[403] In fact, Watson has at times gone on offense at the seduction of using precision medicine in a new "genetics age" to treat cancer. In 2015, he went as far as publishing a "manifesto" declaring that, "The now much-touted genome-based personal cancer therapies may turn out to be much less important tools for future medicine than the newspapers of today lead us to hope. Sending more government cancer monies towards innovative, anti-metastatic drug development to appropriate high-quality academic institutions would better use National Cancer Institute's (NCI) monies than the large sums spent now testing drugs for which we have little hope of true breakthroughs. The biggest obstacle today to moving forward effectively towards a true war against cancer may, in fact, come from the inherently conservative nature of today's cancer research establishments."[404] Watson is not alone in arguing against using specific molecular compounds to treat cancer.

"Cancer isn't space travel," wrote Jarle Breivikmay, a professor of medicine at the University of Oslo, in a blunt op-ed cautioning against hyperbole of the $1 billion moonshot program. "The growing cancer epidemic is not a problem that medical science is about to solve. In fact, it is a problem we are about to make worse. The better we get at keeping people alive, the older they will get, and the more cancer there will be in the population." He rightly notes that "the current optimism stems from recent breakthroughs in the field of immunotherapy. This ability to direct immune cells to seek out and eliminate cancer cells is an astonishing scientific accomplishment and a 'moon landing' in its own right." But cancer is closely linked to aging and "all of our cells, including those that make up the immune system, are subject to aging. We are essentially temporary cell colonies evolved to relay life to the next generation, and as long as we are human, there will always be another cancer." Even those we miraculously cure, Breivikmay notes, "even if they are cured, they live on with an increased risk of getting cancer again."[405]

The few stunning success stories today seem to be suggesting that tools like the dispatch of suites of CAR T-cells, or other cell-based treatments such as "cell-linking moieties," which can train the immune system on surface markers of the cancer cell, are coming to dominate the field in surprising ways. In June 2016, an advisory committee at the NIH approved a proposal for the first human trial using Crispr. Edward Stadtmauer, who was set to lead the trial at Penn, still had to convince US regulators and officials at his home institution to move forward. Carl June told *Nature* that he expected the trial to begin by the end of 2017. In *Nature*, Sara Reardon reported: "The researchers will remove T-cells from 18 patients with several types of cancers and perform three Crispr edits on them. One edit will insert a gene for a protein engineered to detect cancer cells and instruct the T-cells to target them, and a second edit removes a natural T-cell protein that could interfere with this process. The third gene that is being knocked out in the very first human Crispr trial we can identify as Programmed Death (or a gene named "*PD-1*", which we will discuss in the next chapter): it will remove the gene for a protein that identifies the T-cells as immune cells and prevent the cancer cells from disabling them." Immunotherapy was a vaunted new approach that was quickly making in-roads in surprising new ways, in one instance, by treating brain cancer with a stripped down poliovirus. Glioblastoma multiform, among other tumors, include widespread expression of a poliovirus receptor named *CD155*. The gene *CD155* builds a protein on the epithelial cells, a general-purpose cell which lines the cavities and organs, and this protein itself is a component at a junction or bridge between these cells. It is also the doorway by which poliovirus has found a way to slip into cells. Strangely, many types of cancer cells express *CD155* inappropriately, or "ectopically," meaning a gene is turned on in a context where it is not programmed or designed to come on. The coincidence is so striking it almost appears to be an instance of co-evolution, the poliovirus providing an advantage to mankind in the case of cancer, while it also exerts it pathogenic effects. Strikingly, an engineered form of poliovirus which has been stripped of its pathogenic elements has been shown to alert the immune system to the presence of cancer.[406,407,408] By the spring of 2016, the use of poliovirus to treat brain cancer swept through the news.

"Early tests at Duke University have been so successful the FDA will fast track this treatment to hundreds of patients while it's still being evaluated for final approval," declared the journalist Scott Ridley on a CBS broadcast. "The therapy is audacious. It uses the poliovirus to attack a virulent brain cancer called glioblastoma – which is a death sentence of astonishing speed that leaves patients with only months to live."[409] While some scientists had been using HIV, a lentivirus, to create CAR T-cells, these scientists at Duke had been using the poliovirus to awaken the immune system to attack a cancer. It had nothing to do with personalized medicine or genetic diagnostics.

Duke's polio team includes Darell Bigner, director of the Tisch Brain Tumor Center at Duke, molecular biologist Matthias Gromeier, immunologist Smita Nair, and neuro-oncologists Henry Friedman, Annick Desjardins and Gordana Vlahovic. "I thought he was nuts. I mean I really thought that what he was using is a weapon that produces paralysis," Friedman told CBS, about his initial inclination to Gromeier's idea of using polio to awaken the immune system to fight a brain cancer. The poliovirus, as it turns out, binds to a receptor that is found on the surface of cancer cells in most kinds of solid tumor. The trick the Duke scientists pulled was to create a genetically engineered form of poliovirus, called PVS-RIPO, by removing the poliovirus' disease-causing ability by splicing in the genetic code of a rhinovirus, which causes the common cold. According to their website up at Duke, "the receptor for poliovirus (which is used for cell entry) is abnormally present on most tumor cells." Once inside the tumor, the genetically engineered poliovirus infects and kills cancer cells. "Although this tumor cell killing alone may have tumor-fighting results, the likely key to therapy with PVS-RIPO is its ability to recruit the patients' immune response against the cancer... The human immune system is trained to recognize virus infections and, thus, responds vigorously to the infected tumor."

Thirty-eight patients volunteered for Duke University's experiment to use the poliovirus to kill glioblastoma, but the scientists noted on their website that they were planning to rapidly mobilize a Phase II/III trial, and that, given the ability of poliovirus to target virtually any solid state tumor, they had begun investigating its use in treatment of other than brain cancers. In the laboratory, Duke has used the poliovirus to kill cancer cells of the skin, pancreas, stomach, lung, colon and prostate.

In the CBS report, Nair told the journalists that, teasing apart tumors in the lab "what we found were a lot of T-cells in the tumor." This suggested that an immunization with poliovirus might work as a cancer vaccine. "Once immune cells are programmed to recognize a cancer, will they remember and attack the cancer everywhere in the body for a lifetime?" the journalist Scott Pelley asked. Nair responded "if you get a tumor again, these are memory T-cells, they will remember that. And they can eliminate a recurrent or a metastatic tumor."[410]

The CBS segment profiled patients in the glioblastoma trial, including Nancy Justice, 58, and Stephanie Lipscomb, who was a nursing student when she began having headaches. "It's a hell of a thing to be told that you have months to live when you're 20 years old," she told the reporter, on her reaction when a doctor told her she a brain tumor the size of a tennis ball. "So we treated her in May. Then in July the tumor looked bigger, looked really inflamed. I got really concerned, got really worried," Desjardins said. The doctors considered halting the treatment, but Stephanie objected. "Five months after her infusion, an MRI showed the tumor only *looked* worse because of inflammation caused by Stephanie's immune system which had awakened to the cancer for the first time and gone to war," Pelley's transcript read. "It appears the polio starts the killing but the immune system does most of the damage." But, by now, her immune system was awakened, summoned like a leviathan to the task of wiping out her brain cancer.

"Stephanie's tumor shrank for 21 months until it was gone."

On June 21, 2016, Carl June, Joseph Melenhorst and Edward Stadtmauer, three doctors from the University of Pennsylvania, stood before the NIH's Recombinant DNA Advisory Committee, or RAC, as it is known. All three were wearing dark blue suit jackets, but June had a red tie. Melenhorst is tall with self-assured reflection that is nearly risible. Stadtmauer is shorter with a mustache. June is stoic, dignified and yet almost gaunt, as if he has given every ounce he had to fighting cancer, basically nonstop since the 1970s.

The RAC is a pensive sort of inquisition. It's the closest thing to a council of elders that I know of, a panel of experts, scientists and ethicists, who dare to think out loud, a "ponderous" regulatory agency, as Maxine Singer once called it. It's quaint in a sort of way, but it also feels a little bit dangerous, like the conversation could go in absolutely any direction, like a paper airplane flying through the room. Laurie Zoloth, a bioethicist from Northwestern University, Mildred Cho, an ethicist from Stanford, and Lainie Ross, an ethicist and medical doctor at the University of Chicago, were grilling the three doctors. "This is a really exciting moment for the RAC and for the study team," Zoloth noted. "This is the first in-human use of Crispr and the reason for all of the anxiety for how to name it, and what to call it, and how to write the consent form for patients who are taking part in a trial that takes a significant change."

The first human trial using Crispr would rely on a genetically engineered T-cell, but not technically a CAR T-cell, which Penn had licensed
to Novartis. Ross was up in arms that June and some doctors at Penn
might be brushing up against a conflict of interest, since they had
financial interests at stake to see genetically engineered T-cells work,
and hence might have an unconscious bias to take more risks. June
noted that the proposal he had in mind did not, again, make use of a
CAR T-cell, but it did not seem like enough assurance for Ross. Penn,
she noted, had an "infamous history" with gene therapy trials which
were influenced by financial stakes. She was, of course, referring to the
Jesse Gelsinger case, which resulted in the first gene therapy death at
Penn. The RAC spent more than an hour talking about Gelsinger. And
then they talked about it some more. They talked it into the ground.
Penn was the birthplace of gene therapy, and the place where it sum-
marily went into retrenchment.

But, at the same time, Penn has maintained the most sophisticated
apparatus for engineering and scaling up gene therapy trials in the
United States. They are still the best. The trial would enroll up to 18
people to treat relapsed and refractory forms of melanoma, sarcoma and
myeloma, from three centers including Penn, MD Anderson and University of California at San Francisco. All of the manufacturing would be
done at Penn. Speaking to doing both the manufacturing and enrollment
at Penn, Ross said, "I think not only do you have a conflict of interest,
but you're doubling down on your conflict of interest." There was a
static silence in the room. If you listen closely to the tape, you can barely
hear Carl June respond – a mutter – "point taken."

There is more silence. The RAC is not so nice. Cho points out that in
a Crispr trial, patients can't withdraw from a trial, since they have
genomes of a portion of their cells permanently modified. And so that
creates a long-term obligation for the study designers. Zoloth is
hammering the scientists that they are not paying for housing or auxil-
iary cancer treatments for the patients. Ross points out that insurance
may not cover the complete treatment, and they both agree on the spot
that it proportionately benefits wealthier patients. The RAC is perplexed about "off-target effects," which is what happens when Crispr
is deployed and hits an unexpected genomic target and causes an unin-
tentional edit. The Penn scientists explain they tried their method in
cells in a lab and found only one such unintended edit in 148 of their

tests. Off-target effects can never be totally eliminated, since everyone has a unique genome, and there is always a possibility of an idiosyncratic genetic region that is highly similar to the one which you are trying to edit. The experts on the RAC think about this, without knowing exactly what to make of it.

At the end of a very long day, the RAC votes nearly unanimously, with a few abstentions, to approve Penn's proposal for the first human trial using Crispr. Stadtmauer, who was set to lead the trial, still had to convince US regulators and officials at his home institution to move forward. But June told a reporter at *Nature* that he expected the trial to begin by the end of 2017. It was a day of rapprochement between Penn and the RAC, a new moment, and it truly had the weight of new page turning. It was symbolic in that way.

A scientist named Lloyd J. Olds had discovered a protein called NY-ESO-1 which served as an antigen or marker on the surface of many types of cancer cells. It turns out that this protein is not expressed in adult cells in humans, but cancer cells ectopically express it, meaning they begin to express this protein when they should not. Olds and other scientists learned that they could even vaccinate patients with fragments of this protein, and sometimes the immune system would notice it as a "damage associated molecular pattern," and begin to go on attack and fight the cancer cells. In other words, they were introducing it on purpose as a cancer vaccine. The Penn scientists wanted to take this intelligence a step further. They would remove a patient's T-cells and genetically engineer them to express a protein called an NY-ESO-1 receptor, meaning the T-cells would be equipped with a receptor that would sense and focus the T-cells onto cancer cells which expressed this NY-ESO-1 antigen.

The scientists said they would use a lentivirus to insert the gene for this NY-ESO-1 receptor into the T-cells and put it under a constitutive promoter, meaning one that was constantly turned on, called *EF1*. Lentivirus was a safer virus to use as a cargo plane to ship a transgene into a cell. The field had shifted from using retrovirus that Richard Mulligan had engineered in the 1980s to using lentivirus. June explained that there was a problem with adding an NY-ESO-1 receptor to T-cells. It would sometimes create "mixed dimers," or crazy new fusions and adhesions with the normal receptors on the surface of T-cells. That was one reason the scientists wanted to use Crispr-Cas9. They would use it to snip out and disable the natural T-cell receptor, or TCR, so that it would not interfere and bind with the transgenic NY-ESO-1 receptor, also a form of T-cell receptor, they planned to install. In this way, the scientists "could achieve brighter expression of the transgenic TCR," June told the RAC. Secondly, they planned to use Crispr-Cas9 to disable a gene called Programmed Death, or *PD-1*, which was expressed on the surface of T-cells and which cancer cells could activate to kill off the T-cells. Disabling *PD-1* was a defensive move.

What we were about to experience was a watershed moment. Crispr would be used for the very first time in humans. Laurence Cooper, a scientist at MD Anderson had been the first to create a genetically engineered CAR T-cell using an older technology called a "zinc finger nuclease." Now things were moving much faster, ever since Crispr-Cas9 had been fully elucidated by Doudna and Charpentier and colleagues in 2012. It was easier to make gene edits. Penn was in the vanguard, genetically engineering T-cells by altering them with Crispr-Cas9, editing cells in their factories and changing how we do medicine, as we began to contemplate the beginning of the "industrial revolution of the human genome." June was no angel. He had drawn heavily on the work of Dario Campana, and was a competitive man of industry, a Henry Ford of biology. And over the years he stood to profit. But seeing June and the other scientists from Penn standing before the RAC after so many cataclysmic moments, so much grinding bench work, so many false starts and blind alleys, I had to admit, there is something powerful when someone continues to show up and register their presence. And there was Carl June, standing, with his hat in his hand.

9   A Molecular Fairytale

> I want to change the calendars to April 25, 1953.
>
> – RJ Kirk, indicating his desire to change the year 1953 to Year 0,
> resetting calendars to suggest the date of the discovery of the
> structure of DNA by James Watson and Francis Crick, and later
> deciphering the code of its scripture, surpassed the significance
> of biblical scripture.

"Humans don't molt," RJ Kirk tells me. Kirk, 62, is a self-made billionaire who runs his offices out of West Palm Beach, Florida, a balmy land of pelicans and tangled mangroves. He built his fortune on conventional small molecule medications that can be taken as a pill, and I phoned to talk about his newest endeavors in biotech, the most interesting to me being a gene switch for gene therapy. A gene transferred into a human cell would only be expressed if the patient took the pill, establishing an important safety control. Strangely, the system was developed from a molting system in insects. Kirk had offered to fly me down to his estate in Florida to talk with him in person. I was writing a story on his company for *Scientific American* and I asked the editors if it was OK to accept the trip. It is easier to ask for forgiveness than permission – that is the short explanation of how I ended up scheduling a phone interview with Kirk at a Starbucks on a winter afternoon at the end of 2014. I was on the second floor of a hotel at Kendall Square next to The Broad Institute. Snow was halfway melted on the grass outside. I had a damp, drizzly November in my soul, a dwindling hope of achieving any sort of momentary happiness as the six months of overcast in Boston began to set in. His home, wrote Andrew Pollack in *The New York Times*, is "on a narrow stretch of land, has property extending from the Atlantic Ocean to the Intracoastal Waterway. He also keeps a residence in the Four Seasons Hotel in San Francisco and owns a 7,200-acre cattle farm near Radford, VA, where he used to raise falcons, hawks, owls and eagles, tramping through the woods to roust squirrels and rabbits that the birds would eat."[411]

Kirk is self-taught in biology, excelling to the extent that he quickly rose to be a singular force in biotechnology, as his investment firm Third

Security became exceptionally adept at scouting out the prey of emerging technologies. In 1998, Tom Reed, a molecular geneticist, along with his wife Jackie, had founded Intrexon – drawing inspiration for the company's name from introns and exons – as a means to provide constructs for genetically engineered mice. Third Security had begun sinking investment into Intrexon, and by 2004, moved the company to Blacksburg, VA as it grew up to more than 750 employees, filing an IPO in 2013. Kirk thinks of himself as a simple country lawyer, and a falconer who often retreats to his land in Virginia. But he spends much of his time with Reed as they run the company's work out of offices in West Palm Beach.

There is something about the air in Florida in the winter, its balm, its lightness, its lift. I have been there many times. Someone just being on the telephone in Florida lifted my spirits. It reminded me that a place called Florida actually exists. I asked Kirk about this gene switch his company had. I wanted to know how it worked. I wasn't expecting to hear about bugs. But the molting process, in which a growing insect builds a new exoskeleton to replace an old one that no longer fits, turns out to have some very important properties that can be adapted to make gene therapy, still a largely experimental procedure, safer.[412]

Doctors would like to deliver extra copies of working genes to people to treat a variety of hereditary ills. Genes provide cells with the instructions or code for manufacturing proteins or sometimes other compounds, and so inserting a functional gene into the body can, in theory, provide a lasting supply of whatever missing molecules a patient might need. But gene therapy has had a troubled history, in part because scientists cannot precisely control where a new gene inserts into a cell's DNA and how active it is (which determines how much protein is produced) once there. These problems can lead to unwanted side effects – including the development of malignant tumors. A logical solution to the problem of having proteins made in undesirable places and amounts would be to combine a therapeutic gene with a switch that could reliably turn it on or off as needed. As it happens, says Kirk – who is the chairman and chief executive officer of Intrexon – insects routinely use just such a switch to control molting. Here's the thing. Insects do not just sort of molt, starting and then stopping part way; they either do it or they don't. The suite of genes that drive the molting program must be turned off until the time is right. The gene that interests Kirk serves as the master switch for all this activity. It codes for a hormone called ecdysone. As ecdysone surges through the insect, it turns on a raft of other genes to start building the new exoskeleton. After the new exoskeleton is ready, the insect discards the old one. Once molting is nearing completion, the levels of ecdysone fall to zero – at which point the genes turn off again. Importantly, from Intrexon's point of view, the switch is airtight when turned off – in the absence of ecdysone, the genes for molting remain inactive. The scientists at the company realized that they could take advantage of this foolproof characteristic to tightly control any genes transplanted into people.

Imagine equipping each replacement gene with a biological switch that turns on – and thus activates the therapeutic gene – only in the presence of ecdysone molecules that have been adapted to work with human physiology. Patients given low doses of this activating drug (technically known as a ligand), could turn on only a few copies of the new gene, thus producing low amounts of whatever compounds were encoded. Patients given high doses of this activating drug could turn on many genes and thus manufacture large quantities of the related compound. In an unexpected emergency, however, withdrawing the ligand would shut the whole process down. No ecdysone, no activity by the introduced gene. As an added bonus, the ecdysone would not interfere with any biological processes, which biologists call "cross talk," because the human body does not otherwise use, or need, ecdysone. Or, as Kirk puts it, "Humans don't molt."

The system was developed as "Rheoswitch," which borrows its name from a "rheostat," a resistor used in electronic circuits that can adjust a signal that is continuous rather than binary. In this case, the signal is delivered in the form of a pill, a humanized version of ecdysone. A handful of "gene switches" have been tried before, and notably, the ARGENT system from Bellicum Pharmaceuticals, Inc. entered human clinical trials. Bellicum's switch works on a protein, the product of a gene. Rheoswitch is the only true "gene switch" in trials, since it acts on the transcriptional machinery that turns genetic DNA code into an RNA molecule. In 2007, Intrexon obtained its gene switch technology from a company called RheoGene. Since then, it has "wired" up the switches to thousands of human genes, which can be turned on with a dose of activator molecule as a pill. Kirk's group has not only developed a catalog of switches and activator molecules, but "cell-specific promoters," which cause genes to turn on only in specific cells, such as neurons, blood or liver cells, or only in certain conditions, such as in a low-oxygen tumor environment, reducing the collateral damage to healthy cells. Jonathan Lewis, a physician-scientist and a former chief executive officer at Ziopharm Oncology, Inc. which has an agreement with Intrexon, believes the regulation of synthetic genes with switches, "cell-specific promoters," and continuous dial controls, will allow the technology to emerge in the mainstream. "The next phase in gene therapy is control," Lewis told me. "It's all about temporal control and also spatial control, defining which organs and cells genes are expressed in."

Importantly, Kirk's gene switch is emerging in lockstep with new prospects for using an "immunotherapeutic approach" to fighting cancer. This rests on an old dogma that the immune system is perfectly competent, and in fact does wipe out most cancers before we're ever aware they exist. But for whatever reason, the theory goes, it sometimes fails. In the 1890s, a doctor named William Copley injected his cancer patients with a glob of bacteria, after noticing that cancer regressed in some patients with severe infections, possibly due to a ramped up immune response that further proceeded to attack a tumor. A few patients survived, but physicians couldn't explain why. Jorgen Rygaard in the 1970s showed that cancers do not occur at higher rates in mice with knocked-out immune systems, throwing the hypothesis into doubt. But over those decades scientists would begin to gain a more sophisticated appreciation of the immune system, describing hundreds of cytokines, or immune system signals, which either ramp up an immune response, or prevent it from going on the attack, a brake which became called a "checkpoint blockade."[413]

In the 1980s, Stephen Rosenberg at the National Cancer Institute began using a cytokine called *IL-2* to rev up the immune system, but it helped less than 10 percent of patients with late-stage melanoma. Near that time, immunologist James Allison described checkpoint mechanisms, a means by which signals can be used to temper an immune response. A raft of new evidence began to accumulate to show that cancer cells hijack the body's own mechanisms to temper T-cells, which evolved to repress immune defenses under conditions such as pregnancy. For instance, cancer cells can promote the expression of the Programmed Death or *PD-1*, a natural protein on the surface of T-cells. It works as a natural "checkpoint blockade," whereas when it is activated, it leads to the death of the T-cells, creating a check on an immune system response. In fact, cancer cells can hijack this mechanism, pumping out proteins such as Programmed Death Ligand 1 and Ligand 2, which bind to *PD-1* and initiate the blockade, meaning the ligand binds to the protein built by the *PD-1* gene, and initiates a death of the T-cell. In this way, cancer cells can silence the immune response to attack them. At least five major drug companies are competitively pursuing *PD-1* as a therapeutic target for cancer. For instance, Bristol Myers Squibb is marketing an antibody that interferes with *PD-L1* binding to *PD-1*, marketed as Opdivo or Nivolumab. This immunotherapy strategy has been effective in lung, kidney and other cancers, but its effects on patient prognosis appear to be linked to the forms of cancer which have high percentages of cancer cells producing *PD-L1* ligand. The drug company's antibodies seem to have a therapeutic effect, for instance, if 50 percent of the cancer cells are producing *PD-L1* ligand, but not if as few of 5 percent of the cancer cells are. If cancer can disable an immune response, scientists came to believe that maybe they could restore its controls. Maybe, they might even leverage the immune system to the task of the fight. Indeed, biopharma had in short time developed antibodies to *PD-LT* and *CTLA-4*, which neutralize those signals and prevent cancer cells from shutting down the immune system. The antibodies to these two targets account for one of the most able arrows cancer drug makers have in their quiver. Scientists started to believe they could go farther, adding booster signals to arm immune cells in a fight against cancer.

In particular, investigators are studying the switch approach as a way of making cancer immunotherapy less of a harrowing ordeal for patients. Cancer immunotherapies, which have made a lot of headlines of late, aim either to reawaken an immune response that has been lulled to sleep by chemical signals from a malignancy, or to jumpstart an entirely new and more powerful anti-cancer response than a patient's immune system can achieve on its own. The trouble is, a rebooted immune system can easily slip into overdrive, triggering life-threatening fevers and the potentially lethal buildup of fluids throughout the body. Gene switches are now being evaluated, for example, in small trials of carefully chosen patients with recurrent melanoma (a type of skin cancer) and breast cancer. Doctors inject one or two tumors in these individuals with genes designed to boost the production of cytokines – signaling molecules (such as interferon and various interleukins) that the immune system uses to monitor and adjust the fight against tumors. Investigators believe that they do not need to treat all the malignant lesions in each patient because once the immune system is primed to tackle one nest of cancerous cells, it will automatically start searching for others elsewhere in the body without the need for further prompting. So unlike CAR T-cell immunotherapy which is genetically engineered T-cells weaponized to target a specific cancer cell marker, cytokine therapy is deployed under a schema of "treat locally to effect globally," meaning to boost the body's immune system in a broad sense. Cytokines trigger a wide range of physiological reactions – from opening up blood vessels so that immune cells can rush to the scene of an infection to activating ruthless "killer T-cells," which, among other things, specialize in destroying cancerous cells. But doctors to date have not been able to treat patients successfully with one of the most powerful cytokines, known as interleukin-12, or *IL-12*.

This failure stems in part from *IL-12's* propensity for unleashing a "cytokine storm," in which the immune system seemingly goes on a rampage against the body. In the bloodstream, *IL-12* can cause a sharp drop in blood pressure, difficulties with lung function and heart problems that together can easily lead to organ failure and death. And yet, says Laurence Cooper, a physician-scientist at the University of Texas M.D. Anderson Cancer Center in Houston and CEO of the biotech company Ziopharm, "there is a ton of literature on its effectiveness in the tumor microenvironment. *IL-12* is the holy grail of immunotherapy."

The plan is to deliver as much *IL-12* as possible to a single tumor, but not so much that a cytokine storm occurs. Here is where the switch technology could prove revolutionary. Researchers insert the switch-enabled *IL-12* genes into an individual's tumor, where they take up residence in the immune cells that are already there to give them a boost. Because the switch can be activated only by the presence of ecdysone, physicians can increase the levels of cytokine in the tumor very deliberately by slowly increasing the amount of ecdysone they give their patient. If a cytokine storm starts to develop, they can skip the next scheduled dose, thereby averting the worst of the damage. Ziopharm, which is working with Intrexon to develop switch-enabled cytokine treatment in people, reports encouraging results so far. Kirk acknowledges that they might have chosen to test their approach on a cytokine less potent than the *IL-12* gene – where the slightest misstep could prove fatal. But he says, "We chose one of the hardest genes, because we wanted to pressure-test the switch."

Results from two safety studies conducted at several medical centers suggest that the answer is yes, the gene switch works in safety trials and can be applied in humans. Although no one was cured, the switch-controlled regimen appeared to be reasonably safe. As anticipated, a few patients did begin showing signs of a cytokine storm, but it dissipated soon after they stopped taking the ecdysone pills. "We've been able to turn it off and completely reverse clinical symptoms" when "adverse events" of immune overdrive occur, Lewis told me.

The researchers also found hints that the *IL-12* therapy could be helpful in reducing cancer tumors. In one of the studies, they injected the gene-plus-switch combination into 12 people with metastatic breast cancer. Each of them had already endured an average of eight previous cancer treatments, with diminishing hopes of survival. For various reasons, investigators were able to evaluate the new therapy's effect in only seven patients, however. The *IL-12* treatment shrank some of their tumors. In three people, the disease appeared to remain stable during the trial. The second safety study, in 26 patients who had been treated an average of six different times for metastatic melanoma, showed an uptick in cytokine levels and other cancer-fighting activity. In May 2015, Ziopharm initiated another study using switch-enabled *IL-12* as an experimental treatment for glioblastoma multiforme, a particularly aggressive type of brain cancer. Cancer trials were underway at Sloan-Kettering, and trials were starting on glioblastoma multiforme, a brain cancer, spread out over hospitals at Stanford, UCLA, University of Chicago, Harvard at Dana-Farber and Sloan-Kettering.

Richard Mulligan at Harvard Medical School has been working on a different kind of switch. His approach features small, naturally occurring RNA molecules called ribozymes. First described in the 1980s, ribozymes are like enzymes in that they catalyze chemical reactions in the body, but they consist of RNA rather than protein. In the 1990s, Jennifer Doudna was among a number of scientists who began to clarify the structure and function of ribozymes, which fold up into all sorts of jungle-gym structures, including one called the hammerhead ribozyme, which takes its name from its similarity to the hammerhead shark.[414]

Doudna was a Howard Hughes investigator and a major force in science before Crispr. Ribozymes are very much analogous to enzymes in this respect: they are action molecules with catalytic functions, meaning they fold up and carry out the "actions" in the molecular world. Ribozymes are not just a bit of junk RNA, they are critical to the very nature of life. In a feature useful for switches, some ribozymes constitute "self-cleaving introns" and have the ability to cut themselves up and induce any RNA molecules to which they have been attached to self-destruct.

Mulligan's constructs consist of a ribozyme linked not to a classic gene but to a messenger RNA molecule. When cells make proteins, they first copy the DNA in a gene into messenger RNA, a mobile, single-strand transcript, after which the mRNA gets translated into the protein. From the cell's point of view, the injection of a stretch of DNA or its corresponding mRNA should result in the same outcome – production of a specific protein. As a first step, researchers carefully select a "self-cleaving" ribozyme to embed alongside the messenger RNA encoding a selected therapeutic protein. If just this synthetic ribo-mRNA construct were to be inserted into a human cell, the ribozyme would cut itself at a single precise site in the midst of the gene, causing the mRNA molecule to fall apart, and the whole process of building a protein would grind to a halt. It would be as if the gene had been turned off.

In 2002, Ronald Breaker and colleagues at Yale showed how to protect the ribo-mRNA construct by linking the ribozyme to an additional molecule called an "aptamer," which is a kind of sensor that is designed to be activated by a particular drug. In the presence of the drug, and only in the presence of the drug, the sensor changes shape in a way that prevents the ribozyme from destroying the mRNA. With the full length of mRNA intact, the cell makes the protein. When the drug that acts on the sensor is withdrawn, the ribozyme and the mRNA self-destruct. By 2004, in studies initiated by Laising Yen, Mulligan was regularly kitting up his ribozyme switches with carefully customized drug-sensitive sensors, and he continues to hone the technology today. The sensors can be designed with great specificity, he says, further reducing the chances of unwanted side effects. As with ecdysone, the mRNA that is connected to the ribo-switch would work only if the patient swallows the appropriate pill. Take the pill and you have, in effect, turned on a gene. Stop the pill and the gene stays off.

Mulligan's ribozyme switch is one of multiple such tools that were rapidly emerging to turn our genes on or off. Intrexon had put its gene switch in trials, and was hoping to soon market it. Doudna colleague Jonathan Weissman, a scientist from the University of California at San Francisco, and many other top-notch scientists including Stanley Qi and Wendell Lim, had been tinkering with Crispr systems to develop them into switches, creating innovative tools such as Crispri and Crispra, which could turn on or off gene expression.[415,416,417,418] In the words of Doudna and Charpentier, CRISPRi "has been used to repress multiple target genes simultaneously, and its effects are reversible."[419]

Although single gene switches are not yet perfected, investigators can envision a not-too-distant future in which multiple switches become the norm, allowing increasingly precise control of gene therapy. Take a different pill, each of those genes would be turned on separately, or together. Take a pill to turn on one of the genes, and if a cancer found a way to put the slip on that signal, doctors could simply have them take a second or third pill, say to induce *IL-15*, *INF-alpha*, or a gene that represses *CTLA-4*, one of the "checkpoint blockades," which cancer cells use to temper immune response. "In a space of time, you can intervene in a second pathway," Jonathan Lewis told me. "It's precision therapy." And the cell-based cancer treatment of CAR T-cells may be increasingly equipped with cytokines that can be turned on with pills, or multiple pills, flipping a series of switches on cancer. If inserting new genes into our bodies in the 1990s was Genetic Engineering 1.0, some say, then the switch-based control of our genes is Genetic Engineering 2.0.

Lawrence Cooper had begun leading trials by combining a couple of switch-enabled genes with CAR T-cells. The genes contribute the *IL-12* and another cytokine, *IL-15*; laboratory tests suggest that *IL-15* makes *IL-12* even more effective at rallying immune cells. The third part of this experimental treatment – the cells – are a group of genetically engineered CAR T-cells that are better able to direct their firepower on cancerous tissue than naturally occurring immune cells can. Adding switch-bearing *IL-12* and *IL-15* genes to the CAR T-cells should allow

Cooper to boost the cells' potency and effectiveness even higher. Because the gene switches and their respective activators will allow him to adjust the levels of *IL-12* and *IL-15* independently, he should be able to fine-tune the treatment to produce the best results with the least amount of *IL-12*, thereby further reducing the risk of unleashing a "cytokine storm."

Scientists have solved most of the problems of the viruses themselves triggering an immune reaction – by selecting recombinant viruses to use in gene therapy which are less immunogenic, such as adeno-associated virus or lentivirus, and steering clear of viruses which tend to trigger immune reactions, such as adenovirus. CAR T-cells, however, can also unexpectedly shift the immune system into overdrive, resulting in cytokine release syndrome, often throwing patients to the brink of death. To evoke the immune system is to summon a leviathan, one that is often too powerful to control, and summoning it can lead to "adverse events." Old ideas about how to control an overpowering immune reaction due to a cell-based technology include the addition of "suicide genes" which can be evoked to trigger cell death, or apoptotic machinery, killing off all the genetically engineered T-cells, in effect, calling off the war. But there is also a problem with that, which is similar to destroying a large cancer tumor very rapidly, an effect called "tumor lysis syndrome." Unleashing many dead cells in the body at one time may result in high toxicity. In contrast, gene switches may allow attending physicians to "dial up" the expression of CAR on the surface of T-cells and control key cytokines that decide when a T-cell multiplies, and when a cytokine or chimeric molecule in an engineered CAR T-cell comes on. Hence, these are new ways to control the timing and action of gene therapy.

Bruce Levine said he expected to see an increasing use of multiple synthetic genes in engineered cells which can be implemented in conjunction or in series to put a pincer move on cancer. Indeed, the combination of switch-based cytokine therapy with CAR T-cells "could provide substantial improvement, especially in solid tumors," and he and others have been developing a suite of CAR T-cells, which can be dispatched to seek out the molecular signatures of cancers specific to different cell types and organs. Levine imagines having some CAR T-cells that can be dispatched to fight liver cancer, others for pancreatic cancer, others for brain or breast cancer, a complete toolset, "a garage of CARs," he said.

With a touch of whimsy, Cooper calls gene-switch controlled versions of these engineered cells "remote-control CARs."

In 1997, Perry Hackett, a University of Minnesota biologist, was the dashing squire at the heart of a love story, and to my knowledge, one of science's only true fairytales. Did you, reader, think this book would go on without a love story? Of course not. But lest I deceive you further, this is a "molecular fairytale." Still, it might be the greatest love story ever told about a molecule. Hackett, Zoltan Ivics and lab members, woke up a molecule called a transposon from a 20-million-year-old evolutionary sleep. It had been sleeping, or non-functional, in a genome of a salmon fish for all of those millions of years. Once he woke up the molecule, charming it to life, he developed it into a delivery tool for gene therapy. He called it the "Sleeping Beauty Transposon System."

Recall the incredulous finding that up to 10 percent of the human genome is literally a graveyard of viruses that "once upon a time," leapt into the human genome, became compromised and went dormant. The other curious finding was that almost half of the human genome is made up of transposons, "jumping genes" or "mobile elements," artifacts of proto-viruses that literally jump around the genome. Recall that transposons in vertebrates are dormant like jumping beans that have lost their thwack: they've stopped hopping, skipping and jumping. Sleeping Beauty was a transposon that went dormant due to mutations that rendered it non-functional. Transposons are coupled at each end with an enzyme called transposase which makes double-strand breaks into the genome, and armed with it, the hoppy molecules can leap anywhere inside a genome. But once they land at their new hopscotch site, they tend to stay put. "Transposons are designed evolutionarily to hop once in order to limit the damage they inflict on the genome," Hackett told me. And once they do jump into the genome, further accumulation of mutations over evolutionary time ruins their ability to hop anywhere, ever again. The trick that Hackett pulled was to correct all of those mutations, so that after millions of years, a transposon, or jumping gene, would come back to life.

At first, it seemed no more than an intriguing bit of "genetic archeology," but it wasn't long before Sleeping Beauty was identified as an efficient tool for gene therapy, given its preternatural ability to leap into a host genome. It did not have strong switches like promoters or enhancers like retroviruses that could switch on cancer. And scientists could easily pop new gene cargo into Sleeping Beauty, and send it into human cells in a plasmid delivery vehicle. Perry Hackett wasn't a medical doctor, but he did know one, Lawrence Cooper, a pediatrician at M.D. Anderson Cancer Center. It wasn't long before Cooper was leading a clinical trial with Sleeping Beauty for patients with lymphoma and leukemia, bolstered by the support and technology of RJ Kirk's Intrexon, bringing together CAR T-cells, switches to turn on booster signals of cytokines and the entire construct packaged in Sleeping Beauty, which would snap it into the genome of a T-cell.

Although he'd seen no "Lazarus moment," or patients' cancers stunningly cured, as Carl June's group had reported, it appeared the engineered cells had engrafted into his patients, and that the procedure was safe. Cooper likes to joke to his child patients that they are "part fish," since they are true chimeras with pieces of fish DNA sewn up in their genomes. He has now treated 40 patients for B-cell cancers and is setting up trials for solid-state tumors, like brain, breast or pancreatic cancers, which are more complicated than liquid tumors of the blood and immune system. By now, the technologies were accelerating each other, CAR T-cells were equipped with multiple attack weapons, switched-controlled *IL-12* and *IL-15*.

Sleeping Beauty is a gene therapy tool that could be the most accessible, sweeping and cheapest in the field, Cooper told me. "If I pull this off, it will be a system that many people have access to, and that could really change the field," Cooper said. It would effectively make gene therapy "open source." "Suddenly, everyone is going to be able to do gene therapy," Cooper said. "And, the field isn't going to move ahead, we're not going to win, until we have enough brains working on these problems." But, Sleeping Beauty will probably never replace virus engineering as a means to install new genes into cells, because it must be used "ex vivo," meaning outside the body, while viruses containing gene transfer constructs can often be injected into a patient's leg, or the site of a tumor. Many of the pills that doctors give patients may be used to switch on various transferred genes at precisely the right place and time in the body instead of flooding every organ and tissue with the powerful pharmaceutical agents that act both where they are needed and elsewhere, causing side effects. Drugs will no longer be manufactured in giant vats and so-called bioreactors in pharmaceutical facilities. Instead, new gene treatments will allow patients to spit out a molecule exactly where and when it is needed most in the body. Cooper believes synthetic biology is nearing a critical mass. Instead of giving patients a drug, more and more we will engineer our own cells to spit out a drug like a "tiny bioreactor." All of this will enable scientists to "democratize" the field as an "open-access" workspace. He made the analogy that viral vector systems were like Apple, while non-viral systems were like Android, a cheaper open-source platform on which to innovate, which will enable more to work in the field, which anyone could built an "app" on. "It has to happen," Cooper said. "Only when multiple people come together with shared concepts and rigor, only when gene therapy is nimble and cost-effective. Only then will it be worth something."

In December 2013, Intrexon and OvaScience forged a $1.5 million joint venture with stated objectives including gene editing to the germline to stop heritable diseases. David Baltimore's and Jennifer Doudna's letter in *Science* in early 2015 had called for a pause on editing the germline, and it was not clear to me whether this human germline work was proceeding. Intrexon had begun as a company to provide constructs for genetically engineered mice, but Kirk's investment a decade ago came with a grand vision to move the genetic engineering into agriculture, aquaculture and, indeed, humans. I wrote to Tom Reed, the founder of Intrexon, asking him about it. "Intrexon is highly cognizant of the scientific, social, and business issues associated with genome engineering," Reed told me. "As such, our proprietary business strategy becomes revealed through our collaborators' commercial efforts versus premature disclosure via public forums." In other words, the extent of their work in human engineering is a trade secret. At the same time, it was increasingly clear to me through my correspondence with leaders at the FDA that human genome engineering would be regulated as a "drug," and could not proceed without passing through the regulatory bodies at the FDA.

Engineering in agriculture and horticulture was swiftly proceeding. Intrexon's core technology, UltraVector, is a computerized system for assembling snippets of DNA into complex genetic circuits, which was inspired to assist in the creation of genetically engineered mice. The company hasn't published any scientific articles on the technology, seeking to protect its trade secrets, and also making it difficult to determine its value. Intrexon's technology portfolio has been significantly built out in recent years, however. RJ Kirk got his gene switch by snapping up RheoGene, enabling the company to enter a competitive market of human genetic engineering in T-cells; it acquired the company Okanagan Specialty Fruits, positioning it to bring to market a genetically engineered apple, which resists browning when sliced; it bought AquaBounty to bring to market a fast-growing salmon; it snapped up Oxitec to create genetically engineered mosquitos. Kirk and Reed's company put their abilities on stunning display by showing they could even clone your favorite kitten!

RJ Kirk told me we were entering a revolution so profound we might reset the calendars to begin in 1953, the year Watson and Crick published the structure of the double-helix. The journalist Andrew Pollack christened our age a second moment when life began, suggesting before now, "the foods and creatures nurtured by Mr. Kirk would have been found only in dystopian fantasies like those written by Margaret Atwood. But Mr. Kirk's company, Intrexon, is fast becoming one of the world's most diverse biotechnology companies, with ventures ranging from unloved genetically engineered creatures to potential cancer cures and gene therapies, gasoline substitutes, cloned kittens and even glow-in-the-dark Dino Pet toys made from microbes."[420]

In the United States, regulatory bodies were opening up gigantic holes for biotech. In the fall of 2015, the FDA approved the first genetically engineered animal for consumption, laying down a doormat for the agricultural sector to move ahead with a raft of genetically modified foods in the United States. The so-called "AquAdvantage" fish engenders polarizing debates. A third of worldwide fish stocks are overfished or near extinction, while consumption doubled from 1973 to 1997, says the International Food Policy Research Institute. In 2006, the world consumed 110.4 million metric tons of fish. Just under half of that was produced by aquaculture, and the world was poised for land-locked aquaculture, even open-ocean farming technologies to usher in a Blue Revolution of the seas, on a par with the Green Revolution of agriculture that occurred in the US between the 1940s and late 1970s. AquaBounty, a Massachusetts based company – which Intrexon recently acquired a majority stake – generated a construct that includes a "gene cassette" from the Pacific Chinook salmon that it can splice into the Atlantic salmon to give it the instructions to grow big. The construct is called opAFP-GHc2 and it contains two units, one of which is a gene that encodes a protein called a growth factor hormone. The construct also contains a stretch of DNA from the promoter region of an ocean pout, an eel-like creature that lives in extremely cold environments (the promoter is a switch that controls the expression of a downstream gene). Normally, the eel uses this promoter to keep an antifreeze gene turned on constantly so it does not freeze. The promoter is therefore "constitutive," meaning it is always active, and coupling it with a growth factor gene in an Atlantic salmon results in the salmon experiencing a continual growth spurt – since the growth factor is continually produced. Studies have shown that the genetically altered Atlantic salmon's appetite would make it constantly ravenous, meaning that it would eat everything around on sight. In its first year, AquaBounty Technologies' AquAdvantage Atlantic salmon has a two-to-sixfold increase in size – the largest being 13 times bigger than the average natural Atlantic salmon – and it reaches full maturity in half the time.[421]

The British company Oxitec – another acquisition of Intrexon – had hardly attracted the polarizing conversation, as it sought to introduce a genetically engineered "ouchless" mosquito which cannot bite, a favorite curiosity of the evolutionary biologist Stephen Jay Gould. The genetically engineered mosquitos were male with a gene variant which prevents them from biting while retaining the power to mate, thus they pass on this "ouchless" gene, promising to reduce the mosquito population over months. Intrexon was proceeding with the construction of a factory with plans to produce 60 million genetically engineered mosquitos a week in Piracicaba, a city in Brazil, in an effort to cut down on mosquito-borne illnesses. "New Weapon To Fight Zika: The Mosquito" declared a headline in *The New York Times*.[422] "The biotech bugs could become one of the newest weapons in the perennial battle between humans and mosquitoes, which kill hundreds of thousands of people a year by transmitting malaria, dengue fever and other devastating diseases and have been called the deadliest animal in the world," wrote Andrew Pollack. Zika is a virus which is transmitted by daytime-active *Aedes aegypti* mosquitoes; it is spread in the tropics and causes a fever, while outbreaks recorded in 2015 suggested a connection between infection in mothers and microcephaly in newborn babies, meaning a small head size. A genetically engineered *Aedes aegypti* mosquito would not transmit dengue virus, and research had suggested it would also not spread Zika, spring-boarding it to headlines. Kirk argued that an emerging opposition to genetic engineering is "mostly born of fear based on lack of knowledge." Quipped Andrew Pollack, "If that sounds like something Monsanto, the leader in biotech crops might say, it could be because Mr. Kirk recruited Robert B. Shapiro, former chief executive of Monsanto, to be Intrexon's lead outside director."

Kirk was assembling a lobbying team, including the law firm Sidley Austin in Washington, Cesar Alvarez, chairman of law firm Greenberg Traurig, and Jack Bobo, who formerly directed biotechnology trade policy at the State Department. "Dr. Luciana Borio, acting chief scientist at the Food and Drug Administration, told a House subcommittee on Wednesday that the agency was 'greatly expediting' Oxitec's application to test the mosquitoes in the Florida Keys and would issue a draft environmental assessment very soon."[423]

10 Secrets from a Freshwater Fish

> There is only one word that matters in biology and that is specificity. The truth is in the details, not the broad sweeps.
>
> –Aaron Klug

At 34, Feng Zhang has a youthful light-bulbish energy and a laser-like focus. Born in China, he has straight black hair in a bowl cut, pale skin and wire-rimmed glasses. Eric Lander, the director of the institute, told me Zhang is "in my opinion, the most effective genetic engineer today."

When I met Zhang at the Broad Institute, where he is a core member, the highest ranking position at the institute, he was doing a pen trick. It's a trick popular among grade school students. The pen springs over the top of the thumb and lands back in the grasp, using only one hand. I saw him do it at least 30 times without a miss.

I had already read what had become a trove of newspaper articles and press that was compiling on his fast-moving career and life. I was thinking about the article, and I knew he was churning on his next experiment, and all the time we were talking that pen kept springing over his thumb. In his youth, Zhang saw the film, *Jurassic Park*, in which hubristic researchers brought back extinct dinosaurs, and prompted a piece of silver screen magic that "told me that biology might also be a programmable system."[424] As the journalist Sharon Begley commented "a seed had been planted in his mind. An organism's genetic instructions, he realized, could be overwritten to change its characteristics, just as his parents wrote computer code." He sought mentors who would give him a chance to try science, and succeeded in slipping a glow-in-the-dark molecule from a jellyfish called a green fluorescent protein into a human cell. In 1999, as high-school student in Des Moines, Iowa, his mother Shujun Zhou often waited in her car for hours as he worked late in a gene therapy lab. It paid off. He earned third place in the Intel Science Talent Search, which landed him $50,000 in prize money he used toward tuition at Harvard. As a college student, he went on to publish a 2004 paper showing how flu viruses enter cells, using the green fluorescent protein he had practiced with in high school to show

how it is done. But while a college student at Harvard, Zhang come up against the more visceral and troublesome course of biology. "When a close friend and fellow student developed major depressive disorder, Zhang spent hours trying to help and making sure he was not suicidal. The friend was so deep in the abyss of depression as to be unreachable, however, and had to take a year off from Harvard. Zhang was deeply touched and dedicated himself to developing better treatments for mental illness."[425] As Feng Zhang told the writer Michael Specter, "People think you are weak if you are depressed. It is still a common prejudice. But many people suffer from problems we cannot begin to address. The brain is still the place in the universe with the most unanswered questions."[426]

In 2005, at the spritely age of 23, Zhang and colleagues invented a new field in science called "optogenetics," which makes use of genetic engineering to switch on and off neurons with a tiny beam of light. "Deisseroth?" I asked him. "Yes, that was my thesis project," he told me, still flipping the pen around this thumb, with each new turn, perfectly falling back into his grasp. Zhang and Ed Boyden were graduate students at Stanford in the lab of Karl Deisseroth, when the group published the first demonstration of splicing genes for photosensitive proteins, called rhodopsins, into neurons and then using light to turn on those neurons at will. Light information is therefore transformed into electrochemical information in your head.[427] Rhodopsins build cones and rods that transmit light signals into chemical signals in our eyeballs, but they are broadly conserved in nature. One called channelrhodopsin 2 is a light-activated cation channel found in algae, meaning that when light hits the protein it allows cations, or positively charged molecules, into the cell causing it to transmit an electrical signal. The lab engineered channelrhodopsin 2 into a specific subset of neurons. By shining a blue light on these neurons, they found they could actually trigger the neurons to fire and release neurotransmitters. They also found they could shut off neurons by introducing a new molecule, halorhodopsin, which silenced the cells in response to yellow light. The system became a widely used tool to map neural circuitry in disorders such as schizophrenia, depression or autism. Medtronic went on to couple the genetically engineered neurons with a tiny laser unit that could be implanted in the brain to control neuron firing. "Optical deep brain stimulation" was now being explored to control the firing of neurons in brain regions such as Area 25 to treat depression, or in the substrata nigra to treat Parkinson's disease. Scientists were becoming astute at recombining DNA and creating cells which built photosensitive receptors on their cell surfaces, or virtually any protein they wanted, a stunning feat of synthetic biology.

Zhang began his postdoc work as new tools for "genome editing," were emerging to make very precise edits in a sea of three billon bases in the human genome. The first such tool was the zinc finger nuclease, or ZFN, a programmable system to edit DNA. In 2009 and 2010, Zhang became a Harvard Junior Fellow working in George Church's lab, co-authoring papers on genome editing based on a new editing tool called TALEN, which gave some benefits over zinc finger nucleases. Church's lab was also working side-by-side with co-investigator Keith Joung on some projects, holding monthly group meetings during this time. Zhang would build upon his deep bench work in the lab to begin to edit genes, and he was publishing like gangbusters, often leading the charge on new research initiatives and making them work technically. Robert Desimone, director of MIT's McGovern Institute for Brain Research, heard of "this amazing superstar" and soon recruited Zhang to McGovern. "In a collaborative enterprise like science, where it's not unusual for papers to have a dozen authors, you always wonder who did what," Desimone was quoted as saying. The McGovern asked around and was assured "that Feng played a key role" in developing optogenetics, said Desimone. Zhang's list of papers, he added, "was the strongest publication history of anyone [at this stage of a career] in the history of neuroscience."[428] Zhang was hired by the McGovern and the Broad Institutes.

By the time I met him, genome editing was in full swing. He had published a key paper showing a newer gene editing tool, Crispr-Cas9, could work to edit mammalian cells in January 2013. By the close of 2015 he had 40 papers in publication and was often staying at the office until 1 or 2 am "because he genuinely can't wait until morning to know the answer," according to his postdoctoral fellow Naomi Habib.[429] By early 2016, venture capitalists were regularly swinging by his office. Zhang captured a prestigious Canadian award for his work on Crispr, the Les Prix Canada Gardier Award, which he shared with Doudna, Charpentier, Horvath and Barrangou. Eric Lander sent out an email heralding Zhang's promotion to tenure at MIT and setting up a reception with cake and prosecco, a sparkling white wine. Instead of using the moment for self-promotion, Zhang spent a lot of yarn giving credit to his grad students and postdocs for doing amazing work.

Genome editing did not happen out of the blue. It depends on more than 50 years of grinding bench work, being able to culture cells in a lab, learning how to use viruses to slip constructs into cells. The disruptive technology of Crispr-Cas9 was proceeded by first-generation genome editing tools, namely the zinc finger nuclease. Zinc fingers are a string of 30 amino acids, crooked in the shape of a finger and stabilized by a zinc ion; depending on their structure, they are classified as treble clef, gag knuckle and zinc ribbon. In fact, they serve as the clasps and snaps of the genome, assembling protein complexes, including transcription factors and other effector proteins near start sites of genes to initiate the copying of those genes into messenger RNA. We now know there are more than 700 versions in the human body, but it was only in 1985 that the first zinc-finger protein was discovered, in the lab of Nobel laureate Aaron Klug. In the words of Monya Baker, "Zinc-finger binding is subtle, and depends on more than simply matching triplets of DNA to the corresponding finger. Just as fingers on a hand have a certain order – pinky, ring, middle, index, thumb – zinc-finger proteins also fit together in a certain way. For example, a finger could bind tightly to one triplet of DNA when it is in the 'index' position, but have a less-secure grip when it is in other positions."[430] The discovery of these clasping proteins was a piece of happenstance. "Scientists studying the genetic code of the African clawed frog noticed a finger-shaped protein wrapped around its DNA," Baker wrote. Not long after, the "zinc finger nuclease" was invented by fusing together a nuclease, a restriction enzyme that works like tiny molecular scissors, and these zinc finger proteins, which could be assembled into unique combinations to bind and clasp to specific addresses in the human genome. "They soon figured out how to combine that tenacious grip with an enzyme that could cut the DNA like a knife."[431]

Srinivasan Chandrasegaran, or Chandra, in 1985, had spent 10 months in the lab of Nobel laureate Hamilton Smith to learn about restriction enzymes, the molecular scissors that had been identified a couple of decades before. In 1986, he was hired as an assistant professor at the Johns Hopkins University. Smith suggested he try to engineer these enzymes to target specific addresses in the genome, but then cautioned that he might fail. "Just before I moved to my own lab at (Hopkins), I asked Ham Smith what project he thought would be important enough to work on over the next five years," Chandra told me. "He suggested changing the sequence-specificity of restriction enzymes. But he cautioned that many attempts had been made to engineer the DNA-cutting enzymes to recognize and cleave new sequences without much success. And that it has proven to be a burial ground for many postdoctoral research projects." Chandra began to study a class of restriction enzymes in which the recognition and cleavage sites are separated by a few base pairs. In other words, he was looking for an enzyme that was specific enough, where its recognition site (a "DNA binding domain" which binds its molecular target) and its cleavage site (which does the cutting) were only a few bases apart so that it could snip pieces of DNA that were extremely close to the chromosomal address that it was binding.[432] Chandra selected the restriction enzyme *FokI* from a catalog of enzymes, which is derived from a family of bacteria, *Flavobacterium okeanokoites*, which infects a freshwater fish.[433] Chandra had isolated *FokI* which he observed to work as "an indiscriminate nuclease that chomped through DNA without specificity."[434] His stroke of genius was to fuse this chomping enzyme to a zinc-finger protein.

In 1991, Carl Pabo and Nikola Pavletich published the X-ray structure of three zinc finger domains bound to DNA. This work was about to come into collision with Chandra's work on FokI. Chandra paid a visit to Jeremy Berg, a colleague at Johns Hopkins and a former postdoc of Pabo's. As Baker recounted, "Berg walked Chandra to his freezer and handed him two tiny tubes, each containing a plasmid encoding a zinc-finger protein that bound a specific sequence. Chandra used these to create two fusion proteins by combining each binding motif with the cleavage domain of FokI. The hybrid enzymes cut where expected. The first zinc-finger nuclease had been engineered."[435] In 1996, Chandra published his creation of the zinc finger nuclease. Remarkably, this genome editing system came with an address guide and pair of scissors, but no paste to repair the double-strand break that it created in a genome. How our cells pasted back a double-strand break after we hacked into it was a deeply intriguing question with startling new revelations.

Maria Jasin, a molecular biologist at Sloan-Kettering, had done an important experiment in 1994, which I will talk about in a few sentences. Recall that Mario Capecchi had invented "gene targeting," showing that "knockout mice" could be created by introducing a new gene to a cell; often, the genome would magically swap out its original gene for the new gene he introduced. In fact, the means cells did this was by a mechanism called homologous recombination. This feat worked about 0.01% of the time, and it had to be performed in mouse cells which could be selected for and picked out of an *in vitro* plate in the lab. It was by no means efficient. But the implications were obvious. This mechanism, or something like it, could be used to repair genes in a human cell. In a 1985 paper, Oliver Smithies, who would share the Nobel Prize with Capecchi, reported that "a 'rescuable' plasmid containing globin gene sequences allowing recombination with homologous chromosomal sequences has enabled us to produce, score and clone mammalian cells with the plasmid integrated into the human beta-globin locus. The planned modification was achieved in about one per thousand trans-formed cells whether or not the target gene was expressed."[436] Transla-tion: we can swap out a new gene for beta-globin to fix a red blood cell disorder in humans, but it is far from safe or effective.

Jasin performed an elegant experiment to show that by instigating breaks in a plasmid, a circular vector that included a new gene to introduce to the cell, with an endonuclease called *I-SceI*, she could dramatically increase the frequency of recombination at those places. She then did a few other marvelous experiments to show that she could improve the rate of gene transfer into a cell by using an endonuclease to instigate a double-strand break in the actual chromosome of the cell she wanted to introduce a gene into.[437,438,439] In fact, Jasin and colleagues showed causing a double-strand break in the plasmid actually increases recombination events 100-fold, suggesting that causing a break was a critical step for gene engineering. This insight also contributed to an appreciation that cellular machinery pasted a break back up through a mechanism which would be called homology-directed repair. In fact, up to 100 proteins are involved in double-strand break repair. Homology-directed repair is the preferred method when there is an overhang of one strand of the double helix at a break site, a "cohesive" or sticky break, whereby this overhang can be used as a template for a tidy repair. Non-homologous end-joining is an alternative method for repair, which is preferred for "blunt end" breaks, where there is a clean break in the double-helix with no overhang. Since non-homologous end-joining is a repair without a template, it can repair a break in two broken ends of

DNA with non-matching genetic material from far flung regions in the genome, or cobbled together from disparate genes. This is a far more error-prone repair technique, leading to a raft of so-called structural variants, small insertions or deletions, in the broken region. The impacts of these basic science experiments were not lost on technologists or venture capitalists. If scientists could use a zinc finger to guide a nuclease to a site in the genome to create a "double-strand break," they could remove or excise genetic material, or introduce new genetic material to prompt the genome to patch itself back up with their own gene.

Joung, who joined Pabo's lab at MIT in 1998, but now works at Massachusetts General Hospital in Boston, helped to clarify and simplify the methods for engineering zinc fingers. Joung had earned his medical degree from Harvard Medical School in the 1990s, where he did his PhD work on bacterial transcription with Ann Hochschild, before moving on to do postdoctoral work with Pabo. The useful thing about zinc fingers, of course, is that they can be engineered to clasp virtually any sequence of DNA, thus they could be programmed to target specific sites in a sea of three billion nucleotides in the genome. I asked Joung whether he had envisioned in the 1990s zinc fingers having a place in human genetic engineering, or whether he thought it was just a dorky science experiment. "A mix of both," Joung laughed. "It was a cool technology at the time, and we knew we could engineer it to bind to virtually any site in the genome, and that it was potentially very powerful. It is the molecular equivalent to a GPS. You can fuse anything to it, and once you can bring something to that location, there are endless applications for treating a number of diseases."

Pabo, and Aaron Klug, had shown that individual zinc fingers could be re-engineered to a variety of different target DNA sites. But a single zinc finger only binds to 3–4 bps of DNA, an address that is not sufficiently long to be unique in a large genome. Zinc fingers could be stitched together into "arrays" capable of recognizing longer sequences; for example, arrays of three or four fingers could recognize 9 or 12 bp sequences, respectively. However, an outstanding and very difficult problem in the field was that these multiple zinc fingers had to work together in combination to bind to a specific sequence, and elucidating the formula for the right combination was a major research challenge. Joung set out to tackle this by generating varieties of zinc fingers by "evolution in a tube," in short, by generating a number of zinc fingers and then seeing which worked best in combination at binding a specific DNA sequence.[440] And an entrepreneur named Ed Lanphier was soon flying around the globe, talking to anyone who knew anything, sensing the business potential of "genome editing." "If you have a motif that can be engineered, by definition those different proteins will be encoded by different genes," Lanphier said. "So you might have a technology platform here to generate an infinite number of genes."[441]

Lanphier started Sangamo Biosciences in 1995. Klug started Gendaq. Genome editing was emerging, and so much was being learned about the genetics of major diseases. "In 1996, scientists had shown mutations of *CCR5* are present in a subset of healthy humans who are high risk for HIV infection. We felt that *CCR5* could potentially be an attractive therapeutic target for future gene therapy to treat or prevent HIV/AIDs by knocking out both alleles of *CCR5* gene," Chandra said.[442] John Hopkins, which had his patent library, licensed it to Sangamo "for the purpose of refining and developing ZFNs for biotechnology and biomedical applications." In a reflection, Chandra described the "thought experiment" by which many diseases could be treated with genome editing. "As far back as 1999, we had anticipated the upcoming genome engineering revolution in biology... The availability of chimeric nucleases, a new type of molecular scissors that target a specific site within the human genome, will likely contribute and greatly aid the feasibility of genome engineering...."[443]

Dana Carroll at the University of Utah called up Chandra on the telephone, and told him he had the lab and the resources available to push the zinc finger nuclease technology to its limits. Chandra agreed, and before long, Carroll was delivering on his promises, making quick work of the tools. He discovered that zinc fingers had to dimerize, in other words, two of the molecules had to come together to cut a DNA site. He also found he could adjust the distance between the recognition site of the zinc finger and the cutting site of the enzyme to optimize the editing tool. In 2001, Carroll's postdoc Marina Bibikova spent a year in colleague Kent Golic's lab working with the model fruit fly *Drosophila*. The first target the group chose to test the tool was the "yellow" gene, which contributes to pigmentation of the adult cuticle (mutants with a broken copy of the gene are yellow rather than brown). Bibikova used a zinc finger nuclease to snip the gene, making it non-functional.

"Peering through a microscope, Bibikova saw them first: tiny pale splotches on the dark abdomen of a fruit fly. Carroll saw the splotches too but was not sure that he could recognize the phenotype."[444] "When we saw our first apparent mosaic flies, with what looked like small yellow patches on their cuticle, I asked Kent to take a look," Carroll told me. Golic replied, in his typical, rather flat voice, "I'd be pretty excited, if I were you." Carroll's group had performed the first gene editing operation in a living animal, a fruit fly.

Not long after, Carroll coined the term "genome surgery" to codify a new era when scientists would begin performing operations on our genes. It wouldn't be long before scientists began to think in terms of editing genetic variants that cause human disease. Matthew Porteus was a medical student working with patients with sickle cell anemia. At David Baltimore's lab at California Institute of Technology, Porteus was using a reporter system based on a broken "green fluorescent protein," such that double-strand breaks would induce repair of the protein, causing the cells to light up with a garish green glow. He soon obtained a zinc finger nuclease from Chandra to see if he could make a specific edit in human cells and actually see an effect. "I remember it was a Saturday morning... and I started seeing green cells pop up," he says. "I'd done enough experiments not getting green cells to know this was real."[445]

After Porteus published his results in 2003, Sangamo began using zinc finger nuclease technology. Before long, Sangamo had built an extensive library of zinc fingers for unique sites in the human genome, and had a technology platform that allowed them to identify combinations of fingers that work well together in an array to recognize DNA sequences. In 2005, for instance, Sangamo published with Porteus at the University of Texas Southwestern Medical Center in Dallas, the description of a zinc-finger nuclease to target a mutation in a gene called *IL2*-gamma receptor and showed that they could repair the mutation in 18 percent of cells.[446] This was the gene that results in SCID, or Bubble Boy disease, and using a genome editing approach to fix the disease was considered potentially safer than simply dropping a supplementary copy of a gene into a genome using a virus, a method called gene trapping, which resulted, in effect, in creating a random mutation. In effect, those random mutations can, and did, lead to mutagenesis or cancers in gene therapy patients. The zinc finger nuclease emerged as a new paradigm because scientists could now introduce a targeted edit.

So far, gene therapy would be useful for treating enzyme deficiency disorders or recessive diseases such as X-SCID, hemophilia or any disease in which a therapeutic effect can be achieved by editing only a fraction of cells. It would be less useful for "dominant negative" diseases or those such as Huntington's, or breast cancer risk variants, or in any cases in which a disease would loom over a patient, until 100 percent of cells were repaired. In those cases, the gene edit could only truly be effective in the germline, when just an eight-cell embryo could be treated and all cells repaired. Exciting prospects lay in wait. Genome "editing" had application not only to human therapeutics, but to basic science. At the time, all scientists had was RNA interference, or RNAi, a method to introduce a molecule into a cell to clasp onto an RNA transcript and interfere with its success rate at becoming a protein. By using RNAi scientists could test the relationships of networks of genes, by interfering with one, and seeing its effects on a related gene, or suites of genes. "RNAi was ubiquitously available and easy to use, high-school kids were using it," recalls Lanphier. "So we said: 'How can we get this in the hands of every lab in the country or the world that wants to use it?'"[447]

However, zinc finger nucleases were difficult to use and expensive. Sigma-Aldrich began selling kits for $25000, based on techniques developed by Sangamo. Joung wanted to create libraries that were easier to use and cheap enough that academics could get them, and to do this, he and a technician named Morgan Maeder designed a means to identify combinations of zinc fingers from small preidentified "pools" that could work together effectively for recognizing a given target in the genome.[448] After years of grinding bench work, Maeder demonstrated that she had edited a gene called *VEGFA* with a zinc-finger nuclease in a human cell, making Joung the first academic to pull off the feat without requiring reagents from Sangamo. "I remember being relieved the platform was working," Joung told me in his office. "We'd spent two years on it, and I was very scared it wouldn't work." He showed me a framed gel of the experiment, which he still kept in his office, and which showed that the *VEGFA* gene had been edited. Maeder recalled it as "the most exciting thing ever. Even Keith was giddy; he said 'give me a high five' and we were jumping up and down, it was so exciting. For me it's two years' worth of work – for him it's a whole career."[449]

Before this moment, Sangamo was the only group that had demonstrated a mastery over the zinc finger nuclease. Joung turned it into an "open source" tool that any academic could use. But just as this was being achieved, an even more elegant and inexpensive genome editing tool was invented. *Xanthomonas* is a pathogenic bacteria that can infect plant species including pepper, rice, citrus, cotton, tomato and soybeans, causing insidious problems for these plants, like black rot and blight disease. The bacteria do this by injecting a number of effector proteins, including TAL effectors into the plant, which aid in bacterial infection. In fact, TAL effectors have a DNA binding domain, meaning that they can bind to the DNA in plants and switch on a number of plant genes that can lower the plant defenses and aid in the bacteria's conquest of the plant.[450] Adam Bogdanove at Iowa State University was studying TAL effectors that infect rice plants and discovered their structures are similar, except for a unique section in the middle, which is highly repetitive and composed of three dozen amino acids and which was each unique only at two amino acid positions. He noticed the number of repeats in the TAL effector that infected a bell pepper was equal to the number of nucleotides to which it bound. "I thought, 'Could it really be so simple?'," Bogdanove recalled.[451] He and colleague Matthew Moscou suggested that this repetitive sequence held the unique code that bound to repetitive code in the regulatory elements of plant genes. Bogdanove dropped a paper simultaneously in *Science* alongside Jens Boch and Ulla Bonas, whose work provided much stronger evidence and who are chiefly credited with deciphering the TAL code. Boch engineered TAL effectors that bound to predicted targets of DNA, in effect, showing they could easily be engineered to bind to any DNA sequence. "The potential was very clear right from the beginning," says Boch. "I couldn't sleep for two nights."[452]

In 2008, Bogdanove and Dan Voytas at the University of Minnesota fused a TAL effector to the DNA-cleaving domain of *FokI*, the restriction enzyme that Chandra had used to invent a zinc finger nuclease, resulting in a new gene editing tool, the miraculous and amazing TALEN. In 2009, by the time Feng Zhang got to working with George Church, TALENs appeared to be leapfrogging zinc finger nucleases, because of their cheap cost and ease of programmability. Zhang told me that's why there was some excitement when "we described the first system for customized cells using TALENs. It was entirely motivated by ZFN work, but ZFN is difficult to use." It would be a while before TALENs or Crispr-Cas9 made it into clinical trials, but zinc finger nucleases were far along in trials and I was interested to get a report on how they were faring.

In 2013, I called up Philip Gregory, who was, at the time, chief scientific officer at Sangamo Biosciences, Inc. (and has since moved to Bluebird BioSciences). I asked him how it was going and he said, "Very encouraging. One of the patients was aviremic." I did not know it at the time, but scientists rarely say that a patient is cured or free of HIV, because they simply can't check every cell in a patient's body for a stealth virus and declare the patient "cured." Instead, they say "aviremic," which means they can't find any trace of the virus, and they are pretty sure it is fairly under control. Gregory proceeded to tell me about the results of a trial of zinc finger nucleases on patients with human immunodeficiency virus, or HIV. In this case, zinc finger nucleases had been used to make an edit to a gene that builds a receptor in the patients' T-cells, causing them to be impenetrable to HIV. Miraculously, it appeared to work.

In fact, HIV could no longer be detected in one of his patients. A mutation called *CCR5-Delta32*, a 32-nucleotide deletion in a gene called *CCR5*, prevents the HIV virus from infecting people. *CCR5* is a gene expressed in CD4+ helper T-cells of the immune system, and it codes a protein for a co-stimulatory chemokine receptor, which is a lock on the door of a cell. This deletion breaks or jams the lock on the door, and virus can no longer get inside the T-cells. Over time, it is expected that the virus will kill off all the native T-cells and the genetically engineered T-cells will come to reign in the body.

The theory was tested in 2009 when German scientist Gero Hutter wrote a paper describing a US-born patient, Timothy Ray Brown, the "Berlin Patient," who was living abroad and happened to have both acute myelogenous leukemia (AML) and HIV. Brown received a bone marrow transplant to treat his cancer, but in a sly move, doctors selected a donor who also had two copies of the *CCR5* mutation. HIV continued to destroy his native T-cells, but the ones which were implanted with the mutation survived and grew in population. The HIV could no longer enter those T-cells, and before long this population of cells was on the rise. Brown had a fully functioning immune system. Hutter's paper described the only known patient to be functionally cured of HIV. Since these 32 nucleotide deletions in *CCR5* are somewhat rare in nature, Sangamo decided it would try to manufacture the deletion in the gene using tiny molecular scissors. The company built a zinc finger nuclease tool called SB-728 that could edit a specific site in the *CCR5* gene. The engineered T-cells would then be returned to the patients. Gregory began collaborating with Carl June, Bruce Levine and Pablo Tebas at Penn, and hatched a plan to outfox HIV.

Penn enrolled patients into the trial under the direction of Tebas, director of the AIDS Clinical Trials Unit. Levine, director at Penn's vaccine production facility, scaled up methods for genetically editing T-cells. The adenovirus carrying SB-728 was contract manufactured. The scheme was to program the correct address into the delivery system using the zinc fingers (more on this in a moment) which would take the scissors (nuclease) to the right address in the genome to make the tiny edit, removing 32 bases of DNA. The HIV virus was expected to continue to wipe out the native helper T-cells, while the newly introduced cells with the jammed *CCR5* locks blocked HIV's entrance and grew in population. In effect, the engineered cells would be repopulating the immune system. Researchers then planned to do a daring thing. During the trial, they would take their patients off their regimens of antiretroviral medications.

Philadelphia resident Emory Jay Johnson is an African American man who was in his 50s when he became the second patient (Patient Number 202) to get the treatment. He was diagnosed with HIV in September 1991, a couple of years before Tom Hanks starred in the film *Philadelphia*, and the disease was becoming an epidemic. Today, he works as a community director at ActionAids, a community outreach group, and takes a cocktail of anti-HIV drugs, including Trizivir and Isentress. In 2009, Johnson received a transfusion of his own genetically altered CD4+ cells. Ten billion cells that had been targeted for installation with copies of the *CCR5* gene altered with a broken lock that wouldn't allow HIV in the door were infused into his body. The idea was that as HIV destroyed the native CD4+ cells in his body, the population of the cells with the *CCR5-Delta32* mutation would gain a selective advantage and predominate in the population. "I had a severe reaction at the time of transfusion, which I was told is a good sign," Johnson told me. "This is a sign that the altered cells have taken. After a few minutes of the cells being trans-fused into my body, I got chills and rigors, and then severe cramping all over my body." Tebas took Johnson off his antiretroviral prescription for a few months after he received the transfusion of the genetically altered cells, and promisingly, his viral loads were observed to decrease. The engineered cells were working. "I decided to go back on my medications when my viral load became detectable again," Johnson said.

Counts of HIV virus shot back up in all the patients when they skirted their medications for months at a time, but in Patient Number 205, the virus load plummeted below a level of detection. That person no longer takes medications. Sangamo had treated 12 patients, but only Patient Number 205, a 50-year-old male who had lived with HIV for 1.9 years, no longer had detectable HIV. So what's so special about Patient 205? It turns out that 205 had one native copy of *CCR5*-Delta32, meaning he was "heterozygous" for the mutation. Sangamo's editing technique worked about 25 percent of the time, and since each cell contains two copies of *CCR5*, only a small fraction of cells (25 percent ×25 percent, or about six percent) would get the deletion in both copies of the *CCR5* gene needed to all-out slam the door on HIV. Patient 205 already had one copy of *CCR5* with the mutation, so he got a much higher number of cells, about 25 percent, with two broken locks.

"From early on, I thought ZFN could be game-changing, and I always had this feeling. We could see what was coming," Joung told me. But zinc fingers were still complicated to work with. The protocol that Joung and Maeder had published for assembling zinc finger nucleases had been 20 pages long. "It was not a trivial thing to do." And, when these new genome editing technologies emerged, Joung knew that the pace was going to start moving much faster. He developed a technology called FLASH, an automated way to make it easier to build arrays of TALENs, to target specific sites in the genome. In his first try with 96 constructs, he showed 84 out of 96 made edits at the correct site. "It was such a high success rate, and there was no real optimization involved," Joung said. "I was suddenly contemplating the reality that we could modify many, many genes at once. TALENs were so much easier to work with." And, Crispr-Cas9 was even easier to work with and more efficient than TALENs. "Through tireless efforts of numerous scientists around the world, most of the predictions about the applications using custom nucleases have come true," Chandra told me. But the technology was not without its pitfalls, often resulting in so-called "off-target" effects, when you end up editing a hundred other sites, like MapQuest putting you on the right street in the wrong neighborhood.

In 2008, Erik Sontheimer and Luciano Marraffini at Northwestern provided evidence that Crispr systems target DNA and suggested they might have practical applications in genome editing, filing the first of what would become a barrage of patent applications.[453] The Northwestern patent was not approved due to its "failure to describe invention," and was eventually abandoned.[454] We knew it worked – we just could not yet describe how. By the time Crispr-Cas9 emerged in its preparadigm phase 2008–2011, it quickly captured the interest of synthetic biologists. Zhang returned to Harvard, now a member of the Society of Fellows, becoming the first scientist to use TALEN to control the genes in a mammal. Zhang was soon reading papers on Crispr-Cas9. "The more I read, the harder it was to contain my excitement," he told the journalist Michael Specter.[455] "It didn't take Zhang, or other scientists long to realize that, if nature could turn these molecules into the genetic equivalent of a global positioning system, so could we. Researchers soon learned how to create synthetic versions of the RNA guides and program them to deliver their cargo to virtually any cell. Once the enzyme locks onto the matching DNA sequence, it can cut and paste nucleotides with the precision we have come to expect from the search-and-replace function of a word processor. "This was a finding of mind-boggling importance," Zhang said.[456] By now, "working mostly with mice, researchers have already deployed the tool to correct the genetic errors responsible for sickle-cell anemia, muscular dystrophy, and the fundamental defect associated with cystic fibrosis. Inevitably, the technology will also permit scientists to correct genetic flaws in human embryos. Any such change, though, would infiltrate the entire genome and eventually be passed down to children, grandchildren, great-grandchildren, and every subsequent generation. That raises the possibility, more realistically than ever before, that scientists will be able to rewrite the fundamental code of life, with consequences for future generations," Specter wrote.

In 2011, Zhang had been recruited to MIT by Ed Scolnick for a McGovern Institute opening, and wound up securing a high-ranking position at the Broad Institute in a single sweep. Crispr-Cas9 was bursting onto the scene at that time. "Crispr emerged in 2011 and the goal was to see if we could harness a bacterial nuclease to work in human cells," Zhang said. "Can you use this system in eukaryotic cells to edit a specific nucleotide?"[457]

Emmanuelle Charpentier, a medical microbiologist at Umea University, with her student Chylinski, made the first real breakthrough in describing the mechanisms of evolution of the "type II systems" in a *Nature* paper in 2011. "I did not know anyone from the field," Charpentier recalls, when she presented her findings at a conference in the Netherlands in late 2010. "Having said this, I had developed the idea to harness the minimal system of Crispr-Cas9 for a genetic tool and also proposed that it could be useful to treat human genetic disorders. Hence I was the first one to approach Jennifer Doudna (not convinced at first) and Feng ... to convince them to join me to build a company."

"In reality, by that point, Jennifer and I had already been talking with three venture capitalist firms, Third Security, Polaris and Flagship, as well as key co-founders in what would soon become Intellia and Crispr Therapeutics, forged by Charpentier."

Charpentier and Doudna, the powerhouse Berkley biochemist, showed for the first time that it could be used to cut purified DNA in a test tube. By January 2013, Zhang and Church each dropped papers in the same issue of *Science* showing that Crispr could be reprogrammed to edit mammalian cells, including human cells, drawing on the cells' machinery for homology-directed repair. That same month, Jennifer Doudna and Jin-Soo Kim separately published results that the Crispr system could work in human cells. Joung demonstrated its ability to edit the germline in zebra fish. Importantly, Zhang made a molecular tweak to his system by restoring a small hairpin structure to the guide RNA and showed this approach cuts and repairs DNA with higher efficiency, a task accomplished independently by Prashant Mali and Luhan Yang, both in George Church's lab.

In January 2013, "five papers appeared in the space of less than four weeks. It was a virtual five-way tie, for all purposes except those related to patents, where differences of even a single day have to matter. The crucial point is that if any one group had failed or had taken longer, it would have made no functional difference to the rest of the world – it would have still been available to everyone else at the same time, and the Crispr genome editing revolution would still have happened in the same way. All five groups deserve huge credit for showing that Cas9 can work in living cells for genome editing," Sontheimer told me. Crispr-Cas9 quickly leapfrogged zinc finger nucleases and TALENs as a technology of choice for therapeutic applications and basic research. In 2013, researchers in the Netherlands had used Crispr-Cas9 to edit and repair the *CFTR* gene in stem cells, putting the technology on stunning display and showing it might be used to treat cystic fibrosis.[458] Ravenous capitalists were soon swooning over the technology.

Zhang knew people at the venture capital firm Third Rock, and had visited them. Polaris and Flagship, two other firms, then approached him. "I remember Kevin Bitterman and Doug Cole came to visit. I told them I was already talking with Third Rock, and the three decided to work together." A new company was forming, called Editas Medicine, based on the patent wins – but it was forged from a handful of founding scientists who each held expertise, but who frequently clashed, even after the departure of Doudna. However, Joung told me that the perceptions of sour relations between the founders were mostly injected by competitors hoping to spike their punch. In July 2016, David Liu, a founder of Editas accepted a high-paid position as core member at the Broad Institute, strengthening the ties between the venture-backed Editas and the Broad.

Crispr-Cas9 was a programmable system that could be used to target virtually any address in the genome, progressing from a stage where "scientists noticed a bunch of repeats" to one where it's "unambiguously a technology," Church told me. Few targets had been discussed publically. The Delta508 mutation in the *CFTR* gene was being edited to provide a therapeutic benefit for patients with cystic fibrosis. A gene called *CEP290* could be edited to treat the devastating eye disease Lebers congenital amaurosis. Many diseases of hematopoietic lineages such as disorders of red blood cells or the white blood cells of the immune system were being discussed. But it was also becoming clear that Crispr-Cas9 was coming up against the complicated realities of biology.

In April 2016, the great MIT biologist Rudolf Jaenisch and colleagues used Crispr-Cas9 to create a genetic alteration in human pluripototent stem cells in a distal enhancer element – meaning a section of code not in a gene, but which enhances the expression of the gene – and showed it could affect changes in the expression of α-synuclein (SNCA), "a key gene implicated in the pathogenesis of Parkinson's disease."[459] Rather problematically, Jaenisch noted, such changes in the genetic code only accounted for extremely weak effects on the expression of that gene, and that dozens or more of such variants each contributed small effects. The finding was impressive, but the paper clearly impressed the point that Crispr-Cas9 was not so useful at providing a therapeutic mechanism for a complex disease.

The effect on basic research was immediate. Crispr reagents had been ordered from the molecular repository Addgene 50000 times by the close of 2015. Although hundreds of scientists have contributed Crispr reagents to the repository for scientists to order, Zhang's deposits have dominated orders and account for a majority, perhaps up to 75 percent of orders. The Cancer Cell Lineage Encyclopedia which involved a partnership between Novartis and the Broad Institute included a program called Project Achilles, which used Crispr-Cas9 to knock out every gene – one by one – in a thousand cancer cell lines to determine which genes could stop its growth. If knocking out a gene resulted in an abrupt end to cancer growth, that gene might be thought of as a target. "What I love most about the Crispr process is that you can take any cancer-cell line, knock out every gene, and identify every one of the cell's Achilles' heels," Eric Lander told *The New Yorker*. "You can also use Crispr to systematically study the ways that a cancer cell can escape from a treatment. That should make it possible to build a comprehensive road map for cancer... of every trick that cancer cells have – how they form, all the ways you can defeat them, and all the ways they can escape and defeat a treatment. And when we have that we win. Because every cancer cell starts naïve. It doesn't know what we have waiting in the freezer for it. Infectious diseases are a different story; they share their knowledge as they spread. They learn from us as they move from person to person. But every person's cancer starts naïve. And this is why we will beat it."[460]

New applications were being submitted like gangbusters. Zhang, Church and Charlie Gersbach at Duke had been feverishly filing claims for patents around Crispr technology that could be used to edit eukaryotic cells. There was new urgency to file. For years, scientists had sent themselves postcards and self-addressed letters in the mail to establish a timeline under a "first to invent" patent claim, which was a system that weighed evidence regarding the scientist who first had the kernel of an idea, but was also based on demonstration of the technology and "reducing the concept to practice." But the patent laws were changing.

On March 16, 2013, the system changed to a "first-to-file" approach with the United States Patent and Trademark Office (PTO). Zhang filed his provisional application describing a method for eukaryotic genome editing on December 12, 2012, while Doudna and Charpentier had filed a provisional patent application on May 25, 2012,[461] seven months before, and another patent was filed by the Lithuanian scientist Virginijus Siksnys in March 2012.[462] Jennifer Doudna's provisional patent application was filed under "first-to-invent" rules and became an official patent application on March 15, 2013, one day before the rules changed to "first-to-file;" Zhang filed his application on October 15, 2013.

As Jacob S. Sherkow, an associate professor at New York Law School, detailed the patent battle in the Stanford Center for Law and the Biosciences Blog "On October 15, 2013, Zhang filed his own patent application (No. 14/054,414) – months after the first-to-file rules came into effect – but claiming a December 12, 2012 priority date under the old first-to-invent rules. Concurrent with his application, Zhang also filed an Accelerated Examination Request (also known, somewhat comically, as a Petition to Make Special), a request that the PTO make an up or down decision on an inventor's application so long as it's short (no more than three independent claims), directed to a single invention, and under the condition that the inventor won't argue the patentability (or lack thereof) of individual claims during prosecution (i.e., that the inventor agrees to an all-or-nothing decision on his application). Zhang's patent application, unlike Doudna and Charpentier's, however, specifically contemplated adapting Crispr in eukaryotic cells."[463] In fact, Doudna's non-provisional application refers to "genetically modified cells" and she was quick to point out to me that her provisional application articulated that these cells could be broadly applied to include prokaryotic or eukaryotic cells, which could be extended to include plant, mammalian or even human cells, which functioned as a recital or listing of potential applications. Indeed, a search of Doudna's application turns up the word "eukaryotic" a resounding 70 times. In an email, Doudna chastened Sherkow's report that her application did not contemplate eukaryotic cells, calling it "factually incorrect" and stating firmly that "adapting the Crispr-Cas9 system for eukaryotic cells is disclosed and claimed in" her patent filed on May 25, 2012. Sherkow conceded to me in an email that he could have been more careful in his wording, and what he implied was that Zhang had been explicit in specifically contemplating the use of Crispr in eukaryotic cells, while Doudna wrote in broad terms of using Crispr on "genetically modified cells" and then covered all of the possible meanings in her application. Doudna and Charpentiers' patent may, or may not, be an example of "threadbare recital," a claiming of patent disclosures that don't describe the practice in enough detail that those of ordinary skill could pick it up as a practice in eukaryotic cell type— although five independent groups did just that, rapidly within months. Doudna told me she objected to media coverage suggesting that she had not "specifically contemplated" using Crispr-Cas9 in human cells. But Sherkow noted it's not the media, but the courts and lawyers, who will impart a legal interpretation on the language of the patents. "Reasonable minds could disagree," Sherkow told me in an email. "Whether Doudna's disclosures were sufficient to award her a patent is a legal issue, not a factual one. It's not like there's some scientifically correct answer." This issue – whether Doudna disclosed eukaryotic applications in her patent application – is precisely the issue in dispute in the interference right now. A little more granularly, the interference currently centers on whether that information related to eukaryotic cells in Doudna's application was legally sufficient to adopt Doudna's CRISPR system to eukaryotic applications. It may be sufficient; it may not be. That's what the interference is all about." The patent office issued Zhang his first Crispr patent on April 15, 2014,[464] stoking a fierce conflict over who had the legal authority to use the technology in therapeutics.[465]

"Even though Doudna had both an earlier invention date and filing date – Zhang won the initial patent race, and with specific claims covering profitable eukaryotic applications," Sherkow wrote. "Doudna and Charpentier's patent application languished" at the patent office for that year owing to deficiencies in the ownership of the patent due to co-inventor Charpentier's agreements with several European institutions. Her initial application described only "genetically modified cells that produce Cas9," the enzyme critical to the Crispr reaction and "Cas9 transgenic non-human multicellular organisms" and noting that "the present disclosure further provides methods of site-specific modification of a target DNA" and "methods for modulating transcription of a target nucleic acid in a target cell." Doudna was retooling her application; competitors were submitting counterweight. Sherkow writes, "In addition, on September 5, 2014, a mysterious third party submitted a 66

page report of prior art – including one of Zhang's patents – in an effort to
sink Doudna's application." Doudna's attorneys amended her claims on
January 9, 2015, canceling 155 of her previous claims, while banking on
nine claims covering applications of using Crispr as a gene editing tool
including eukaryotic cells. "But this, too, spurred a response from a
mysterious third party, who submitted more literature – including UC
Berkeley press releases – to sink Doudna's application."

It was a game of battleship. On April 13, 2015, Doudna's attorneys
amended her application once again, cancelling all previous 164 claims,
and submitting 82 new claims directed to "a desired cell type," which was
"presumably an effort to include both prokaryotic and eukaryotic cells."
Importantly, Sherkow wrote, "Doudna's attorneys filed a 114 page
Suggestion of Interference, claiming that ten of Zhang's issued patents were
interfering with their patent application. Two days later, Antonio Regalado
of theTechnology Review quoted Paul Goldsmith of the Broad Institute
saying that the Institute had made "repeated efforts and trips since the
beginning of 2013 to resolve this situation outside the legal system."[466]

Joung was continuing to test the limitations of Crispr-Cas9 in his lab at
Mass General. A decade before he turned down a job interview at
Sangamo, telling them he was a scientist, not a man of industry. But
he had been taking responsibility not only for innovation, but for doing a
lot of the hardcore bench work to demonstrate how safe Crispr-Cas9 is
to use, exploiting its technical limitations and propensity to cause off-
target effects, or unintended mutations. As 2013 pressed on, capitalists
kept showing up at his office, knocking on his door.

The technical limitations of the technology were dropping off the
radar *even as I was writing*, making the moral and regulatory questions
more and more urgent. But there is a lot more to evaluating the safety
and efficacy of a genome editing tool and bringing it to market as a
therapeutic, than simply getting the technology operational. It can't
cause unintended problems. Joung realized the FDA was never going to
give Crispr-Cas9 a pass without metrics and a surefire way to quantify
its technical problems. He came up with a clever method called "GUIDE-
seq (Genome-wide Unbiased Identification of Double-strand breaks
Enabled by sequencing)," a means to insert a "shortdouble-stranded
oligo," or molecular tag, anywhere that a nuclease causes a break in a

cell's DNA. With that tag, he could locate all of the "off-target effects" anywhere in the 3-billion-base genome. Prior to that, scientists only looked for off-target effects where they suspected they might occur. "The old analogy we always use is looking for your car keys under a streetlamp," Joung said. "Well you could have dropped your keys in the dark someplace else. We needed a way to quantify and localize the risk."

Joung tested Crispr-Cas9 targeted to ten different gene targets, and he found some had as many as 130 or 150 "off-target effects," although some had less than 20; one of the genes he targeted had none that could be detected. Just a few mistakes in the editing tool counted in the tens or hundreds doesn't seem like much. "Don't assume this doesn't matter," Joung said. "In a cell culture, even if you hit the wrong target in 1 in 1,000,000 edits, if you are modifying hundreds of millions of cells, you may still have some off-target hits. And if you hit a tumor suppressor (cancer-related gene) then the consequences could be catastrophic." Joung came up with a few clever solutions. One was to trim the 20-nucleotide programmable sequence of the Crispr system down to 17 bases.[467] The other thing that Joung did was to create mutant forms of the Cas9 protein which were more precise. "There's always a risk with any drug," Joung said. "However, if the number of off-targets is low and has little deleterious effect, if the disease is severe, and if we have that data to measure all of this, we can make a stronger case to the FDA."[468]

On January 6, 2016, Massachusetts General Hospital released a press release stating that "High-fidelity Crispr-Cas9 nucleases have no detectable off-target mutations: Team develops improved version of important gene-editing tool." The statement said that, "A new engineered version of the gene-editing Crispr-Cas9 nuclease appears to robustly abolish the unwanted, off-target DNA breaks that are a significant current limitation of the technology, reducing them to undetectable levels." Keith Joung, Benjamin Kleinstiver, Vikram Pattanayak and Michelle Prew discovered a variant in a Cas nuclease that was highly discriminating against mismatched target sites, while retaining full on-target activities in human cells. The variant was called SpCas9-HF1,[469] and it made correct alterations 85 percent of the time using GUIDE-Seq. deep-sequencing experiments.[470] These molecular scissors were precise. Soon there were new nucleases being discovered that cut with even more precision and resulted in cuts that left "sticky ends," which resulted in cleaner repairs based on homology-directed repair. In September 2015, Feng Zhang and colleagues published a paper in the journal *Cell* showing that another protein, Cpf1, might be easier to use than Cas9. The endonuclease Cas9 lands like a shoehorn on a specific code called a "proto-spacer motif" or PAM, which begins with two guanine nucleotides such as NGG where the N can be any random letter, while Cpf1 first contacts genetic code at two thymines, or NTT. Importantly Cas9 makes a "blunt ended cut" meaning it snaps the double helix without leaving any overhangs, and that makes a subsequent repair much more likely to occur through the mechanisms of non-homologous end-joining, which results in insertions and deletions, a cobbled patch. By comparison, Cpf1 leaves an overhanging strand, sometimes called a cohesive or "sticky end." It turns out that the sticky end with an overhang provides a template that makes it more likely to apply a repair by drawing on its apparatus of homology-directed repair.[471,472]

Derrick Rossi had meanwhile been collaborating with Fred Alt, a geneticist at Harvard, who developed his own means to test for off-target effects called "high-throughput, genome-wide translocation sequencing," or HTGTS, to test off-target effects, or mutations, caused by Crispr genome editing systems. In an elegant study using Crispr-Cas9 in hematopoietic stem cells, Rossi and colleagues found only a single mutation.[473] "The important point is we've been able to empirically determine the frequency of off-target effects in a clinically relevant cell type, and we found very little off-target activity – actually we found only 1 off-target mutation from 6 different experiments on human hematopoietic stem cells," Rossi told me. "The current standard for gene therapy trials that the FDA has deemed acceptable involves at least 1 large mutagenic event per cell because that is what occurs when you use viral vectors such as retroviruses or lentiviruses to introduce therapeutic transgenes into cells. From this perspective, I'd say that getting too hung up on the exceedingly rare off-target effects of Crispr-Cas9 strikes me as alarmist." Furthermore, there will always be unintended off-target mutational effects using Crispr systems, because each human genome is a unique sequence, so there is no way to establish a means without risk. Church told an audience at a talk that off-target effects occur as infrequently as 10 events per million cells, while the spontaneous mutation error rate in a cell division in the body is 0.1 to 10 events per each cell division. In fact, Church argued, the rate of such off-target mutations is "far below spontaneous error rate. I'm a scientist. I'm for setting the bar high, but I wonder how high we are aiming."

The techniques of using Crispr systems for editing was increasingly sophisticated with new variants of Cas9 and Cpf1 which could improve the rate of homology-directed repairs. The earliest versions of Crispr-Cas9 systems favored non-homologous end-joining, which essentially allowed scientists to create gene "knockouts" by causing a double-strand break which was fixed by the cell's machinery for non-homologous end-joining. Zhang and colleagues' revelation that Cpf1 could create "sticky ends" of double-strand breaks with an overhang meant the system could be used to cause a break which resulted in a preference for homology-directed repair. In doing so, scientists not only had a means to create a knockout in a gene, but they could now add customized genetic variants by including a template for homology-directed repair. Rossi had discovered another way to tip the cells' preference to use homology directed repair in hematopoietic stem cells. Non-homologous end-joining is the dominant repair mechanism during the G1 phase of the cell cycle, while homologous recombination, or homology-directed repair, is preferred in the S and G2 cycles. By applying a set of molecules to a plate of hematopoietic stem cells, Rossi was able to sustain the growth of these stem cells and expand their numbers exponentially, "something that had been notoriously difficult to do."

By maintaining the growth cycle, he was able to tip the repair strategy in favor of homology-directed repair. Over the course of several dinners and meetings with Harvard colleague David Scadden, and with backing from Third Rock, Rossi hatched a plan to start a new company called Magenta Therapeutics, which couples a suite of technologies focused on transplantation medicine, including the stem cell expansion technology developed in Rossi's lab. Another technology that Scadden had developed involving an antibody targeting strategy to wipe out specific hematopoietic cells in the body, allowing safe and effective stem cell transplantation. Existing strategies make use of a full body irradiation to zap all the bone marrow cells in the body followed by an allograph bone marrow transplant or cord cell transplant, but this results in a lot of collateral damage to the body, including to sensitive tissues like reproductive organs. And there is a mortality rate of 15 to 20 percent associated with current transplantation approaches, limiting the use of this life-saving treatment to only the sickest of patients. If Magenta's vision is realized, collateral damage and transplant-related mortality would be a thing of the past, opening up the possibility of introducing Crispr-engineered blood-forming stem cells into patients to treat a wide range of diseases. It was a powerful demonstration of how Crispr-Cas9 was changing the landscape of medicine in the clinic.

As of January 1, 2016, the United States Patent and Trademark Office (USPTO) has issued 23 Crispr and Cas9 patents, including a robust portfolio of 13 Crispr patents to the Broad Institute, MIT and affiliated groups for inventions from Zhang. The patent office has also issued four Crispr patents to Harvard University relating to George Church and David Liu, three Crispr patents to DuPont, one to Agilent Technologies, one to the University of Georgia Research Foundation and one to Institut Pasteur. In February 2016, another Crispr patent was awarded, this time to Caribou Biosciences, a company founded by Doudna which extends its expertise to gene editing in agriculture and livestock. "Engineering any genome, at any site, in any way," declares Caribou's website. The Cas 9 licencing agreement between the Broad Institute / MIT / Harvard and Editas is issued exclusively for therapeutics, with a "clawback clause," which means, as Zhang told me, "if you're a third party, and no one else is working on a particular disease application, you can say: 'let us work on it.' It's very expensive to make a drug, and no one can tackle drug development all by themselves," he noted, pointing me to a recent *Boston Globe* article that cited an average cost of $2 billion for a single drug. Patent wins can be huge. "Just by way of example: In 1983 Columbia University scientists patented a method for introducing foreign DNA into cells, called cotransformation. By the time the patents expired in 2000, they had brought in $790 million in revenue."[474]

Church, Doudna, Joung, Zhang and David Liu founded Editas Medicine with backing from Third Rock, Flagship, Polaris and the Partners Innovation Fund (a venture fund run by Partners Healthcare, the parent organization for Massachusetts General Hospital and other local Boston hospitals). Doudna withdrew from Editas, and along with Rossi, Marraffini, Sontheimer, Barrangou and others, she started Intellia Therapeutics with backing from Atlas Ventures and Novartis, and in partnership with Caribou Biosciences (another Crispr company that Doudna had co-founded in Berkeley in 2011, even before the advent of genome editing). Caribou's icon looks like an antler shape, which is designed to depict a folded RNA molecule, but as Church told me "the cool Easter egg is that it contains the word "ribo."

Charpentier, Shaun Foy and Roger Novak had started Crispr Therapeutics with funding from Versant Ventures, while Chad Cowan,

Matt Porteus, Dan Anderson and Craig Mello joined as scientific co-founders. Doudna's attorneys kept fighting. On December 21, 2015, "the primary examiner responsible for Doudna and Charpentier's patent application, Michelle K. Joike, along with an interference specialist (likely Brandon Fetterolf) issued an Initial Interference Memo, a recommendation that the Patent Trial and Appeals Board (the PTAB) conduct a procedure known as an 'interference proceeding' between Doudna's and Zhang's patent applications," which has "the potential to decide who owns the core Crispr intellectual property, possibly stripping Zhang of his near-dozen patents, and shaking up hundreds of millions dollars of investment in their respective companies."[475] On January 11, 2016, the office initiated a declaration for an interference proceeding.[476]

THE BROAD INSTITUTE, INC., MASSACHUSETTS INSTITUTE OF TECHNOLOGY, AND PRESIDENT AND FELLOWS OF HAVARD COLLEGE,
(PATENTS 8,697,359; 8,771,945; 8,795,965; 8,865,406; 8,871,445; 8,889,356; 8,895,308; 8,906,616; 8,932,814; 8,945,839; 8,993,233; AND 8,999,641),
Junior Party,

v.

THE REGENTS OF THE UNIVERSITY OF CALIFORNIA, UNIVERSITY OF VIENNA, AND EMMANUELLE CHARPENTIER
(Application 13/842,859),
Senior Party.

In STAT, the journalist Sharon Begley wrote that the declaration of an interference hearing set up "a winner-take-all intellectual property brawl that will begin in March." But Church tempered that assertion to me in an email, noting that "some of the fundamental Crispr patents are uncontested, and that in most engineering fields, patents from many teams are needed to produce a real-world product. So, Crispr is unlikely, in my opinion, to be a winner-take-tall or zero-sum legal case."

If interference is declared, an assignment of a three patent judge panel to hear the case. Such an interference proceeding, as Sherkow writes, "will likely – or at least – discourage the possibility of a settlement between the parties. The interference declaration is a Rubicon, of sorts, beyond which the parties must compete for territory." And further he notes that "interference proceedings are famous for their formalistic complexity – an almost Soviet-style detail to bureaucratic rules that gives even seasoned patent prosecutors the shudders. With that said, the proceedings look somewhat like an actual trial, with the interference divided into two phases: the interlocutory phase and the testimonial phase. At the interlocutory stage, the three judge panel will set a motions calendar: a timeline for when the two parties – Doudna, the 'senior party,' and Zhang, the 'junior party' – can present initial briefs. Those initial briefs will likely include preliminary substantive statements about the patentability of the inventions at-issue, whether there is truly an interference in-fact... motions often come down to inventor testimony – notarized notebooks and the like – as well as affidavits called Rule 131 Statements," such as statements, "Of course I invented that two years earlier than I originally claimed!" "Whether Doudna and Zhang – two of the most well-liked and seemingly honest scientists in any field – will engage in this priority dispute through Rule 131 Statements will be interesting," Sherkow writes, "I'm only saying that the procedure has a bad reputation among patent attorneys. It'll be like watching Nobel Prize winners defend themselves in traffic court." In addition, the proceedings could include inventor depositions and cross-examinations. "That's right: Doudna and Zhang may be required to take the stand."[477]

11   Gene Hackers

> Consider God's handiwork; who can straighten what He hath
> made crooked?
>
> –Ecclesiastes 7:13

"Can Neanderthals be Brought back from the Dead?" screamed a headline from *Der Spiegel*. The German magazine had just published an article quoting synthetic biologist George Church saying that scientists had collected enough DNA that now only an "adventurous" woman was needed to bring a Neanderthal into this world. *Technology Review* printed a similar story titled "Wanted: Surrogate for Neanderthal Baby." But now he was backpedaling a bit. Saying it's possible is "certainly very different from taking out a want ad," he told the *Huffington Post*. The plausibility of reviving *Homo neanderthalensis* had been deduced since the Neanderthal project was launched in 2006 to elucidate the genetic sequence of the extinct hominid. Birthing one is credible since the extinct species shares 99.7% of its code with modern people, and it's known the two species interbred due to a genetic property called admixture.

A pale winter was coming to a close in Boston. Red and yellow tulips had popped up in the white marble quadrangle at Harvard Medical School. Students were stalling outside. I was on campus to talk to Church about a paper he recently published on a new gene editing tool. He had been suggesting he could use it to do wondrous things, which included springing extinct species back to life. Church studied under Walter Gilbert and was one of the first scientists to demonstrate direct genome sequencing. In the 1990s, he helped create startup Gendaq (later acquired by Sangamo). He has a backwoods beard, which makes him look like a lumberjack; and hair that is soft, silky white. He is a gigantic man at 6 feet, 6 inches tall, and is usually well dressed, in a sport coat, usually tweeds, browns, old-school Harvard style dress, and he is an old soul, as they say, there is this sense that he is solidly in his shoes. He is also light on his feet, sometimes dashing up the stairs at the New Research Building, a glass-cased building at Harvard that houses his offices.

As of late, Church was acting as much P.T. Barnum as he was pioneering geneticist, which is why he can evoke cant, even outrage from a scientific community which counts understatement among its most guarded etiquettes. But he can also be quite reserved and circumspect, and at times when he speaks, his tone is dismissive, slow paced and exceedingly cautious. The cult of personality that has built up around Church is a study in its own right. It is most certainly partly due to his success as an innovator and a provocateur and up-ender of things trusted and orthodox – he definitely has a love for staking counterintuitive position; he wants to bring back the passenger pigeon and the mammoth for Christ sake. But when Church does stake positions, such as editing in a human embryo, or in eggs or sperm, he usually couples it with a lucid argument, in this case, that fewer mutations or risk are actually incurred when editing the germline than in somatic cells, since it involves fewer cells by orders of magnitude. In the case that Church gets in a room with Eric Lander, who is roughly his same height and who has the unbuttoned stature of a brawler, Lander can push for consensus, while Church will demur, digress and be difficult, and revel in discourse. Lander notes there are few cases of rare or orphan diseases in which genome editing may actually apply, and Church will counter that in many circumscribed subpopulations of the world, such as Pennsylvania Dutch, those rates are precipitously higher. And it can go on like this, Lander carefully constructing a reasonable consensus, and Church punching holes.

Genome editing will get "pushed to younger and younger ages" as the technology progressed, Church said. Editing in the germline should in many cases be considered more effective and safer. "Many of the two thousand or so gene therapies, including precise gene editing, being tested in clinical trials around the world today are already curing patients, and some are being approved for general use. As with all new therapies, we need to pay great attention to the effectiveness, safety, reversibility, and cost of gene editing. In some cases, genetic counseling is more effective than gene therapy, but in other cases, both parents carry only the high risk genetic types, or do not want to harm embryos, and so they might choose gene therapy of somatic or germ cells," he said. "The effectiveness of gene editing can depend on age. To cure some types of blindness, it may need to be performed in a young child. Other disorders might require gene editing even earlier, just as some surgeries need to be performed on children in the womb. Doing gene editing in sperm or egg cells can greatly improve both the safety and effectiveness of the procedure. One potential problem with gene editing is the occurrence of "off-target" mutations that can affect the treated cell in possibly unpredictable ways. Correcting a problem in liver or retinal cells may require gene editing in millions of cells. Even if the risk of off-target mutations is low, with so many cells involved the chance of it happening is not insubstantial. Gene editing in a single sperm or egg cell, could lower the risk of off-target mutations by a million-fold."[478]

Church holds more than 50 patents and has helped to start or advise scores of companies, he commands deep knowledge of genetics and synthetic biology, and his office is cased with books on microbiology that go back through the decades. When we met in his office, little red lights on his telephone were blipping, and conversation was interpolated with a barrage of incoming calls, and pauses, as he drifted on the brink of sleep. For all his charismatic appeal, Church is narcoleptic, lapsing into periods of slumber amidst the daylight hours. A British reporter called about ten minutes into our conversation, asking him to clarify comments he made to *Der Spiegel*. "Any question but that one," he demurred, wincing." I've been a good sport for six years." Church had become a statesman for the field, and reporters had been calling to draw on his authority on all matters DNA. But this was one case where fiction got the better side of fact. By now, Church had a stack of letters from a hundred applicants to be surrogates to carry a Neanderthal into this world. The letters were "very earnest, inspired and touching," he told me. Couples, who had been saving for a trip, wrote in saying a Neanderthal birth was a more inspiring way to spend their savings. "I don't do work on Neanderthal, in any shape or form. There were a lot of lessons to be learned from this," Church said, "mostly for me."

Genetic engineering was emerging from the plausible to the real, and the press was railing for more. Everyone, it seemed, from the editors at *The New York Times* to the magazines in Europe, was enamored with his "de-extinction" plans to bring back fleets of large-tusked woolly mammoths, flocks of passenger pigeons. It was so *close* to real. Twenty years before, in the 1993 sci-fi action adventure film *Jurassic Park*, Richard Attenborough played an entrepreneur who built a theme park which features dinosaurs that he brought to life under the auspices of genetic engineering, and which he believes are well contained. A mathematician played by Jeff Goldblum then discovers an anomaly which allows the dinosaurs to begin breeding, escape the control and go on a rampage. Now it seemed like it was finally possible. Church was downplaying the hype, but, at the same time, hosting "fireside chats" to drum up the conversation. Indeed, Church's 2012 book *Regenesis* featured a painting by Eustache Le Sueur of a bearded God creating the world. Soon, it seemed, we'd be racing among extinct species, armed with elephant guns, building Jurassic Parks. Church suggested the return of the mammoth (which he *was* working on) as an example of a way to improve diversity and resuscitate keystone species.[479] While bringing back species of charismatic megafauna such as saber-toothed tigers and prehistoric bears was probably out of the question, a hairy, large-tusked cold-weather elephant would not only be cool, it might graze on spring grasses and preserve tundra in a frozen state, helping to ease global warming. But more importantly, it would be a sort of moonshot for science. "Why was it necessary to put a human footprint on the moon? The fact is that it inspired generations of engineers," he said.

The biologist Richard Dawkins once said that groups and individuals mingle in loose federations, like "clouds in the sky or dust-storms in the desert," while "genes, like diamonds, are forever." If the publishing of the first draft of the human genome in 2001 was like decoding an ancient, antediluvian script, Crispr-Cas9 now existed to rewrite the Tablets of Stone. Unlike methods of "gene insertion" which made a cargo drop of a gene at a random site in the genome, scientists could use Crispr-Cas9 to make a highly specific edit to a gene adrift in a sea of billons of nucleotides in a genome. Duke biologist Charles Gersbach summed up the state of affairs to *The New York Times*, in which he noted the tool not only makes germline alterations feasible, but allows for "customizing the genome of any cell or any species at will." The writer Matthew Herper exalted the technology to the highest order. "This Protein Could Change Biotech Forever," he trumpeted in his blog post for *Forbes* magazine.

Certainly it was emerging as a "disruption" to modern medicine, redefining the field of options since they can edit DNA with a one-time treatment. It appeared to work with more efficiency and precision than the other pair of molecular scissors on the market, the zinc finger nuclease, which Sangamo and Penn had been demonstrating with great panache in human trials. So far, the zinc finger nuclease appeared safe in humans, at least for *ex vivo* therapies, genetic engineering performed in blood and immune cells outside the body and then reintroduced into patients' bloodstreams. Church was hemming and hawing in his office that Sangamo's success in HIV trials beckoned an optimistic future for gene therapy. Sangamo's tool "would fly through the FDA. The FDA is regarded as a bunch of Luddites, but they're not," Church said. "They only care if it works." Meanwhile, the Europeans were backing gene therapy.

Glybera, that spring, became the first gene therapy drug to gain approval by a major western regulatory body – the European Commission. The construct is delivered as a shot to the leg to treat a disease known as lipoprotein lipase deficiency by delivering the *LPL* gene using a viral vector known as adeno-associated virus. Not long after the "drug" went to sale, a group of scientists at Harvard University showed that they could use this virus to deliver a gene to mice to restore their hearing.[480] Those scientists, led by Charles Askew and Jeffrey Holt, used the virus to install a gene called *TMC1*, or transmembrane channel-like 1, into deaf mice, restoring their hearing. In a trick of engineering, they wired the gene to a switch, or promoter region, from a gene in a chicken, so that the gene would have gentler expression. Jim Wilson at Penn was now a scientific advisor to RegenexBio, which was also engineering adeno-associated virus into constructs for gene therapy. Importantly, adeno-associated virus slips into cells, but does not integrate into the chromosome, unlike lentivirus or retrovirus, which do integrate into our genomes at random locations, in effect creating a random mutation in each cell that the construct is deployed into. Many scientists were arguing that the FDA's threshold for mutations, one per cell using integrating viruses such as lentivirus or retrovirus, was vastly riskier than using a genome editing technique such as Crispr-Cas9, which when deployed into a plate of tens of thousands of human cells usually creates a handful of "off-target effects," staggeringly fewer mutations than one per cell. This is a technical argument. The controversy of editing the germline is that these mutations will stay with us, interrogating the "sacred" space of human genome was primarily framed as a moral argument. Many people wanted to cure deafness, and there's not much controversy here, although it's important to note some people in the deaf community do not see their status as a disability, but as a unique advantage. But the germline is a hot button issue, because the mutations continue in future generations and are therefore suggestive of a "transhuman" or GMO people, even summoning out imagination for new kinds of racism. As the cognitive scientist Steven Pinker noted, the conservatism over GMO foods probably foretells a conservatism over engineering GMO children. "With each enhancement providing a trifling benefit and a non-negligible risk, and with the editing process itself imposing risks, it's unlikely that today's morbidly risk-averse helicopter parents will take a chance at enhancing a child. They won't even feed their babies genetically modified applesauce!"[481]

Church and other biotech entrepreneurs were highly conscious of the parallels and concerned that reactions in the popular press could lead to activists obstructing gene therapy trials in humans, as they once rung out loudly in protest to the genetically modified crops introduced by Monsanto Corp. in the 1990s. "These controversies over genetic modification will stay with us for a while. Vaccines have been contentious since the days of Jenner and Pasteur, and still are, and today people keep coming up with reasons to be against vaccines, which are often emotional." Public perception was a tangle of contradictions. "We now have genetically modified Europeans, intermixing with people who won't eat genetically modified food," Church noted.

As we continued to talk, Church was at work like a kid, tinkering with colorful plastic models of proteins and nucleotide structures, tiny models of life scattered on a round wooden table in this office. If the genome was an arrangement of molecules, then scientists should be able to rearrange those molecules to change the outcome of diseases. It was an idea that had been gaining traction, as our molecular nature was further revealed. In January 2009, Church introduced the Personal Genome Project, a project to publish the genomes of 100000 volunteers. Steven Pinker joined as one of the first ten guinea pigs and wrote about it in *The New York Times Magazine*. It was an ambitious work to put the molecular signals of many diseases in sharp relief. Church has a vested interest in such open-access data since he cofounded the personal genome sequencing and interpretation companies, Knome, Inc., and Veritas Genetics, which take clients' saliva and generates prognostic data on their likelihood for attaining any number of diseases. Presumably, more data would mean more reliable signals to diagnose diseases. Church's genome was the fourth whole human genome sequence published (*Science* 2009) and by 2010 there were about a dozen. Not long after, as Church was about to give a talk in Seattle, someone sitting in the front row told him they'd seen his genome online and suggested he get off statins, since they can cause muscle damage and might not help his cholesterol. Church consulted with his doctor, and the advice was valid. Church stopped taking statins, and lowered his cholesterol from 285 to 205 mg/dL with a vegan diet.

Personal genomics concealed important secrets, but federal regulators were wrestling with how genomics should be used. In early 2013, the FDA made a much publicized and controversial decision to stop the personal genomics service 23andMe from selling its interpretive services. "23andMe made two tactical errors," Church said. "First, they did not follow the clinical route and weren't providing true medical genetics. For instance, they were testing only three alleles for the *BRCA1* and *BRCA2* (breast cancer) genes, and in reality, hundreds of variants exist which could alter the prognosis. Their second mistake was that they didn't stay engaged, and while the FDA had tried to contact them for six months, there was nothing but radio silence." Just how reliable personal genomics was, and importantly, how to disclose genetic data, was increasingly under fire. The FDA was playing it safe. "I believe, emphatically, that there is a lot you can learn from your genome today," Church countered. "The anti-determinists want to say that DNA is a little side-show, but every disease that's with us is caused by DNA and can be fixed by DNA."

In June 2013, around the time I was in Church's office, the Supreme Court struck down the rights to a patent held by Myriad on *BRCA1* and *BRCA2*. (The Court allowed the company to maintain patents around so-called copy DNA, or cDNA.) Since Myriad has genetic data on more than four million people, and tests for hundreds of variants in the breast-cancer-related genes, the decision had barely eroded Myriad's virtual monopoly on the gene, Church told me. Indeed, the American Civil Liberties Union or ACLU had called Church to testify, due to his open access work on the Personal Genome Project, but backed off when they learned he supported genetic patents. The patenting of genetic variants "encourages innovation. A lot of observers believe open access will result in free and open and shiny things, but the alternatives to patents are trade secrets. In biology and medicine, trade secrets are particularly dangerous; biological obfuscation, you can call it." But there was an elephant in the room. Personal genomics would remain stuck, if there were no tools to edit the mutations in our DNA. The open secret was no one really wanted a report from Knome or 23andMe predicting a chance of a serious disease, if nothing could be done about it. It was like having a Chilton's manual for auto repair, and no socket set. Despite the prodigious work of genetics, despite the cache of data on more than four million patients that Myriad held, the actress Angelina Jolie had been pressed into the most unfortunate, and also courageous, decision of surgical intervention – so what good is it? It is a blunt warning you may get breast cancer or Alzheimer's. What the field needed was a tool like Crispr-Cas9, which instead of surgically removing a breast, could surgically remove a disease-causing snippet of DNA.

Something like a genetic variant that disposes us to breast cancer might be best tackled through the germline, since editing those cells could eventually enable all cells in the human body to carry the editing fix. To be sure, Church is high on imagination, and whether he could get his Crispr-Cas9 system to work in living humans was an open question. Talking to him involves tact. It's a circular type of dialog, as conversation pauses, and he drifts on the brink of sleep. You can tell when he's starting to nod, and learn to modulate your voice to maintain the dialog. And you pick up conversations where you left off, after he tells the British reporter to take a hike, and snaps back from a brief nod. Church was telling me a story, in the fold of narcoleptic daydreams and handling telephone calls, about how his latest ideas marked a departure from the standards of hypothesis-driven science. Scientists were looking back to Mother Nature, mining her for drug ideas, so-called "discovery science."

In fact, it was in his office that I first grasped the significance of finding a useful mechanism for editing human genomes in the unfathomable sea of the microsphere. Craig Venter, one of the authors of the first draft of the human genome, had been trolling the oceans of the Earth, mining the sea for strange microbes, sometimes called "extremophiles," which can be developed for biotech purposes, and that scientists stumbled on a number of apparatus in these microbes that could be adapted for medicines suggested that because of the vast populations of microbes in the sea and soil, more wicked things this way would come. Crispr-Cas9 was surely only *one* of a multitude of tools that science would stumble upon. Through its eons of tinkering, evolution had engendered a raft of apparatus that we might use, as if stumbling into an ancient and vast scrap yard that contained parts and models from curious histories past, and extinct forms of life. It is like going into an old rummage yard, the odds and the ends, and then, the narcotic moment when you hit on a piece of genetic archeology that will stun the world, an Arc of the Covenant. If something like Crispr-Cas9 occurred naturally in mammalian cells, "we would have stumbled on it by now," Church told me. Not long after, scientists did stumble upon something similar in mammalian cells, pieces of retroviruses which enhance or turn on interferon genes in response to the invasion of viruses. In short, mammalian cells had incorporated bits of virus directly into their own genome and used those sequences to enhance the expression of genes which interfere with viruses.[482] Evolution is fascinating because it can involve one structure being repurposed for a second task – it's called *exaptation* – and it's one of the answers to the argument that there was not enough time for evolution to create such a panoply of organisms. Not every invention in nature was built from scratch! If we are now doing the inventing, it suggests the possibility of escalating the rate of evolution.

In October 2015, Church's lab did a fantastic thing, worthy of his reputation. In work with pig cells, he used Crispr-Cas9 to edit 62 separate genetic regions at one time, putting on a stunning show of the ability to manipulate a vast constellation of genes. It turns out pig cells include 62 retroviruses – called PERV, or porcine endogenous retrovirus – lurking in their cells that can cause havoc when intermixed with human cells.[483] Church showed that by using Crispr-Cas9, he could hunt and delete those 62 retroviruses, enabling pig cells to be used as a crop that might be used to develop organs for transplant to humans. Indeed, Church and colleagues at Harvard Medical School soon set up eGenesis, Inc. which sought to use Crispr-Cas9 to snip out pieces of PERV code in pig organs to make them inert to immune response in humans. "This work brings us closer to a realization of a limitless supply of safe, dependable pig organs for transplant," David A. Dunn, a transplantation expert from the State University of New York at Oswego, told *The New York Times*.[484]

Engineering multiple genes at once also appeared to cross a critical threshold that might allow scientists to engineer "complex traits," such as athletic potential, height and intelligence. Intriguing possibilities were arising over how far it would go. If we are able to make genetic engineering work, for instance, for the sake of transplants, or editing of disease risk variants, or use it in ways to reduce social costs, it can be coupled with a utilitarian argument to do so. Genetic engineering is a separate function than social engineering, which can leverage group dynamics to present a "rational choice" to an individual; for instance, genetic diagnostics tells us you have a genetic variant, and it's in the interest of all of us, if you and your family make an alteration to this gene. The message we see in fiction, again and again – from Crichton to Shelley – is one of sanctity. Art, films and literature often deliver far-fetched scenarios, but tell us things in subtle ways. Genes have a long and layered history, and making a single gene edit almost certainly has three or four effects, while biology gives us no superior genes, but genes and traits give us advantages in some niches at the expense of disadvantages in other niches. The subtle message of sanctity is it's not right or wrong to alter the code of life – that's not the issue – instead it's the insistence that engineered organisms *maintain their sanctity* or will to survive.

In *We Ate the Children Last*,[485] the writer Yann Martel tells the story of a surgeon who operates on a 56-year-old male who was suffering from colon cancer, by performing a transplant with a colon from a pig. "The French medical team felt vindicated. Until then, the success rate of full-organ xenografts was zero; all transplants of animal organs to humans – the hearts, livers and bone marrow of baboons, the kidneys of chimpanzees – had failed. The only real achievement in the field was the grafting of pigs' heart valves to repair human hearts and, to a lesser extent, of pigs' skin on to burn victims. The team decided to examine the species more closely. But the process of rendering pigs' organs immunologically inert proved difficult, and few organs were compatible." But it appeared to work, and the surgeon was able to transplant a pig colon into the human. Then, the patient began acting strange. "A nurse reported that one morning she found him eating the flowers in his room... When asked about what he ate, he was evasive. A visit to his apartment three months after the operation revealed that his kitchen was barren; he had sold everything in it, including fridge and stove, and his cupboards were empty. He finally confessed that he went out at night and picked at garbage. Nothing pleased him more, he said, than to gorge himself on putrid sausages, rotten fruit, mouldy brie, baguettes gone green, skins and carcasses, and other soured leftovers and kitchen waste. He spent a good part of the night doing this, he admitted, since he no longer felt the need for much sleep and was embarrassed about his diet. The medical team would have been concerned except that his haemoglobin count was excellent, his blood pressure was ideal, and further tests revealed what was plain to the eye: the man was bursting with good health. He was stronger and fitter than he had been in all his life."

The Les Bons Samaritains, an advocacy group for the poor, sought to make use of the unexpected effect of a human being able to eat garbage. "What better, more visionary remedy than a procedure that in reducing food budgets to nothing created paragons of fitness? A cleverly orchestrated campaign of petitions and protests – 'Malnutrition: zéro! Déficit: zéro!' read the banners – easily overcame the hesitations of the government... The procedure caught on among the young and the bohemian, the chic and the radical, among all those who wanted a change in their lives. The opprobrium attached to eating garbage vanished completely. In short order, the restaurant became a retrograde institution, and the eating of prepared food a sign of attachment to deplorable worldly values. A revolution of the gut was sweeping through society. 'Liberté! Liberté!' was the cry of the operated. The meaning of wealth was changing. It was all so heady. The telltale mark of the procedure was a scar at the base of the throat; it was a badge we wore with honour."

Things soon turned dark. "Little was made at the time of a report by the Société protectrice des animaux on the surprising drop in the number of stray cats and dogs... Then old people began vanishing without a trace. Mothers who had turned away momentarily were finding their baby carriages empty. The government reacted swiftly. In a matter of three days, the army descended upon every one of the operated, without discrimination between the law-abiding and the criminal... There were terrible scenes during the round-up: neighbours denouncing neighbours, children being separated from their families, men, women and children being stripped in public to look for telling scars, summary executions of people who tried to escape. Internment camps were set up, nearly always in small, remote towns... No provisions were made for food in any of the camps. The story was the same in all of them: first the detainees ate their clothes and went naked. Then the weaker men and women disappeared. Then the rest of the women.

Then more of the men. Then we ate those we loved most... I escaped. I still have a good appetite, but there is a moral rot in this country that even I can't digest. Everyone knew what happened, and how and where. To this day everyone knows. But no one talks about it and no one is guilty. I must live with that."

Martel's story is a warning not of the potential failures of science and industry, but a presentation of problems that emerged when the science does what we hope it to. The lesson is not one of failure, but of fantastic accomplishment. We are not to take literally the idea of cannibalism and garbage eating, but asked to awaken to reality. Technology that disrupts our social and biological order does not obviate divisions, but merely creates new "in-groups" of biologically enhanced patients who enjoy a competitive advantage and income generation for venture capitalists who fund the creation of GMO crops and animals; it also creates new "out-groups," of people who do not.

That the acceleration of technology can lead to improved lives is often true, but acceleration exposes new risks and pitfalls, never achieving a "technological salvation," which is why almost all versions of a technologically enhanced future are dystopian. In a blog, the philosopher Roy Scranton made the distinction between bio-conservatives and "accelerationists," who portend that technology can solve any social problems of inequity, issues with global warming and food shortages, and medical and infectious diseases.[486] "The Western world has been grappling with radical nihilism since at least the seventeenth century, when scientific insights into human behavior began to undermine religious belief. Philosophers have struggled since to fill the gap between fact and meaning: Kant tried to reconcile empiricist determinism with God and Reason; Bergson and Peirce worked to merge Darwinian evolution and human creativity; more recent thinkers glean the stripped furrows neuroscience has left to logic and language... Scientific materialism, taken to its extreme, threatens us with meaninglessness; if consciousness is reducible to the brain and our actions are determined not by will but by causes, then our values and beliefs are merely rationalizations for the things we were going to do anyway."

Scranton explains that Friedrich Nietzsche was not a nihilist, but rather believed "there is no ultimate, transcendent moral truth" rather that truth is a "mobile army of metaphors, metonyms, and anthropomorphisms," which was part of his complex philosophy of perspectivism. "This is different from relativism, with which it's often confused, which says that all truth is relative and there is no objective reality." Nietzsche believed a human being could learn "amor fati," the love of one's fate: this was his much-misunderstood idea of the "over-man." Nietzsche labored mightily to create this new human ideal for philosophy because he needed it so badly himself. A gloomy, sensitive pessimist and self-declared decadent who eventually went mad, he struggled all his life to convince himself that his life was worth living. Scranton believes, like most philosophers, that a soul is something that you have to earn, and to endure, rather than a situation that can be solved or fixed through appeal to a higher authority, be it God or Google.

"In a nation founded on hope, built with 'can do' Yankee grit, and bedazzled by its own technological wizardry, the very idea that something might be beyond our power or that humans have intrinsic limits verges on blasphemy... Right and left, millions of Americans believe that every problem has a solution; suggesting otherwise stirs a deep and often hostile resistance..." Instead, he suggests another choice for a mature society: willing our fate, learning to find meaning in coping with the micro-moments of life, rather than technological salvation. The implication is a heady one: technology will give us some small advantages and improve lives, but we still have to grapple with relationships, cope with the fallout of love and tragedies, and succumb to an organic death.

The instinct to engineer life is in some ways tied to our instinct to control or overcome our fate, and the subtle difference that Scranton makes is that coping or mastering life is different from control. But we have the Yankee instinct (and ability) to tweak genes not only in our own bodies but also within the kingdoms of nature to usher us into a new age of biotechnology. As the ethicist Hank Greely argued, "To me, the biggest likely change in our world from Crispr-Cas9 and other genomic editing methods won't be in humans but in the non-humans we use the methods to modify. As it gets cheaper and easier to modify genomes, non-human genomes offer freedom from a lot of regulation, liability, and political controversy, while offering plenty of opportunities to improve the world, become famous, or make money – with combinations of all of the above... Want to end malaria? Come up with a modified version of *Aedes aegypti* that can't transmit yellow fever, dengue fever, or chikungunya viruses to humans and will outcompete and eventually eliminate the wild type. Want to make a really economical biofuel? Take an algae and modify its genome in thousands of ways to optimize it for producing hydrocarbon fuel. Want to bring back the passenger pigeon? Use Crispr-Cas9 to modify the genomes of existing band tail pigeons to match, more or less, the genomes sequenced from specimens of the extinct passenger pigeon. Want to corner the market in high-end gifts? Start playing around with horse genomes adding in bits and pieces from other species in an effort to produce actual unicorns. Want to make a splash as an artist? Use Crispr-Cas9 to make a warren of truly glow-in-the-dark rabbits."[487]

Crispr-Cas9 was being applied to make genetic alterations to agriculture, aquaculture and livestock, poised to engender sweeping changes to our biosphere, begging nothing short of a bio-industrial revolution. Investors were throwing down cash. Intrexon had introduced a form of genetically modified "ouchless" *Aedes aegypti* male mosquito, which was designed to control mosquito populations, since any offspring could also not bite, meaning they could not serve as a vector to transmit a disease to humans. In the words of the journalist Claire Ainsworth "the mosquito has long held the title of the world's deadliest animal. The *Anopheles* genus causes hundreds of thousands of human deaths annually by transmitting malaria parasites. Editing *Anopheles* genomes – as well as those of *Aedes* mosquitoes, which spread viral infections such as yellow and dengue fevers – brings with it the possibility of new research and control methods."[488]

Eric Marois of France's National Centre for Scientific Research in Strasbourg and colleagues had shown they could use genetic engineering to disrupt the gene *TEP1*, which helps *Anopheles gambiae* resist infection by malaria parasites.[489] Ben Matthews, a mosquito specialist at Rockefeller University used Crispr-Cas9 to delete parts of a gene in the *Aedes aegypti* germline.[490] Those were tricks pulled in a lab. Intrexon was the first to unleash its "ouchless" male *Aedes* mosquitos into the wild in a ploy to spread a defective gene and quickly reduce the mosquito population in Brazil, sparing local populations from the threat of Zika without ever casting a mosquito net.

Church and colleagues were working on a genetically engineered mosquito, which would continue to propagate, but which would contain a version of a gene which is preferred in selection, meaning scientists could *accelerate the rate of evolution* in a mosquito species. In fact, "gene drives," is a mechanism of putting an allele under strong selective advantage by equipping it with Crispr weaponry to outcompete other alleles, or versions of the same gene, basically by equipping some genes with enzymatic scissors to chop up all similar looking genes – their competition.[491,492] In the words of Ainsworth, "during normal inheritance, there is a 50% chance that offspring will inherit a modified gene carried on one chromosome. The gene-drive system, however, cuts the partner to this chromosome and, during the repair process, the mutation is copied to the partner chromosome so that an edited organism will transmit the altered gene to almost all of its offspring."[493] In a July 2014 blog post in *Scientific American*, Church and colleagues noted "the offspring will now have two copies of the edited version plus Crispr. This insect will mate with other insects in which the same process of turning the normal genes into edited genes will be repeated. Given enough generations, Crispr will spread the edited gene through the entire population of mosquitoes and this is key *even if the edited gene reduces the odds that each mosquito will reproduce*. Since Crispr can be directed to cut essentially any gene at a precisely determined location and works in every organism we've tested, Crispr gene drives may allow us to spread nearly any type of genome alteration through many sexually reproducing populations."[494]

The proposed uses of gene drive did not stop with bugs. The conversation soon shifted to small mammals. In June 2016, Kevin Esvelt, an evolutionary biologist at the Massachusetts Institute of Technology, gave a presentation at a public meeting for the citizens of Nantucket, a 10000 resident island off the coast of Massachusetts, which has been plagued by Lyme disease. The island is home to deer populations that carry ticks, which are a vector for the Lyme pathogen. For years, residents have been struggling with whether to cull the deer herds, but Esvelt proposed a novel idea upstream in the chain of events, which was to focus on white-footed mice, which ticks often feed upon while still larva. Esvelt proposed creating and releasing genetically engineered mice on Nantucket that are immune to the Lyme pathogen, or to a protein in the tick's saliva, to stop the transmission of Lyme early in the chain of events. He proposed to use a method of vector to introduce an antibody, and a second technology – gene drive.

Consider the first technology in the couplet – the use of a vector to get an antibody into an organism. In 2011, David Baltimore's lab demonstrated an ability to use an adeno-associated virus to insert an antibody into humanized mice which would protect them from a form of HIV. Despite decades of research scientists had yet to develop a vaccine for HIV, a strategy, in short, to use a defanged version of HIV to prep the immune system to respond to it. However, along the way, numerous antibodies had been identified that can neutralize most circulating strains of HIV. "These antibodies all exhibit an unusually high level of somatic mutation, presumably owing to extensive affinity maturation over the course of continuous exposure to an evolving antigen… it remains uncertain whether a conventional vaccine will be able to elicit analogues of the existing broadly neutralizing antibodies." The strategy he introduced, he and colleagues called, "vectored immunoprophylaxis," and described it as a means which in "mice induces lifelong expression of these monoclonal antibodies at high concentrations from a single intramuscular injection." Stunningly, the humanized mice appeared "fully protected from HIV infection."[495] Such a strategy could also be used to insert an antibody into a mouse to make it immune to a Lyme-carrying tick.

Gene drive could be used as a second technology to promulgate the antibody throughout the population. And not long after, on June 8, 2016, the Committee on Gene Drive Research in Non-Human Organisms, which was established by the National Academies of Sciences, released a report which endorsed continued research into gene drives, with a caveat that any such testing undergo a laboratory phase, followed by "carefully controlled field trials" before being released into the wild.

An accompanying press release summed up the report noting that "gene-drive modified organisms are not ready to be released into the environment." The committee noted that no ecological risk assessment has been conducted for a gene-drive modified organism, and that at present, the regulation of gene drive research does not fit within the purview of any of the US agencies involved in the Coordinated Framework for the Regulation of Biotechnology, which includes the Food and Drug Administration, US Department of Agriculture, and the US Environmental Protection Agency. The Academies explained, "Gene drives are systems of biased inheritance that enhance a genetic element's ability to pass from parent organism to offspring. With the advent of new, more efficient, and targeted gene-editing techniques such as CRISPR/Cas9, gene modifications can, in principle, be spread throughout a population of living organisms intentionally and quickly via a gene drive, circumventing traditional rules of inheritance and greatly increasing the odds that an altered gene spreads throughout a population. Preliminary evidence suggests that gene drives developed in the laboratory could spread a targeted gene through nearly 100 percent of a population of yeast, fruit flies, or mosquitoes." It also instantly cast a thought experiment into everyone's mind – gene drives for humans.

"It's these kinds of uses of genomic engineering that could reshape the biosphere," Hank Greely noted, while begging for some caution not to treat the mosquito as a kind of software for every kid to build applications on. "As the ability to make carefully engineered genomic changes becomes more widely accessible, the possibility of insufficiently controlled or considered experiments increases dramatically."[496]

Ainsworth identified a parallel with antibiotic resistance in that gene drives might confer immunity to mosquitoes against pathogens, only to trigger a new kind of arms race in which pathogens such as malaria and Zika simply become smarter: "an edit succeeds in making an insect immune to infection, it also creates a strong selective pressure for the pathogen to evolve a means of getting around the modification."[497] Harvard's Wyss Institute for Biologically Inspired Engineering was already on the march, outlying prospects for using gene drives for achieving pesticide resistance in insects, herbicide resistance in weeds, and for engineering and limiting populations of rats, and kudzu, an invasive tree-climbing plant. As Ainsworth cautioned, gene drives do not come for free, but may "destroy a key segment of a food web, facilitating the invasion of another species."

UC Berkeley researcher Maywa Montenegro noted a subconscious awareness that we tend to particularize genetics and its effects, while throwing out the window the reality that species exist in full-tilt competition, in the context of other life. "In what scholar Donna Haraway calls the 'god-trick,' we thought of genetics as the key to scientific mastery of nature, as if there was no context, no agency in the object, no imperfection in human knowledge. Molecular science somehow licensed us to treat genes as separate from ecology and bodies. Now we are fathoming intricate interactions between genes and environments, and ecosystems whose changes aren't smooth or predictable, but that bristle with threshold effects and emergent properties. We've come to appreciate the inseparability of nature and culture in complex systems," Montenegro wrote.[498] But by now, the biotechnology companies were already lifting us off our feet and carrying us across a new threshold. In an authoritative essay in *Nature*, Jennifer Doudna wrote about the spate of Crispr advances, modified plants, altered butterfly-wing patterns, pest-resistant lettuce and fungal strains with reduced pathogenicity.[499] Crispr-Cas9 editing had been demonstrated in crops such as rice, wheat, sorghum, sweet orange and liverwort.[500,501,502,503,504] It had been used to genetically modify salamanders to study limb regeneration and tissue repair[505] and to knock out a gene in frogs to study albinism and eye development.[506,507] In the words of Jill Wildonger of the University of Wisconsin–Madison, Crispr-Cas9 "really opens up the genome of virtually every organism that's been sequenced to be edited and engineered."[508] Biotech was looking for profits, but at the same time pressing the case for sustainability.

"According to projections by the United Nations, the world's population is set to soar from the current 7.3 billion to 9.7 billion by 2050," Ainsworth wrote. "Agricultural output will have to increase to feed more mouths, even though the amount of fresh water available for irrigation is decreasing, and most of Earth's arable land is already under cultivation. Add in the effects of climate change – crop-damaging higher temperatures, drought and flooding, not to mention a rise in agricultural pests and diseases – and it is no surprise that food security is top of the international political agenda."[509]

Chinese scientists created a strain of wheat resistant to a powdery mildew. Caribou Biosciences, one of Doudna's companies, began collaborating with DuPont to grow "corn and wheat strains edited for drought resistance" with "field trials set to begin in spring 2016."[510] In 2015, San Diego-based Cibus introduced the first gene edited crop, an oilseed rape altered for herbicide resistance so that farmers could effectively spray it with weed killer. Intriguingly, Cibus was marketing the crop as a non-genetically modified organism, since it technically did not introduce a new gene; instead it disrupted an existing gene in the rape. Cibus' website noted the company was also working on potato, rice, canola and flax, and argued its genetic alterations "produce precise and predictable results with beneficial traits that are indistinguishable from those developed through traditional plant breeding, but with faster results."

As the journalist Gina Kolata wrote, "A lot hangs on how governments around the world decide to regulate agricultural products that have had their genomes edited. The decisions will influence the types of edited crops and animal products that are developed. To US regulators, Cibus's oilseed rape is an example of mutagenesis, not of genetic modification. This is a relief to the company because preparing for regulatory approval of a GM organism in the United States can take more than five years and cost tens of millions of dollars. Europe is even stricter, and the European Commission has yet to publish its legal interpretation of how genome-edited crops, such as the Cibus oilseed rape, should be regulated. Several political groups are lobbying for a hard line."[511]

In early 2016, neither the European Commission nor the US Food and Drug Administration had decided how to regulate Crispr crops or animals. "To U.S. regulators, most organisms currently under development may not be considered genetic modification," Montenegro wrote. "This is because U.S. policy is product-based, and with many types of Crispr edits, the product will not include foreign genetic material. In cases where editing introduces sequences from close crop wild relatives, the product might even be genetically indistinguishable from the results of conventional crossbreeding – and, say researchers, could even qualify as organic. But the rules are different in Europe, where the term 'GMO' is defined not by verifiable characteristics of a product but by the process used to create it. As long as methods of genetic engineering are used somewhere in the production process, then the label would apply."[512]

In the US, 93 percent of soybeans and 86 percent of corn is genetically modified, often to enhance growth or reduce blight, a disease caused by fungi such as mildews, rusts and smuts. Nina Fedoroff, a plant researcher and emerita professor at Pennsylvania State University, noted that chemicals and radiation cause mutations all the time, and many genes in nature automatically undergo spontaneous mutation, so when Chinese researches made a bread wheat resistant to rust not too long ago, it was not so much different from putting crops under selection. Bread wheat plants, Fedoroff was quoted as saying, are "genetic monstrosities created 3,000 years ago" with three different genomes.

Montenegro wrote the difference this time is that "scientists knew which gene they had to knock out to make wheat rust-resistant. But because wheat has three genomes, it is impossible to use crossbreeding to knock out that gene in all three at once. So the researchers used Crispr, a gene-editing technique, to surgically remove the gene."[513] Technically, "they did not create a transgenic plant," Federoff was quoted as saying. "They knocked out a gene that makes a plant susceptible to rust." Whether or not a gene from another species, a "transgene," is added to an organism is a subtle difference in the hot new debate around genetically engineered crops.

In 2000, the British biochemist Peter Bramley reported the creation of "golden rice," after he discovered a relationship of communalism in a tomato, such that a single bacterial gene, *CrtI*, can convert a compound, phytoene, into a second one, lycopene, which then goes on to be converted into beta-carotene, a red-orange pigment, which is then converted into vitamin A. In a set of elegant experiments, Bramley introduced genes from bacteria, daffodil and cauliflower to introduce "the entire beta carotene biosynthetic pathway into a rice plant."[514] A deficiency in vitamin A is estimated to kill 670000 children under the age of 5 each year. In 2005, a new version of the genetically engineered rice, "golden rice 2," was introduced and produces 23 times more beta-carotene than the original golden rice.[515] But, activists stonewalled golden rice due to its splicing of genes from multiple organisms, despite its value to the malnourished. Cibus' oilseed rape doesn't contain any added nutritional benefit, but instead allows farmers to spray weed killer over their fields – purely a financial move. Crispr can be used not only to "knock out" genes, but to shuttlecock genes from other organisms into a cell, creating genuine "transgenic" organisms.

"Using Crispr, wheat, corn, pigs, bananas – any agricultural organism, really – could be engineered to include gene sequences from a range of donors: microbes or fungi or fish," wrote Montenegro. "Meanwhile, even Crispr edits that don't intentionally involve genes from other organisms are turning out to include exactly that. The way researchers usually get Crispr technology working in a plant cell is to use a pest bacterium, *Agrobacterium tumefaciens*, to shuttle in the genes that code for Cas9. As a result, bacterial DNA can wind up in the plant genome." The journalist David Cyranoski noted that even when *A. tumefaciens* is not used "fragments of the Cas9 gene may themselves be incorporated into the plant's genome," creating organisms that continue to breed and contain foreign DNA.[516]

Forays into Crispr-Cas9 agriculture and aquaculture were moving just as fast. Scientists had already shown they could improve the growth rates of carp and tilapia. China developed a cow that produces human breast milk. An "Enviropig" was designed to generate eco-friendly manure. Many of the engineering tricks seemed to be altering the zoology of life for the sheer novelty of it. "Chinese researchers have produced meatier cashmere goats that also conveniently grow longer hair for soft sweaters, miniature pigs lacking a growth gene to be sold as novelty pets and bulky beagles lacking a muscle-inhibiting gene, an edit that could make for faster dogs," Harmon noted.[517] More often than not, the argument to do engineering was based on global health and shrinking resources. "The resulting animals and plants could potentially yield more food with less pressure on inputs such as water and land. A Crispr-tweaked farm system could have a smaller environmental footprint and even humanitarian benefits, if it means farmers don't have to dehorn cattle or cull their male bulls," Harmon reported. "Today's chickens, for instance, produce nearly 80 percent more meat for the same amount of feed as the chickens of the 1950s; if chicken breeders had had access to genome technology over that time, said John Hickey, a quantitative geneticist and a co-author of the paper, farmers would have been able to achieve that increase and also be able to grow chickens on half the land."[518]

Dairy cattle were being developed to resist a parasite that causes sleeping sickness in sub-Saharan Africa, creating an animal that might reduce the overuse of antibiotics. The University of Edinburgh's Roslin Institute genetically engineered Pig26 to have resistance to African swine fever. Bruce Whitelaw, a leader of the study, believes a gene called *RELA*, part of an innate immune complex called NF-kappaB, is more effective in wild pigs, leading to an effort to genetically modify this gene into the version seen in wild pigs. Ainsworth noted this project would benefit rural farmers, but most cases of gene engineering were pitched to industrial-scale farming. "The prospect of tough regulation and consequently an expensive market-approval process has meant that a much more common goal among livestock-focused genome editing has been to generate higher-profit cattle, pigs and sheep with increased muscle mass – often by disabling the *MSTN* gene, which restricts muscle growth."[519] Recombinetics, Inc., a Minnesota-based company, was using "new tools of gene editing to swap out the smidgen of genetic code that makes dairy cattle have horns for the one that makes Angus beef cattle have none."[520]

The rapid advance of Crispr-Cas9 into agricultural and animal husbandry is not without precedent since Monsanto Corp conducted its first field trials of genetically engineered crops in 1987. The dynamics and what we might expect, then, are already known. At the time I was writing this, 30 years had passed. *The Financial Times* wrote of an emerging rift between the biotech giant and India's regional farmers. Monsanto's "biotech arm transformed India's cotton industry with the introduction in 2002 of genetically modified, pest-resistant cotton seeds" by tripling cotton production. However, controversy ensued when Prime Minister Narendra Modi's administration "slashed the royalties paid to Monsanto's local joint venture, Mahyco Monsanto Biotech, by 70 per cent" on every 450 g pack of seeds sold, a move that "effectively cuts Monsanto's royalty to just 6 per cent of the seed price, from 20 per cent previously – a significant windfall for the Indian companies." Monsanto warned it would "reevaluate every aspect of our position in India."[521] The conflict between corporate power and regional farmers is not unique to India, but sprawls across the Americas. Pope Francis soon jumped into the mix, suggesting genetically engineered crops and animals meant "productive land is concentrated in the hands of a few owners due to the progressive disappearance of small producers, who, as a consequence of the loss of the exploited lands, are obliged to withdraw from direct production" and who "become temporary labourers, and many rural workers end up moving to poverty-stricken urban areas. The expansion of these crops has the effect of destroying the complex network of ecosystems, diminishing the diversity of production and affecting regional economies, now and in the future."[522]

"Genetic evolution is about to become conscious and volitional, and usher in a new epoch in the history of life," evolutionary biologist Edward O. Wilson declared in his book *Consilience*. The current epoch was the Holocene. That was until a group of scientists in 2008 announced that we had entered a new epoch, called the Anthropocene, to emphasize the human-centered effects on the geosphere. The term had not yet been formally adopted by the Geological Time Scale, but many scientists had bandied it about as if it's already stuck. The writer Andrew Revkin famously characterized it as a "geological age of our own making," and delineated the start of the new epoch at the Industrial Revolution, with its effects of fossil fuel-based economies and reduction of biodiversity. E. O. Wilson was pointing to the reality that the Anthropocene was soon to take a surprising turn inward, as humans would begin, as the first species in four billion years of evolution, to take a role in engineering our own genetic code. The stakes could not be higher.

The National Academy of Sciences, The Innovative Genomics Institute, The Royal Society and The Chinese Academy, in collaboration with international bodies, had prepared a major conference modeled after the 1974 Asilomar conference for the fall of 2015 at the National Academy of Sciences in Washington. David Baltimore, who had attended Asilomar, would be master of ceremonies. Hundreds of scientists were set to gather in Washington to strike the hot button issues, suggesting we were entering a revolutionary new age, but also harkening upon themes that were cyclic and timeless. I began to see genetic engineering opening up with undulations, or cycles, in its development. In the 1970s, Berg performed the first gene splice, leading to the initial debates on the morality of editing the code of life, and which could be thought of as the "first axis," in the field, while the events leading up to the period roughly circa 2000, which included Gelsinger's death, the first trial in humans and publishing of the first draft of the human genome, could be thought of as a "second axis," while as we approach the 2020s with the emergence of Crispr-Cas9 and the impending approval of the first gene therapy drugs by the FDA, we are on the cusp of the "third axis," which instantiates a mastery of the technology along with its accepted use within proper delineated legal confines. It had been less than two decades since the first draft of the human genome was published. Scientists had not only deciphered its code and elucidated much of its function, but we now had a tool set of tiny molecular scissors to make virtually any alteration to its sequence with high precision. If you consider that deciphering the double-helix, sequencing the human genome and then engineering the human genome all in a single lifetime – it's almost scary to think of the potency that is about to be unleashed in medicine and biotechnology. If I were to make a wager, the biggest game-changer and threat will be the simplification and democratization of the technology to the extent that virtually anyone can use it and engineer life. Atomic energy has been regulated to an extent that it is very tough for any non-specialist to do, and difficult to acquire enriched uranium. Our ordinary environments, by comparison, are teeming with life, making it inevitable that almost anyone will be able to do genetic engineering on themselves or their ecosystem for the purposes of terrorism, or for entrepreneurial purposes such as writing new code into life, or perhaps even to themselves within a century.

Jennifer Doudna reported an existential awakening of sorts. "Some 20 months ago, I started having trouble sleeping... By the spring of 2014, I was regularly lying awake at night wondering whether I could justifiably stay out of an ethical storm that was brewing around a technology I had helped to create." Since the Napa, California meeting held by David Baltimore and others just 12 months before, Doudna had given more than 60 talks about Crispr-Cas9 "at schools, universities and companies, and at some two dozen conferences across the United States, Europe and Asia. I have spoken about it before the US Congress; talked to staff members at the White House Office of Science and Technology Policy, which provides science advice to the US president; and answered questions from the governor of California, among many others. These discussions have pushed me far outside my scientific comfort zone."[523] The meeting scheduled for the fall was seen as an opening to a larger public discussion and institution of formal mechanisms for advising and regulating genome editing. Doudna told *Technology Review* that "it cuts to the core of who we are as people, and it makes you ask if humans should be exercising that kind of power. There are moral and ethical issues, but one of the profound questions is just the appreciation that if germ-line editing is conducted in humans, that is changing human evolution." She added in that interview that, "Most of the public does not appreciate what is coming."[524]

In her interview with Michael Specter for *The New Yorker*, Doudna went deep into the thickets. "I have always been a bit of a restless soul. I may spend too much time wondering what comes next. I lie in bed almost every night and ask myself that question. When I'm ninety, will I look back and be glad about what we have accomplished with this technology? Or will I wish I'd never discovered how it works?" As Michael Specter described his interview: "her eyes narrowed, and she lowered her voice almost to a whisper. 'I have never said this in public, but it will show you where my psyche is,' she said. 'I had a dream recently, and in my dream' – she mentioned the name of a leading scientific researcher – 'had come to see me and said, "I have somebody very powerful with me who I want you to meet, and I want you to explain to him how this technology functions." So I said, Sure, who is it? It was Adolf Hitler. I was really horrified, but I went into a room and there was Hitler. He had a pig face and I could only see him from behind and he was taking notes and he said, "I want to understand the uses and implications of this amazing technology." I woke up in a cold sweat. And that dream has haunted me from that day. Because suppose somebody like Hitler had access to this – we can only imagine the kind of horrible uses he could put it to.'"[525]

12 Washington

Evolution has been working toward optimizing the human genome for 3.85 billion years. Do we really think that some small group of human genome tinkerers could do better without all sorts of unintended consequences?[526]

– Francis Collins, director of the National Institutes of Health

I was in the newly reconstructed 670-seat auditorium at the National Academy of Sciences. It looks like what I imagine the inside of an icosahedral viral capsid would look like. The interior shell of the dome is suspended from trusses, isolating the shell from the auditorium floor and exterior structures, and it is made up of 70 adjoining diamond-shaped projections covered in plaster, and arranged along cycloid-shaped curves, which optimizes the acoustic qualities in the room. I was sitting way in the back. There was no coffee allowed in this auditorium. There were audio people in the center; the downside was that if those audio people struck up even a soft conversation, you can hear everything they said. The acoustics really were that good.

I could see the ethicists Hille Haker from Loyola University in Chicago and John Harris from the University of Manchester in England on stage, engaged in a civilized rift, the kind of ultra-smooth academic debate where an insult is always inverted into a compliment. And you can tell the tension and disagreement is growing when the politeness escalates. I could see them both, up on the stage. Harris was taking a pro-biotech stance, and he was in lockstep with Church's assertions that the genetically engineered, nutritional crop golden rice, which was enriched with vitamin A, was blacklisted for untenable reasons and that there is an irrational, knee-jerk reaction to GMOs. Harris was making the point that inaction on gene engineering, not appropriating and making use of the technology, was a kind of moral sin. "Golden rice is a wonderful technology, would have saved millions of lives, why has it not? Because of absurd and obscene prejudice against modified foods. European regulations are too complex to attend to it, and that is shaming."

The philosophers were staking camps around critical divides. One of those divides applied to using gene editing to engender agriculture, aquaculture and livestock that is cheaper to grow, contains key nutrients and is more resistant to blight, and can be grown in difficult terrain; GMOs such as golden rice – which can synthesize vitamin A. The World Health Organization estimates 250000 to 500000 children go blind each year – half of them die – because they aren't getting enough vitamin A. If not a controversial rice, how about a banana. Researchers had now developed a banana that could produce high quantities of vitamin A.[527]

Opponents respond to GMOs negatively because they believe that biotech companies like Monsanto gain leverage over basic resources, or because the natural is intrinsically more wholesome, while the artificial, or genetically modified, is corrupt. If history is any lesson, people can suffer the same visceral reaction to artificial modes of human reproduction, such as "test tube babies," and I would suspect, GMPs, or "genetically modified people," would usher in a special new kind of racism. *In vitro* fertilization, or IVF, has been widely adopted, and has undergone a steady progress. Combined with genome editing, it will enable genetic alteration of the germline, which carries along the heritable code. But this begs further questions about whether insurance agencies and taxpayers have a duty to pay for genome editing treatments, so-called "positive rights," which account for a "freedom to" something, or whether they can block or take away rights to genome editing, so-called "negative rights," meaning a "freedom from" a restriction.[528]

Neoconservative positions on gene editing are exemplified by Francis Fukuyama and his call for regulation, suggesting that one way to interpret negative rights is that private entrepreneurs should not be able to use technology to constrain resources and control life, a form of biopower which introduces GMOs and designer babies, and creates dependencies on technology. It can be difficult to interpret negative rights since it can refer to a public's protection from biotech's invasion of our supermarkets and hospitals, or the government's intrusive regulation over property rights, and the impulse is that government should not limit entrepreneurship. Bill Kauffman, one of America's great men of letters, exemplified a defense for negative rights when he wrote "my solution is no more 'practical' than a Dorothy Day prayer or a Henry Thoreau spade. It is this: No statesman's coercive power should ever extend over people he does not know." There are plenty of statesmen. GreenPeace has voiced dissent, but on June 30, 2016, 107 Nobel laureates signed a letter in support of "precision agriculture GMOs," primarily speaking to the nutritional value of golden rice.

I realized just how polarizing the GMO issue was when I had run into Emmanuelle Charpentier, one of the happier scientists I have met, in the hallway during one of the breaks while a television camera was in her face. She has dark curly hair, a thick French accent, and was dressed in black with silk scarves. She had secured a job at the Max Planck Institute for Infection Biology. "My life is very busy," she said. "I am moving a lot. I am setting up in Berlin, but I am taking it in a very relaxed fashion." Charpentier was trying to get back to doing some basic science research in Germany, and overseeing her company Crispr Therapeutics, when "I got a letter. Some activist against GMO. It said I'm garbage. It said other things. It was scary. I turned it over to the authorities, which I was required to do." The letter made this philosophy discussion sink into my bones. GMO opponents are extremely ferocious when it comes to defending their right to organic and natural foods, which are based on arguable fears that biotech companies may sweep through and control the food chain. By comparison, those strong advocates come up against people who believe in the democracy of genome engineering which owes something to the net neutrality movement, and has a strong libertarian bent. Strangely, some libertarians want freedom from gene engineering and some want freedom to engineer genes. The idea of transforming life – and an individual's right to do it – is a provocative movement in the arts, which has been leaking into reality.

In 2009, the French artist Eduardo Kac[529] created a Gattaca-type piece of visual art called Cypher, which imagined a DYI or do-it-yourself transgenic kit, which opens as a "portable minilab." It measures "approximately 13 × 17" (33 × 43 cm) and is contained in a stainless steel slipcase" and contains "Petri dishes, agar, nutrients, streaking loops, pipettes, test tubes, synthetic DNA (encoding in its genetic sequence a poem Kac wrote specifically for this artwork), and a booklet containing the transformation protocol – each in its respective compartment." Among Kac's other works, a performance piece and my personal favorite, is a transgenic rabbit, which glows a bright fluorescent green in the dark. Kac created the glowing bunny by adding a green fluorescent protein, and then released it to hop around a dark room in an art gallery, calling it GFP Bunny (2000). Kac made it clear in his description that the glowing green bunny should be treated with immense respect, but his work makes it all too clear that such a bunny would not survive in the wild.

By the end of 2015, a "biohacker" named Josiah Zayner, a PhD and former NASA scientist in his 30s, with a peacock crest of blue hair, had raised more than $65000 in a matter of months on a crowd-sourcing platform called Indiegogo to begin selling do-it-yourself genome editing kits. Zayner provides standard kits which sell for between $25 to a few hundred dollars to allow anyone to do genome editing in their own houses to make edits to bacteria or yeast, to create glow-in-the-dark bacteria, or hack to add genes to bacteria to control them with blue light, a technique in neuroscience called optogenetics. For $130 and up, he provides a complete kit to use the Crispr system on bacteria or yeast. "My motivation is to democratize Science because I think that everyone should have a chance to be able to explore and build genetically engineered organisms," Zayner wrote me in an email. "Maybe one day I will provide kits to work with mammalian cells but they are much more complicated and so require special conditions." But he noted that human cells are harder to culture and require more sophisticated calibrations of carbon monoxide concentration, humidity and media, which "currently prevent them from being very DIY."

Anyone can order DNA on the Internet and it is as cheap and available as water. It raises questions of who should be allowed to tell any of us we can't genetically engineer a houseplant, our gardens, our goldfish or our own cells. How far should we side with the libertarian argument – to what extent – becomes dangerously real when we begin to consider how easy gene engineering may become, and that we might have access to it.

Reproductive technology, too, has been a hot button issue since the destruction of embryos was required to make embryonic stem cell lines for broad utility in the human population, as advocated in a utilitarian stance, and opposed to the sanctity of the individual, a deontological stance. Oddly enough, technology is changing the state of play so that much of the cell engineering we are doing – or which some would like to do – no longer requires the destruction of a human embryo. But the issue of who is to pay for, or have access, to such treatments goes beyond the issues of germline engineering, and even into somatic cell engineering which doesn't affect future generations. Not only do we need to decide whether to pay for expensive therapies, but governing bodies will be wrestling with whether citizens should be allowed to make alterations to their own cells for cognitive or athletic enhancement, and whether to take those rights. Barbara Evans of the University of Houston Law Center, is at least one ethicist who has argued that it is better to leave draft regulations up to local controls to enable legislative tinkering, rather than enact homogenizing global standards on gene engineering. She suggested that homogenization or unified world governance does not allow enough lateral movement to test our assumptions and engage in test practice. By comparison, a risk of leaving governance to local controls is that some states may be especially lenient. Nature does not obey state boundaries, seeds drift where the winds take them, young adults are on the move. We are at the mercy of the most permissible legislation. If Monsanto showed us anything, it's how difficult it is to keep genetically modified seeds on your own futuristic farm field. Lines were being drawn, despite these realities. These issues go to the heart of our open-ended political discussion on whether to lean toward rugged Yankee individualism and the right to patent, or lean to co-operation to defend our resources as a "public trust" against the privileged elite.

John Harris is permissible, individualistic; he wants to quicken the pace of innovation. "We all have an inescapable moral duty to continue with scientific investigation of gene editing techniques," he argues. But, like all tough judicial tests, and moral duties, the answers emerge as a matter of degree. The largest item at stake at this conference is a moratorium on germline genome editing, nothing of which has happened in science for 40 years. In 1974, Paul Berg, David Baltimore and colleagues published a letter in *Science* initiating such a call for moratorium and culminating in the Asilomar conference. In an uncanny series of events, Berg, Baltimore and a new cast of modern colleagues also signed a letter that spring, also published in *Science*, which penned in halting language and gave fair warning to summon the scientific community for a similar conference, being held now in Washington. It was history at its most circular. I also had the eerie sense, I think everyone did, that Washington wasn't even close to an authoritative end to this story; instead, it was an open denouement, an expression of concern about the opening, rather than the narrowing, of options which were certain to expand into a kind of Big Bang of genetics. That we make laws to govern science and business is one thing, that a broad apparatus of biotechnology and marketing will exploit any advantage for gain is another.

Harris was objecting to a moratorium now. "Consideration of moratorium is the wrong course. Research is necessary. As to embryos, we must consider, what would be in their interest, what has happened to them in that petri dish?" And he was making the case, again, that inaction is a kind of moral slight, especially if an embryo has a risk variant. If we did not take action when we have the information and technology to make edits to their genomes, "their rights are violated and interests irreversibly denied." Harris noted that there were a few common objections to genome editing in the germline; firstly, there was the argument that the germline is sacred and mustn't be interfered with; secondly, there are those who suggest an unacceptable risk to future generations; thirdly, the inability to attain consent from those future generations. He noted that it is often safe enough, and that safety is context dependent, continuing to press the audience that "justice delayed is justice denied." In response to the first point, he cited the UNESCO declaration on human rights, "rushed through in 1997 absurdly endorses the preservation of the human genome as the constitution of humanity." He noted that 7.9 million children, or 6%, are born with a serious birth defect with genetic or partially genetic origin. If natural selection was a technology, "it would never have been permitted or licensed, it is far too dangerous. If that is the appropriate test, if the gold standard is sexual reproduction, it wouldn't have to be very safe at all."

He has a fair point. The more we learn about the human genome, the more we realize it is not a carefully constructed piece of architecture, but rather more like the Milan Cathedral, which Steven Jay Gould presented as an opening salvo in *The Structure of Evolutionary Theory*; the cathedral, having been built in baroque style in the sixteenth century, was given a retro-gothic third tier, and then, "wedding cake" pinnacles were added in the first years of the nineteenth century after Napoleon conquered the city. Our genomes – and there is no single one human genome – are like any house continually falling apart and undergoing reconstruction, both literally, and in evolutionary theory. As Matthew Porteus of Stanford University pointed out during the conference, each cell in our bodies takes on between one and ten mutations a day, which considering all of the trillions of cells in our body, translates to one million mutations per second! And those are just random monkey wrenches flying around. A targeted genome editing strategy would evoke a kind of mutation that is at least based on some limited knowledge.

Technical issues aside, an important moral issue on germline editing is that a child cannot give consent to altering his or her own genetic makeup. In fact, "no one is capable of giving consent to their germline. All might-be parents make numerous decisions for their children, in cases of sexual reproduction." Children never give consent to being born, the act of love is not only hostile ("all is fair in love and war"), but to some degree a piece of roulette. As George Bernard Shaw might have told Isadora Duncan (he said it to an actress, but denied who) after she asked, "Why don't we have a child together with my looks and your brains" to which he retorted, "but what if it had my looks and your brains?"

Harris argues that the act of procreation often involves hasty impulsivity, and a good deal of randomness – due to shuffling of alleles between chromosomes in "homologous recombination," and the crap-shoot of X and Y sex chromosomes, means that much of reproduction amounts to throwing caution to the wind. At least with genome editing, alterations are under some sort of guidance and direction, Harris argued. "Those who raise issues of consent, only do so, when they wish to claim that, they could or should not have consented, that children should not be, or should not have been, born," he said, while it is our parental duty not only to focus on the negative aspects of reproductive rights, we can no longer ignore the procreative duty "to create the best possible child, for the best."

Hille Haker was taking a more cautious approach, suggesting a moratorium on germline editing until 2017, until scientists could secure a ban through the United Nations. Between science and society, "trust is the confidence that we are all in this together, and do it responsibly. Scientists interact with patients, to decipher their motive, their aims, to help couples have a healthy child. For instance, the information we gain through medical (genetic) counseling motivates us to come to a responsible conclusion. The intrinsic assessment of goals and methods, of societal needs and priorities, is guided by normative principles.[530] The biggest concerns of parents about the health of children are based on personal goals and decisions. We are talking about women and men, and not mice here. The goal of the social sciences and society is to analyze social transformations on parenthood over the past few decades." Haker thinks like a laser and she's hitting on the right issues. A member of the Society of Reproductive Medicine stands up and says that parents have a right to use Crispr and *in vitro* technologies to have a "genetically connected child," but Haker argues that there is a difference between a freedom right, or a negative right, which is a "freedom from," such as the freedom from harm or tyranny, and a full positive right, which is a "freedom to" access or gain some benefits. I take this distinction to be consistent with most philosophers, who believe that a soul is something that has to be earned, and that positive rights in society must be earned. Haker explained that having a healthy child is a negative right, meaning nothing that someone can take away from you (spare the Chinese government) but it is certainly not a full positive right. If it were, society would be hidebound in debt to pay for all of its citizens to have children, and properly apply genetic tests and *in vitro* fertilization techniques to anyone who wants one, but almost no one would agree that society has a responsibility to pay for this, she argued.

"You may disagree with me, but as an ethicist I put the consequential assessment in terms of rights and obligations. There is no right to a genetically related child, it is a high value, not a right. Future parents have a right to respect the human dignity of the human embryo, because germ-line editing neutralized this status, but not future children's health rights." Haker is compelling when she evokes issues of the imagery between parents and genetically engineered children. An emphasis on genetics has contributed to "The transformation of social imagery of parenthood. Parents are not responsible for the genetic composition of their child. Over the years, it has become the standard, to think in terms of biology, which reduces parenthood to the transmission of good and bad genes, but that is not what parenthood is about. In the assisted reproduction market, this imagery guides us to believe that future children resemble products of design, rather than counterparts of children who may surprise them."

She continues to evoke the "landscape of imagery" between parent and child and how making genome edits to an offspring suggestive or effective at creating changes to eye or hair color or athletic or mathematical ability sets up the child as a "projection" of the parents' ideals which may garner unexpected resentment, duty, obligations and even blow-back from the child. Furthermore, genome editing to an embryo is likely to carry with it a lifetime requirement from the participants to undergo regular monitoring by physicians to ensure there are no unintended consequences, a lifetime burden few people may want to accept. As Eric Lander once quipped, if a Crispr variant turned out to have unexpected effects, people with that given mutation might be called back in to the clinic, "Don't reproduce until you've been re-Crisprized."

Arguing the issues in this conference hall were the true pioneers of gene splicing, Maria Jasin, Matthew Porteus, Jennifer Doudna. I recognized Maxine Singer sitting in the front row of the auditorium. In the hallway, at one point, I was talking to Keith Joung about a monograph he was going to write, when I glanced to my right and saw an old German fellow, with grey hair and blue eyes, and a penetrating gaze. His nametag said "Klaus Rajewsky," recalling that when I first started writing there was a chair at Harvard Medical School with "Rajewsky" written on the back in marker. "Yes, it's me," Rajewsky said, blankly, and wryly, as if anyone should think it was so surprising. He had moved back to Germany. I asked him what he was most proud of, and it was the "conditional gene targeting" he developed using the Cre-Lox reporter system. In that moment, I had a sense of gravity, that science was embodied by its living scientists. Dana Carroll and David Baltimore had been at the rustic retreat of Asilomar sparring in a similar conversation 40 years ago. If there was something new in these modern times, it was the ease of use and incredible accuracy of Crispr-Cas9, and also a deeply funded broad apparatus of biotechnology, which could finance, test and market a genetics tool at the drop of the dime. In the earlier age, scientists simply did not have next-generation deep-sequencing data and powerful tools to disprove their hypotheses or calm any runaway fears, and it led to rumination and thought experiments over the prospects of gene splicing. We now had a lot of tools and scientific ideas were quickly mobilized by a deeply financed biotech apparatus which could turn on a dime. Despite our best intentions, I could see that things were about to move fast.

"What you are talking about is a major issue for all humanity," Merle Berger, a co-founder of Boston IVF, a network of fertility clinics, told Antonio Regalado at the *Technology Review*. Berger suspected genetic enhancement would cause a public uproar because "everyone would want the perfect child": people might pick and choose eye color and eventually intelligence. "These are things we talk about all the time. But we have never had the opportunity to do it." Jennifer Doudna added that, "Any scientist with molecular biology skills and knowledge of how to work with [embryos] is going to be able to do this." Regalado then spun some of his own yarn. "Critics cite a host of fears. Children would be the subject of experiments. Parents would be influenced by genetic advertising from IVF clinics. Germ-line engineering would encourage the spread of allegedly superior traits. And it would affect people not yet born, without their being able to agree to it. The American Medical Association, for instance, holds that germ-line engineering shouldn't be done 'at this time' because it 'affects the welfare of future generations' and could cause 'unpredictable and irreversible results.'"[531] The AMA position dates to 1996, and the positions, which have enjoyed wide consensus, were coming up against a new reality of the potent and highly efficient Crispr-Cas9 technology. "A lot of people just agreed to these statements," Hank Greely noted. "It wasn't hard to renounce something that you couldn't do."[532]

In the 1970s Princeton theologian Paul Ramsey staked a bio-conservative camp, urging caution on tampering with life, an intellectual tradition supported by Francis Fukuyama, Leon Kass, a strange mix of conservatives and activists like Bill McKibben. The Christian ethicist Joseph Fletcher argued for the moral imperative to intervene in our own biology, a camp that draws its current line to Julian Savulescu, John Harris and other accelerationists, and in the often surreal movement of transhumanism and the curious ramblings of Ray Kurzweil. In his circa 2000 Foreword to *Frankenstein*, entitled "The Future of Frankenstein," New York University literary scholar Walter James Miller compares accelerationists to bio-conservatists.

"By 2035 – several experts prophesy – gene manipulation will feed the hungry Third World, cure cancer, and even death: gene manipulation may make us immortal. We'll have low-cost solar energy and super-supercomputers. Maybe even before 2035, we'll be served by machines not only intelligent, but sentient, by gadgets that maintain and repair themselves, by totally automated factories: that is, factories that even manage themselves... But other scientists warn that humanity may be hurtling toward mass suicide. These rapid advances can, like the Frankenstein experiment or the development of certain antibiotics, simply boomerang, bringing new types of accidents and destructive conditions.

The long-range effects of gene manipulation are unpredictable. Super-intelligent machines can evolve with humanity, compete for our resources, 'squeeze human beings out of existence.' Some scientists file suits to stop a physics lab from creating an artificial black hole that could – they fear – devour the earth in a few moments. A perennial fear is that some experiment, like creating super-bacteria for benevolent purposes, might leak out of the lab into the hands of terrorists and provide them with new bioweapons. And everyone remembers that Frankenstein himself imagined he could make a creature immortal."

Marcy Darnovsky described the human genome as a kind of tinderbox for instigating social divisions. She envisioned "enhancement genetics" sold to the public "for a once of the lifetime opportunity to give the best start in life, because those are the traits that society values, tallness, good looks, pale complexion, technical and mathematical intelligence." What is at stake is a society, through marketing, which puts pressure on us at a genetic level to achieve what are prescribed social traits such that we begin comporting with social pressures from birth, "fostering the least attractive, or techno-scientific." She suggested that sweeping these objections under the rug would be a "deep denial of devastating social inequality" and that John Harris' argument that we should use technology "to escape our limits, is a kind of market-based eugenics."

Darnovsky hit her strongest note of resonance when she identified her concerns over perceptions and marketing. Eric Lander agreed the biggest pitfalls might not derive from the work of scientists and academics, but instead, through a market-driven economy, based on television commercials at half-time of football games, and other marketing strategies that pull at the heart strings of consumer desires. Daniel Kevles, a legal historian from New York University, noted in the new millennium "neo-eugenics has several forces that animate it, including economic forces of reducing medical costs. There is a hazard not of racism, but racial genotyping for specific diseases, stigmatization, and an over-confidence of selecting advantageous or deleterious traits. The problem is that this is largely driven by consumer demand, for some kind of genetic improvement or control." Church reiterated that "there is a very strong drive among a subset, to use all sorts of adjacent technologies that are extremely valuable medically, and which they are lured into using for small gains and advantages."

Darnovsky further signaled her concern over the "off-label use of drugs, which in this case could spread to germline gene editing for enhancement, do absolutely need to take them into account." In other words, if a genome editing technique is approved for a medical reason, it may also have an alternate performance enhancing effect. Everyone at the conference was in agreement that sociopaths would market the technology for misuse and false promise. "What we need to be concerned about are unscrupulous clinics," Church said. He was talking about unlicensed stem cell clinics that anticipate what may soon happen in the genome editing space. Authors of a recent paper noted "stem-cell clinics in the United States and abroad have capitalized on this confusion (about the therapeutic value of stem cell therapies) by selling treatments that are not approved by the Food and Drug Administration... since insurers don't cover unapproved stem-cell treatments, patients pay out of pocket for procedures that cost anywhere from $5,000 to $50,000... Because FDA guidelines are ambiguous, stem-cell clinics have in effect been operating without regulation."[533,534]

As I was typing up my meeting notes, I was aware of concern over an emerging Wild West of biotech. As US Representative Bill Foster noted, "It's rare for prominent members of the academy to warn of technological breakthroughs that the public may not be prepared for. In Congress, for many members, Crispr is an unknown term. Then, panic over-reaction. Attack from the future on our humanity. Treatments not reserved for only rich and privileged in this world. Cannot be reserved for our individual countries. Verge of technological breakthrough that could change the future of mankind." John Holdren, a senior advisor to President Barack Obama on science and technology, said that "it continues to be the position of the Obama administration, that editing human germline for medical purposes lacks medical justification, and raises ethical considerations; what is done in the vein of one country will have consequences in another. Propagation through generations. Also, exciting therapeutic gene edited somatic cell therapies can and will continue."

The Stanford legal ethicist Hank Greely in a blog post to *The Stanford Review* was quick to point out that germline modification isn't the most immediate concern. "Frankly, although the fuss has been about human germline genomic modification, I think that attention is misplaced. I don't expect engineered human germline modification to be a big issue – as a practical matter – for a long time, if ever, for several reasons. First, the safety issues are enormous. That's not to say anything bad about Crispr-Cas9 or other genome editing techniques, but the stakes are enormous ... a human baby... You'd have to be criminally reckless, or insane, to try to make a baby this way unless and until we've had a decade or more of preliminary research, with human tissues and with non-human animals (including certainly primates and maybe even some of the non-human apes), showing that it is safe. If the moral risk isn't enough of a deterrent, the potential legal liability should be."[535]

The article with co-signers from Napa in *Science* had called for a moratorium on germline editing, and as Greely reiterated, he agreed; but he had taken the position, also adopted by Eric Lander, that, if the technology becomes precise and safe enough, in democratic societies decisions are entrusted to the public. "Perhaps not surprising, I would do what the *Science* piece called for. While reminding people that making babies this way is illegal or heavily regulated in most of the world, I would call for a moratorium on even trying it until both further scientific research (mainly on its safety) and public discussion and study (mainly on ethics) had been attained... In the long run, I believe the permissibility of using germline genomic modification to make babies will be, and should be, a political issue. Right now, I suspect I would opt for regulating it on a safety/benefit basis, allowing it only when the potential benefits outweighed the risks. But I might change my mind, either because of newly discovered facts or well-made arguments. Importantly, though, I do not think that my view should govern. The people, through their governments, should govern. If South Dakota, or Germany, wished to ban it and California, or Singapore, wished to encourage it – preferably, in all cases, after free, open, and active debate – so be it."[536]

I admire confidence in the democratic process. As Steven Shapin wrote in the Boston Review on the problem of "resurgent scientism is less an effective solution to problems posed by the relationship between *is* and *ought* than a symptom of the malaise accompanying their separation... The idea that scientists are priests of nature, that they are morally uplifted by the study of God's Book of Nature, may be dead – as (Max) Weber suggested, that is central to what modernity means – but the question of whether scientists are selflessly dedicated to truth remains alive." As Robert Frodeman and Adam Briggle accurately recapitulated Shapin's arguments in their blog post at *The New York Times*, "The individual scientist is no different from the average Joe; he or she has, as Shapin has written, 'no special authority to pronounce on what ought to be done.' For many, science became a paycheck, and the scientist became a 'de-moralized' tool enlisted in the service of power, bureaucracy and commerce. Here, too, philosophy has aped the sciences by fostering a culture that might be called 'the genius contest.' Philosophic activity devolved into a contest to prove just how clever one can be in creating or destroying arguments. Today, a hyperactive productivist churn of scholarship keeps philosophers chained to their computers. Like the sciences, philosophy has largely become a technical enterprise, the only difference being that we manipulate words rather than genes or chemicals. Lost is the once common-sense notion that philosophers are seeking the good life – that we ought to be (in spite of our failings) model citizens and human beings. Having become specialists, we have lost sight of the whole. The point of philosophy now is to be smart, not good. It has been the heart of our undoing."[537]

Alta Charo, an ethicist at the University of Wisconsin, noted that "sunlight is the best disinfectant" and may be the best means "to create pressure to alter direction or speed of voluntary self-regulation." Charo echoed the concern of many scientists that early on "a single high profile failure could set back the whole field, as it was set back by years before in the Gelsinger death in 1999." That message was reiterated by a number of speakers including Jonathan Kimmelman of McGill University, who said "I am not in doubt" about the capabilities of genome editing and its efficiencies, but argued that "what is the appropriate reference class? Catastrophic events can destabilize the entire field."

In the US, Charo noted there is competent legislature and rules, which can already be used to regulate genome editing, and the oft-cited aphorism that technology is outpacing our moral and legal aptitudes is not true. The question, she begged the audience, is how to interpret and use the existing law. An issue, she pointed out, was whether to regulate genome editing as a technology or a product. In the United States, gene therapy is regulated by the Food and Drug Administration and subject to the Public Health Service Act, which is largely focused on purity and potency, and by laws governing drugs and devices. There are strong premarket controls, in fact, she said, "very strong controls in pre-saleable levels, but the control becomes weaker once a drug is in the market, since it can be used for off-label use." The use of gene therapy is subject to review by the NIH Recombinant DNA Advisory Committee as adjunct to FDA review. So there are regulatory mechanisms in place. The advantages of regulating Crispr-Cas9 as a technology are that it's "easier for the public to understand. You offer a consistent approach to overarching issues, such as human dignity or genetic heritage of human-kind, but it needs supplemental legislation to focus more closely on specific risks and benefits of specific products or contexts." The advantages to regulating Crispr-Cas9 as a drug is it "contextualizes the technology risks and benefits per application. This draws on existing deep expertise and statutory policy choices concerning regulation of various products, but it can be confusing to the public, and there may be unintended conflicts, gaps or redundancies among laws."

Barbara Evans, of the University of Houston Law Center, argued that ethicists don't suggest using the "alpha max-min" or worst-case scenarios in bioethics to drive decisions. "Banning a technology may consign a number of people to harsh circumstance. The problem is that we can't agree what a catastrophe looks like. We need to be precise about what we are trying to prevent. Unedited genes are a catastrophe happening now. Catastrophe has global or broad effects, patients are suffering in standard care. Is it a catastrophe if patient harms pass to the next generation? I prefer a definition that highlights global impacts, such as the destruction of an important food crop. We are more likely to get a catastrophe from corn genomes, or microbes." And she noted that most post-apocalyptic post-human scenarios are not that realistic, since most humans (spare Genghis Kahn) are not that promiscuous, so we are unlikely to spread our genes like wildfire. "Most of us don't have that good a social life," she noted, raising crackling laughter from the audience. Evans further noted that we are "all concerned about off-label use" and that you "go to war with the regulation you have, not the one you wish to have." She reiterated Charo's message that the FDA has excellent tools for regulation of genome editing, not just for regulating the technology, but for regulating products. The key question, she noted, again, was whether to regulate it as a drug or a device?

Many technologies could be regulated either way; and if it could be either, the FDA tends to classify it as a device. A device is classified as an intervention that "does not achieve its primary intended purposes through chemical action within or on the body of man or other animals and... is not dependent upon being metabolized for the achievement of its primary intended purposes."[538] Products that meet the definition of device also meet the definition of drug, due to the broader scope of the drug definition, and "if a product is shown to meet both the drug and device definitions, the Agency generally intends to classify the product as a device."[539] Evans argued that characterizing gene editing instrumentalities as devices rather than drugs may allow better regulation of research involving germline gene editing and better control over off-label uses of approved gene editing products. People who receive somatic gene editing are "human subjects" who are protected by the FDA's investigational new drug regulation; however, people who provide embryos or gametes for germline gene editing do not seem to qualify as "human subjects" under this regulation. But they would be "human subjects" under the FDA's investigational device exemption regulation, which includes people "on whose specimens" an investigational device is used.[540] But we are entering even more complicated social terrain, she noted. "Do you have the right to know if people who you procreate with have a modified genome? Social implications, would it become the norm, if go on date, I've had my genome edited. That goes back to tort law, someone arguing something wasn't disclosed, and should have been."

By the end of the conference, I was in spins over the workings of US drug and device regulation. I decided to write to Peter Marks, deputy director of the Center for Biologics Evaluation and Research at the US Food and Drug Administration. I was surprised when he wrote back. "Thank you for your inquiry.

Significant thought has been given to this topic, and at this time products made using Crispr would be regulated as biologic drugs. Though one could conceive that the enzymatic activity is like a device, ultimately the relevant effect results in chemical modification within a cell – DNA editing – which is a defining property distinguishing a drug from a device. The Office of Cellular, Tissue and Gene Therapies in the Center for Biologics Evaluation and Research regulates gene therapy products and human tissue, including reproductive tissue, intended for transfer into humans. Oversight responsibility includes gene editing technologies currently under IND in somatic cells, using zinc finger proteins, or on the horizon, using Crispr. I hope that this information is helpful."

✢

"Gene Editing Offers Hope For Treating Duchenne Muscular Dystrophy, Studies Find," was a headline at *The New York Times* on December 31, 2015. "Duchenne muscular dystrophy is a progressive muscle-wasting disease that affects boys, putting them in wheelchairs by age 10, followed by an early death from heart failure or breathing difficulties. The disease is caused by defects in a gene that encodes a protein called dystrophin, which is essential for proper muscle function." A trio of papers published in the journal *Science,* in the last week of the year, demonstrated how scientists had used an adeno-associated virus to traffic Crispr-Cas9 into living mice, snipping out a part of a gene that produces dystrophin.[541] Charles Gersbach at Duke had injected the virus into the leg muscle of an adult mouse with Duchenne, splicing a mutated copy of a malfunctioning dystrophin gene to render it into a shorter version which was functional. Gersbach showed that the mice had restored protein, and an improving muscle strength. Importantly, when he injected the construct into the blood, it had a restorative effect on heart tissue. The finding was so splashy because scientists had previously succeeded in using Crispr on mouse embryos to treat the disease in the germline, but the delivery of Crispr in an adeno-associated virus into *living* adult mice, showed they could treat the disease in broadly dispersed tissues throughout the body in a living organism. Hank Greely also lauded the promise of somatic cell therapies, while cautioning against historic hyperbole. Such "somatic cell genomic modification in humans – your basic gene therapy – is, in fact, a likely huge use for genomic editing technologies. About 35 years after gene therapy was first tried by Martin Cline, it is finally approaching clinical use. In fact, one gene therapy, called Glybera, has already been approved in Europe. Others are in phase 2 and phase 3 trials around the world. I would be surprised if FDA did not approve a few in the U.S. in the next year or two... changing the genes of one person, who will die without passing those on to anyone else, just hasn't raised deep questions."[542] Chad Cowan stood up and said he thinks gene therapy has "a very bright future for somatic cell therapies."

Fyodor Urnov, a scientist at Sangamo, explained that his company is moving into beta thalassemia and sickle cell disease. "As is clear from its name, sickle cell disease is characterized by the presence of sickle shaped rigid red blood cells, caused by the hemoglobin gene or protein defect."[543] Babies need lots of oxygen, and they use a special form of fetal hemoglobin that is a product of the gamma globin gene, but just like baby teeth, they grow out of it, switching to a form of adult hemoglobin using the beta globin gene. It is only once the switch occurs that sickle cell disease becomes apparent, since it is a defect in the beta globin. But it has been suspected that reactivation of the fetal form of the complex could stop the "sickle problem" "since the fetal hemoglobin gamma could replace the mutated hemoglobin beta."[544] Sangamo identified a binding site for a transcription factor called *GATA1* as key to enhancer function in erythroid-specific *BCL11A* activation and fetal globin suppression. In short, by causing a disruption to this genetic region, it caused a drop in the expression of *BCL11A* and an increase in fetal hemoglobin, fixing the "sickle problem." "I cannot tell you what the future is with regard to genome editing in the germline, but I really think it is a really, really bright one for the treatment of monogenic diseases, and from a public heath perspective," Urnov said.

Kyle Orwig, from the University of Pittsburgh, reported there had been success in the field and that genome editing of germline cells could be used to treat infertility. In fact, 12% of men in the US are sub-fertile or infertile, often due to a failure in the process of spermatogenesis, meaning the creation of sperm. In some types of male fertility, this can be fixed. Mice with a selective ablation of the androgen receptor in Sertoli cells (a supportive "nurse" cell that helps in the process of spermatogenesis) has led to the creation of so-called SCARKO mice, which display a complete block in meiosis, or cell division of these cells. In other words, they are infertile. "This type of gene defect can be repaired through gene therapy to enable infertile mice to produce offspring. Meanwhile, other genetic defects have been repaired in the sperm, treating heritable conditions in mice. For instance, mutations in a gene called *CRYGC* can cause cataracts, correction of which resulted in mice pups who were spared cataracts and could see.[545,546]

Some scientists were arguing that such techniques therefore should be used for human patients. Sperm and eggs are "gametes" or "germline" cells which carry heritable information to future generations, while an embryo arises from a fusion of gametes from each parent. The outcry over gene engineering at the level of the germline has mostly focused on the fertilized eggs or embryos, the destruction of embryos for research purposes and the genetic testing of those embryos by way of *in vitro* fertilization and subsequent "preimplantation genetic diagnosis" to screen or select for clumps of cells which appear to demonstrate healthy traits and lack genetic variants that are evidenced to cause a disease, and now the surreal prospect of using Crispr-Cas9 as an alternative to selecting favorable cells *in vitro* and instead engendering alterations to embryos by purchase or order. But when cultivating embryos in a lab prior to pregnancy there is a collateral effect of "destruction of embryos" that may be deemed "unfit" by some standard and which gets tempers roiling from certain quarters of the public. But Crispr-Cas9 might be used to edit the gametes, meaning the sperm and ovum cells, drawing us back a step before the embryos are even created, and still allows us to carry out germline engineering. "A sizable fraction of our population don't like harming embryos, so if/when couples get to Crispr-ize sperm, they might consider that much less endangering of embryos than IVF-PGD. We kill a million sperm per day even when we follow the rules of conventional reproduction," Church noted to me in an email. "But most of the ethics debates have focused not on 100% accurately edited spermatogonial stem cell clones (SSCC), which Church's lab has deftly demonstrated and published in Nature Medicine and Nature Methods, but ineffective or botched attempts to Crispr-ize embryos."

Church believes that a quick strike method of Crispr-Cas9 on sperm cells may not only be the best method to treat infertility, but may also be a preferable method to treat a number of diseases. When I saw Church at the conference he was standing in the entryway, a man solidly in his shoes, in his browns and tweeds, surrounded by about ten journalists feverishly scribbling down everything he said in their notepads. He had repeated his oft-cited notes that there are more than a thousand genes which are "medically actionable" and he often carries a list of genes with him that can be interrogated to achieve very predictable effects in a patient. "There are two lists," Church corrected me. "One is of Mendelian deleterious alleles which are actionable via genetic counseling and the other list consists of rare 'protective alleles' which are not currently part of genetic counseling, but are relevant to near future 'augmentation gene therapies' – for example, preventing viruses or reversing, preventing age-related diseases, including cognitive decline." All told, those genes include *CCR5* and *FUT2*, which can provide pathogenic resistance; aging is affected by *GFD11-MSTN*, *TERT-CDKN2A-TP53* and cognitive function is affected by genes including *NGF*, *NEU1*, *GRIN2B* and *PDE4B*. And the list goes on.

"One makes your bones so hard they'll break a surgical drill. Another drastically cuts the risk of heart attacks. And a variant of the gene for the amyloid precursor protein, or APP, was found by Icelandic researchers to protect against Alzheimer's. People with it never get dementia and remain sharp into old age."[547] As the journalist Dina Fine Maron concisely wrote: "Take the *DEC2* gene. Tweaking it could make a person function like the rare individuals who are born with a variant that allows them to function well with just a few hours of sleep. That trait is not necessary for most people, but it could be useful for a soldier in the battlefield, for example. Ultimately, enhancements of many kinds will 'definitely' happen in the future, says Fyodor Urnov of Sangamo BioSciences, a company that is working in the gene editing space. The bigger question, he says, is when it will happen."[548]

Peter Braude, a reproductive doctor at King's College in London, noted that to intervene on all genetic loci in all people is not realistic or affordable. "It would be a monumental task to develop a new set of primers for every new patient," he said. Braude summoned Bertrand Russell to note that we simply don't know that much about how genetic variations in cells translate into phenotypes in a fully formed child. "The extent to which beliefs are based on evidence is very much less than what believers suppose," Russell famously said. In fact, there are a number of studies, Braude pointed out, in which chromosomal abnormalities, or mosaicism, meaning a mix of normal and abnormal chromosomal or genetic variants leads to healthy children being born, questioning whether the benefits can truly justify the risk and cost.[549,550] But to others, this sort of mystery was precisely the point, begging the question of why to suspend developmental embryonic research when so much study is needed. Janet Rossant of The Hospital for Sick Children and the University of Toronto, said that she believed that there were enough "spare embryos I don't believe it is necessary to create embryos" for research purposes. She noted that we have "learned a lot from the mouse, structure of mouse blastocyst, but differences with humans." In humans, once a sperm and egg fuse, a single cell begins to divide into an embryo, which divides into eight, then sixteen, then thirty-two cells. In humans, once the embryo gets to a size of about 0.1 mm and consists of 64 to a couple hundred cells it is called a blastocyst.[551]

In 2006, Shinya Yamanaka showed that he could reverse the process of differentiation of an adult cell to create "induced pluripotent stem cells" by adding a few genes including Oct4, Sox2 and Klf4 to differentiated cells, turning them back into pluripotent stem cells and largely freeing us from the debate on whether or not to destroy embryos. Only one year later, Rudolph Jaenisch at the Massachusetts Institute of Technology used induced pluripotent stem cells to cure mice with sickle cell anemia. He later showed he could use Crispr to create mouse pups in which 80 percent of cells had both alleles accurately edited.[552] And in a second study, was able to add a "reporter gene" such as green fluorescent protein, into genes such as Oct 4, Sox 2 and Nanog, which are among the genes triggered for inducing pluripotent stem cells.[553] Strategies such as that would allow scientists to study the genes that come on in an embryo at specific times in embryo development, and this would be needed to study human embryogenesis, which can only be definitively studied using human embryos. Scientists are actively pursuing the use of stem cell therapies for medical purposes, although the state of the science remains quite immature. Jaenisch called attempts to edit human embryos "totally premature" saying "it's just a sensational thing that will stir things up." He emphasized technical limitations. "We know it's possible, but is it of practical use? I kind of doubt it."[554] Greely said the germline issue is "close to silly, it doesn't matter if it's in the germline, or not germline; within a decade, it will be safe enough to do." Of the ethics, Greely noted, "We will muddle through it, but some things may not be worth muddling through."

Regarding the engineering of complex traits, Greely noted "I think this is the real fear of most people – genetically engineered superhumans. But it turns out that, after hundreds of billions of dollars spent, we know surprisingly little about the genetics of disease. We know almost nothing about the genetics of 'enhancement.' I cannot think of a single non-disease trait where we can say confidently that one non-pathogenic allele is highly likely to confer a substantial advantage over another. That will change, of course, but how much and how fast? My guess, in both cases, is not very." Greely notes the "promise" that we would not try human germline modification is "of course, an easy promise to make when it was impossible, like promising not to try human reproductive cloning when it seemed impossible." George Q. Daley of the Boston Children's Hospital, echoed that in the current state of play, complex diseases are monumental and often seem insurmountable, while "compelling cases for genome editing where there are no alternatives, are so vanishingly rare." One such case, he offered, may be a child with X-linked NEMO immune-deficiency, who is seeking a second "savior" child, a sibling born with immune-matching cells for donation.[555] That second sibling could have genome editing done at the pre-implantation stage so as not to present the disease. Daley noted he was skeptical of using gene editing to alter "most of the large complex traits, intelligence, courage, which are multifactorial and depend on small effects, and dramatic interactions between genes and environment." He further noted the "collective feeling of scientists, including those in Napa, that it is not safe or prudent to move forward with clinical application"[556] and noted "somatic gene therapy, after decades of investment, was driven by ultra-rare conditions, and then it was applied to more common disorders" and germline editing may apply to rare diseases. Church disagrees that Crispr-Cas9 will be limited to rare diseases. "For complex traits involving polygenic loci, many of my colleagues (e.g. Eric Lander) say that we will have a very tough time developing therapies, ignoring the fact that many polygenic traits are treated successfully with single gene products with acceptable collateral damage" such as growth hormone or insulin. "The point is that common diseases might not be as reliably fixed" by genetic counseling or PGD-IVF "as by germline gene therapy using an uncommon protective DNA variant."

Germline editing has been instigated in monkeys. Jinsong Li, Shanghai Institutes for Biological Sciences, talked about his work on using genome editing to alter the germline of *Macaca fascicularis*, or cynomolgus monkeys. So far researchers have edited the germline code of a few genes, *PPAR*, which has a function in fat cell production, and *RAG-1*, which has a role in B-cell and T-cell development.[557,558] Genetically modified monkeys are not new, and have been around since ANDi – which stands for "inserted DNA" spelled backward – was born in 2000.[559] Guoping Feng, a professor of neuroscience at MIT and Feng Zhang of the Broad and McGovern Brain Institutes have been collaborating with Chinese researchers (this monkey research is going on in China, not the United States) to try to knock out a gene called *SHANK3*, which in humans causes a genetically inherited form of autism (a small percentage of people with autism have the *SHANK3* mutation). In another study, which was later published in January 2016, Zilong Qiu, a leader of the research at the Institute of Neuroscience at the Chinese Academy of Sciences in Shanghai, and colleagues, created genetically engineered monkeys by adding an additional copy of a gene called *MECP2* that exhibited behaviors similar to autism.[560] As it was reported in *The New York Times*, "The overarching cause of autism is still unknown, and cases have been linked to about 100 mutations, some inherited and some developing spontaneously. The monkeys in the newly published research did not exhibit every aspect of autism or even every aspect of the genetic autism-like disorder the scientists were seeking to mirror. That disorder, *MECP2* duplication syndrome, occurs when people, especially boys, inherit two copies of the *MECP2* gene."[561] The monkeys the researchers were creating through genetic engineering were more likely to demonstrate social disconnection as they got older, stress and defensive behavior, and were "less likely to be social by sitting with, touching or grooming other monkeys."[562] Just when I was wondering how far we'd actually go with this, Weizhi Ji of the Kunming Institute of Zoology from the Chinese Academy of Sciences was showing a video. In the video, one monkey appeared friendly and engaging, hopping around the cage and trying to engage a second monkey. The second monkey was hiding his eyes, avoiding contact. "He does not like social communications," Ji explained. "This is the avoidance test." One monkey with a genetic variant for social aversion was caged with a normal control. I know this is science but in that moment, I felt a sense of sadness that I can't quite describe. Guoping Feng told Antonio Regaldo he approves of germline engineering, suggesting actual gene-edited humans are "10 to 20 years away."[563]

Ismail Serageldin, director of the Library of Alexandria in Greece, was at the Washington conference and among the majority who saw genome editing as bittersweet. On the one hand, Serageldin was cautioning against the reduction of humanity to the digital and mechanized, suggesting the genome editing may be one more way which allows us to capture our reflection in the aegis of technology ideals, summoning the poet T. S. Eliot, who presaged the Information Age: "Where is the life we have lost? Where is the life we have lost in living? Where is the wisdom we have lost in knowledge? Where is the knowledge we have lost in information?" That we live in an age with accelerating technology and risk diminishing insight is a message I heard continually repeated. Serageldin suggested we would press forward and persevere. We would learn to live with it for the better. "From fire to the kitchen knife, we have been playing God ever since we domesticated animals, or turned on the lights and turned night into day. It is important to reflect on dark chapters of our history. We need knowledge, but we also need wisdom. Does anyone really doubt that we are infinitely better with the Internet than without?"

The concern over technologies defining our lives goes back at least to the German philosopher Martin Heidegger. In the words of Jonathan Moreno, while technology reveals "some aspects of the world, these human activities conceal others. The technological worldview is particularly problematic for Heidegger, as it was for Nietzsche, because manipulating the world obscures the fact that doing so is only one of many ways of viewing it. Science and technology seek to explain everything, leaving no room for other means of explanation." Heidegger wrote, "Technology threatens revealing, threatens it with the possibility that all revealing will be consumed in ordering."

In fact, one of Heidegger's keynote ideas was the "dasein," or "being there," the presence of life. His famous example of negating the dasein, was reaching for a hammer, while grabbing the hammer in hand, the hammer gets taken up into the world, into "kinesis," or movement. Nature is thus committed to be something specific, a technology, through its use, at the expense of other ways of being. Through such an action, it attains its order in time. Robert Pogue Harrison explained further in *Juvenescence*, "In Creative Evolution (1907) the French philosopher Henri Bergson exposed our 'tendency to conceive of time geometrically rather than organically,' but it was Heidegger 'who thought more radically about time than any philosopher before or after him, teaching us that time is a kind of movement, or kinesis.'"[564]

In a blog, philosopher Lawrence Berger wrote that "Heidegger's approach is to inquire into the nature of 'being,' which is simply understood to be how things in general come into presence and then withdraw. This means that attention is the human side of a universal process of manifestation of entities, with an associated effort that is referred to as *vigilance* in the cognitive science literature. This effort of *staying with* the entities that we encounter is crucially important for Heidegger, for if attention is how we gain access to anything at all, then staying with an entity would enable a deeper revelation of its nature. In this regard he emphasizes the fact that entities are made manifest over the course of time (hence his famous 1927 work, "Being and Time"). The idea is that staying with an entity as it unfolds affects the manner in which it is made manifest."[565]

As science and technology distracts and abstracts us from nature, Heidegger says, it has the potential not to strengthen, but ironically, to weaken, our sense of reality. In a vignette, Heidegger "considers what it is to stand before a tree in bloom in a meadow" and considers the "supposedly superior physical and physiological knowledge" of systemically analyzing the particular components of the tree, but then considers that science and its categories are not required for the tree to exist, concluding that "thought has never let the tree stand where it stands."

Berger interprets this passage to be relevant in contemporary life in which science is supposed to be fundamental to reality. "We have come up against a deeply ingrained view of what it is to be a human being (which lends credence to views that our experience ultimately does not matter), which is that subjective experience takes place in a private realm that is cut off from the rest of reality. But Heidegger does not even make the distinction between the mental and the physical; for him our experience is an event in the world... The being of the stone and our relation to it cannot be conceived independently of the whole context in which we arise. The prevailing view is that the universe consists of discrete entities that are ultimately related by physical laws. We relate to other entities by way of mental representations of the whole – something like scientific observers who don't really belong here. Heidegger, on the other hand, offers a holistic view of all that is. We belong here together with the trees and the stones, for we are made manifest together. Rather than being discrete entities, the relation comes first, and the extent to which we are related matters for what we and the stone ultimately *are*."[566]

These are not trivial thought experiments, but one reason the emphasis on STEM (Science Technology Math and Engineering) fields have contributed to a dogma of eliminativism, invalidating subjective experience as unofficial, demoting the humanities and social sciences to pleasant distractions of yesteryear. The modern impulse is that the techno-scientific is closer to reality than the humanities, but the reality is that analytic components are emerging properties which will be reabsorbed into organic substance like our bones will someday be. For a long time, I have been obsessed with space and time, and when I see a tree on the sidewalk, I have this sense, that it is not a *part* of anything, but that it a single tree in outer space.

The idea of using genomic editing to create more perfect species is therefore a part of our impulse to isolate nature as a component, like Heidegger picking up a hammer. In doing so, technologists risk an overemphasis on the value of science and technology as a fundamental key to our salvation. The philosopher Nick Bostrom defines transhumanism as the doctrine that "current human nature is improvable through the use of applied science and other rational methods, which may make it possible to increase human health-span, extend our intellectual and physical capacities, and give us increased control over our own mental states and moods." And yet, each time we focus in on an isolated biological feature or trait, we risk a reduction of our being to those ends. In seeking to control or make permanent our image in technology, we may be sacrificing our very coping mechanisms, our vigilance.

These are not just thought experiments, but active research programs. Google purportedly aligned itself with the Kurzweil singularity movement in a bid for a life extension program. In 2013, the *Time* magazine cover story "Can Google Solve Death" became part of that spectacle when it noted that, for CEO Larry Page, solving cancer "may not be a big enough task." But the suggestion of building better humans comes up against resounding skepticism, both in the ability to actually execute on these technical abilities, and secondly, on the ability to manage such rapid changes with maturity. That science and technology may not hold the key to our future, salvation and survival, is a contrarian view that few would dare to espouse aloud, except in some of our deepest quarters. As Jonathan Moreno noted, "A stirring lack of confidence in the human ability to manage the Promethean power of science characterizes neoconservative writings."

But such a lack of confidence in science and technology also characterizes much of our literature. Aldous Huxley's masterpiece *Brave New World* centered on John, an illicit son of Linda and the Director of Hatcheries and Conditioning. The World State now controls reproduction through "Bokanovsky's Process" of human cloning which "is applied to fertilized human eggs *in vitro,* causing them to split into identical genetic copies of the original. The process can be repeated several times, though the maximum number of viable embryos possible is 96." The process further allows for engineering techniques to engender several different classes of embryos based on a kind of caste system, each of which belongs to a "Bokanovsky group," members of which "usually work together doing a single task, and by manipulating the *in vitro* chemicals, various subclasses can be created from a Bokanovsky Group," which consist of lower casts of Gamma, Delta and Epsilon citizens and upper casts of Alpha and Beta citizens developed to their fullest extent. All of this is controlled by a Human Element Manager, who explains that each Bokanovsky group is responsible for specific tasks in society, such as cold-pressing, cutting screws, driving delivery trucks, an entire civilization with its duties and tasks defined by its birthright. Emotion and romantic relationships are obsolete. The State controls population and encourages consumption and productivity through specified modes of work in its command economy. John learns he was born through a tryst between his mother and the Director during an excursion to a reservation of savages who still practice marriage, natural birth and family life. He is caught between two worlds, that of the savages and the State, which disallows his romantic impulses and personal ambitions. He reads nothing but the complete works of William Shakespeare, quoting it throughout, thus his allusion to "Brave New World" is a reference to *The Tempest*.

In fact, Shakespeare's *The Tempest* is set on an island, where a native resident, the lowly and grotesque Caliban, is seen as a monster. Prospero, a magician and his daughter Miranda, are stranded on the island for a decade. Miranda grows up with Caliban and the spirits, but has seen no other humans. When she sees a shipwrecked party from Italy, she exclaims "O wonder! How many goodly creatures are there here! How beauteous mankind is! O brave new world / That has such people in't!" The division between Caliban, as an ordinary being, and the glorious shipwrecked party, signifies the prospects between an existing genome and one that might be repaired or enhanced. And yet, at the end of *The Tempest*, Prospero is rescued and returns to civilization to reclaim his place as the rightful Duke of Milan. Miranda, just a child when they were stranded, is naïve and sees civilized people with awe and wonder as superior, while Prospero is able to regain perspective. He recounts his story of island life, and at its close, he breaks his magic wand. As George

Annas wrote of the snapping of the wand that "this gesture has properly been seen as the author's commentary on the relationship between art and life, art, or at least an enchanted island is no place for man to live, but rather a place through which we pass in order to renew and strengthen our sense of reality."

This interpretation – that one of the main functions of literature is to strengthen our sense of reality – suggests the importance of the humanities to grow in lockstep with our accelerating technologies. It raises the question once more, of whether science and technology bring us closer to reality, or have the potential to do, as Heidegger warned, to abstract us from our sense of coping with the enduring situation of life, developing an adult character which is our rite.

In *Brave New World*, John lives by the code of Shakespeare and the ways of the savages, but his experience is naïve and the narrative of his life is as much imparted into his own consciousness as the hypnotic messages of the World State. He can only articulate his desires, superficially, through the modes of Shakespeare. Traveling back to London to re-enter the State, he is astounded by its technology, but gradually comes to condemn its high-tech life as a poor substitute for individual freedom and personal integrity. He chastens his new love, Lenina for dealing out a narcotic drink called soma to kill any sense of pain or love and failing to live up to his Shakesperean ideals. He absconds to live on an abandoned hilltop to pursue ascetic values. But it is upon the hilltop that he comes to realize that his courtship with her has failed, and he chastens her, calling her a strumpet. "Pain's a delusion," she tells him. "Oh is it?" John replies, picking up a thick hazel switch and pummeling her to death.

His violence derives from a deeply suppressed and subordinated will. John's violence represents a reality that goes deeper than the science and technology that defines him, and it inevitably emerges, rupturing to the surface. In effect, John is a creation of the World State, and he wanders in the countryside, the full force of his repressed subconscious comes back full force upon the State – which is haunted by its repression. Digging in his garden, a couple of weeks later, he also thinks about his mother, Linda's, death and Shakespeare, again, flashes through his mind. He thinks of the character Gloucester in *King Lear*, who makes contradictory statements about the gods being gentle, and then careless manipulators of men. These technologists are manipulators, and here again, instead of locating a metaphysical God, the characters locate God in technology. He thinks of *Hamlet*, whose climatic line, "To sleep, perchance, to dream," refers to his despair that his agony will exceed beyond the grave in a dream, indicating his wish for a "dreamless sleep," a death which ends his strife. In this brave new world, as in *Hamlet* with its ghost, the dream signifies intent as it is abstracted, in the apparition, or in the technology of the World State. The main character is agonized by the separation of a duty that is no longer his own.

The effect achieves its reification in our own contemporary life when it emphasizes that the actions and decisions that guide information technologies, genetics technologies and the engines of finance are valid or reasonable or smart to the extent that they are evaluable in their outcomes or results. The overemphasis on results and outcomes defines the hyper-rationalism of our times and the rise of utilitarian ethics, and the decline of deontic and virtue ethics. The unquestioned belief that science and technology are good and bring us closer to a truth signifies our separation from the dream as intent and its expropriation by industry. What anyone wants is the right to self-organize, the right to dare, the right to adventure, the liberty to a life they've dreamed up all by themselves. In so many ways, today, we freely abdicate our right to dream. If it is not data-driven or results-driven, it is not official and certainly not modern. Virtue goes into decline and existential despair returns in our subconscious desire for a "dreamless sleep." Near the end of the story, Huxley locates this character on a hilltop after he has mercilessly thrashed his love, which signifies his subconscious defiance against technology and its demands, a death drive, which has eliminated any ability he had to be a self-made man, to build a love based on hard-won trust. Precisely because technology has become so sensible in guiding humanity's outcomes, he cannot locate a purpose. "He was digging in his garden – digging, too, in his own mind, laboriously turning up the substance of his thought. Death – and he drove in his spade once, and again, and yet again. And all our yesterdays have lighted fools the way to dusty death. A convincing thunder rumbled through the words. He lifted another spadeful of earth. Why had Linda died? Why had she been allowed to become gradually less than human and at last... he shuddered. A good kissing carrion. He planted his foot on his spade and stamped it fiercely into the tough ground. As flies to wanton boys are we to the gods; they kill us for their sport. Thunder again; words that proclaimed themselves true – truer somehow than truth itself. And yet that same Gloucester had called them ever-gentle gods. Besides, thy best of rest is sleep and that thou oft provok'st; yet grossly fear'st thy death which is no more. No more than sleep. Sleep. Perchance to dream.

Notes

CHAPTER I

1 Begley CG, Ellis LM. Drug development: Raise standards for preclinical cancer research. *Nature*. 2012 Mar 28; 483(7391):531–533. doi: 10.1038/483531a.

2 Prinz F, Schlange T, Asadullah K. Believe it or not: how much can we rely on published data on potential drug targets? *Nature Rev. Drug Discov.* September 2011; 10:712. doi: 10.1038/nrd3439-c1. See also: News and Analysis by Arrowsmith.

3 Thompson PM, Ge T, Glahn DC, Jahanshad N, Nichols TE. Genetics of the connectome. *Neuroimage*. 2013 Oct 15; 80:475–488. Published online 2013 May 21; doi: 10.1016/j.neuroimage.2013.05.013.

4 MacArthur D, Manolio TA, Dimmock DP *et al.* Guidelines for investigating causality of sequence variants in human disease. *Nature*. 24 April 2014; 508:469–476. doi: 10.1038/nature13127.

5 To illustrate one of their points, they described a study on autism in which researchers found four de novo, or new, mutations in the gene TNN. But, it turns out the TNN gene is the largest coding gene in the human genome, and just by chance, we might expect to find two mutations. Finding four, then, is not so surprising. The researchers in that study dropped that gene as an autism candidate. But these are only best practices.

6 Goldstein DB, Allen A, Keebler J, *et al.* Sequencing studies in human genetics: design and interpretation.*Nature Rev. Genet.* 2013; 14:460–470.

7 Open Science Collaboration. Estimating the reproducibility of psychological science. *Science*. 28 Aug 2015; 349(6251), doi: 10.1126/science.aac4716.

8 Hart J, Chabris CF. Does a "Triple Package" of traits predict success? *Personality and Individual Differences*. May 2016; 94:216–222.

9 Baker M. Over half of psychology studies fail reproducibility test. *Nature*. 27 August 2015. doi: 10.1038/nature.2015.18248.

10 James W. *The Will To Believe*, Dover Publications, 1956 (originally published 1897): 21, 25.

11 Bloom P. The baby in the well: *The case against empathy*. A Critic at Large, *The New Yorker* May 20, 2013.

12 McGregor J. Why this Wharton wunderkind wants leaders to replace their intuition with evidence. *The Washington Post* April 9 2016.

13 Kozubek J. Love is not algorithmic. *The Atlantic* September 24 2014.

14 Comfort N. Genes are overrated. *The Atlantic* June 2016.

15 Goldberg N. *Writing Down the Bones*. Shambala. 1986.

16 Cells are discussed in terms of lines or lineages. Stem cells are basically at the root and are very general-purpose, meaning they can give rise to a number of types of cells. In fact, first they give rise to slightly more specific types of "progenitor cells" that give rise to even more task-specific cells, which are adult cells, say, a red blood cell, or a T-cell of the immune system. It turns out that cancer cells have a lot of the same properties as stem cells, such as being highly mobile, slippery and "dedifferentiated," meaning they regress to an earlier general-purpose, stem-like state. Intriguingly, stem cells can remain in a dormant type of state for a long time between cell divisions, and while they do this, they pick up all sorts of molecular debris, called "adducts," chemical compounds from smoking or other sources, which land on their DNA. The classical theory holds that stem cells are specially protected, or "cyto-protected," from acquiring mutations (the prefix "cyto" just means cell), but it may be acquiring adducts during their long periods of dormancy actually cause them to be *more* prone to acquiring mutations once they start to divide, since all of this molecular debris lays in the tracks of their DNA. Enzymes run down those tracks, and the debris may trip them up.

17 Phages, or more technically "bacteriophages," are viruses that infect bacteria. Like the viruses that infect human cells, they have, in general, either lifecycles that are lysogenic, meaning they invade a host cell and replicate along with it, or lytic, meaning they burst the cell and destroy it, releasing packets of new virus.

18 Selective breeding traces back at least to Genesis 30:43: "So the man became exceedingly prosperous, and had large flocks and female and male servants and camels and donkeys," while genetic engineering has roots in the 1930s, when scientists had learned to bombard insect eggs and seeds with x-rays, riddling their genomes with mutations and then selectively breeding the cells that, just by chance, picked up the traits they wanted. This gave us barley for modern beer and red grapefruits. But this kind of havoc could not be gainfully perpetrated on mammalian cells. It was not precise enough. Once restriction enzymes were discovered in the late 1960s, scientists could begin splicing different pieces of genetic code together, which allowed them not just to select, but to *create* specific genetic variants. This was the emergence of "gene

splicing" or "recombinant DNA." Decades after that, scientists would learn to do "gene editing," which is highly precise alterations to single nucleotide bases in a genome.

19 Ishino Y, Shinagawa H, Makino K, Amemura M, Nakata, AJ. Nucleotide sequence of the iap gene, responsible for alkaline phosphatase isozyme conversion in *Escherichia coli*, and identification of the gene product. *Bacteriol*. 1987; 169:5429–5433.

20 Lander E. The heroes of Crispr. *Cell*. 14 January 2016; 164(1–2):18–28. http://dx.doi.org/10.1016/j.cell.2015.12.041(accessed June 2016).

21 Lander. The heroes of Crispr.

22 Mojica FJM, Juez G, Rodríguez-Valera F. Transcription at different salinities of *Haloferax mediterranei* sequences adjacent to partially modified PstI sites. *Mol. Microbiol*. 1993; 9:613–621.

23 Halophilic means "salt loving."

24 Mojica FJM, Ferrer C, Juez G, Rodríguez-Valera F. Long stretches of short tandem repeats are present in the largest replicons of the Archaea *Haloferax mediterranei* and *Haloferax volcanii* and could be involved in replicon partitioning. *Mol. Microbiol*. 1995; 17:85–93.

25 Those include a microbiological zoo including *Mycobacterium tuberculosis*, *Clostridium difficile* and the bacterium *Yersinia pestis*, which uses rodents as a host and is the organism that causes bubonic plague.

26 Mojica FJM, Díez-Villaseñor C, Soria E, Juez G. Biological significance of a family of regularly spaced repeats in the genomes of Archaea, bacteria and mitochondria. *Mol. Microbiol*. 2000; 36:244–246.

27 Jansen R, Embden JDAV, Gaastra W, Schouls LM. Identification of genes that are associated with DNA repeats in prokaryotes. *Mol. Microbiol*. 2002; 43:1565–1575.

28 Eukaryotes and prokaryotes (bacteria and Archaea) are two major kingdoms of life.

29 Mojica FJM, Garrett RA. *Discovery and Seminal Developments in the Crispr Field*. Springer, 1–31.

30 Lander. The heroes of Crispr.

31 Eukaryote cells which build humans, for instance, also are invaded by viruses. In fact, almost 10 percent of the human genome is a graveyard of viral artifacts called long terminal repeats, but these viruses probably burrowed into ancestral eukaryotic cells eons ago. It's possible that a similar immune system once functioned in the ancestors of eukaryotic cells, which are the sort of cells that build higher mammals like us. An intriguing prospect is that mammalian cells later repurposed such a mechanism to cut and tailor their own RNA

as a means to fine-tune their own gene expression. The idea is that an original biomechanical code or structure can repurposed for a secondary function is called *exaptation*.

32 Lander. The heroes of Crispr.

33 Lander. The heroes of Crispr.

34 Mojica FJM, Díez-Villaseñor C, García-Martínez J, Soria EJ. Intervening sequences of regularly spaced prokaryotic repeats derive from foreign genetic elements. *Mol. Evol.* 2005; 60:174–182.

35 Bolotin A, Quinquis B, Sorokin A, Ehrlich SD. Clustered regularly interspaced short palindrome repeats (Crisprs) have spacers of extrachromosomal origin. *Microbiology.* 2005; 151:2551–2561.

36 Pourcel C, Salvignol G, Vergnaud G. Crispr elements in *Yersinia pestis* acquire new repeats by preferential uptake of bacteriophage DNA, and provide additional tools for evolutionary studies. *Microbiology.* 2005; 151:653–663.

37 Pourcel *et al.* Crispr elements in *Yersinia pestis.*

38 Maxmen A. The Genesis Engine. *Wired* July 22 2015.

39 Barrangou R, Fremaux C, Deveau H *et al.* Crispr provides acquired resistance against viruses in prokaryotes. *Science.* 2007; 315:1709–1712.

40 Bolotin *et al.* Crisprs have spacers of extrachromosomal origin.

41 Makarova KS, Grishin NV, Shabalina SA, Wolf YI, Koonin EV. A putative RNA-interference-based immune system in prokaryotes: computational analysis of the predicted enzymatic machinery, functional analogies with eukaryotic RNAi, and hypothetical mechanisms of action. *Biol. Direct.* 2006; 1:7.

42 The nucleotide sequence of Crispr repeats had the property of a palindrome, which are words like "racecar," which spell the same thing whether read forward or backward. This suggested the code could fold up into a secondary structure such as a hairpin.

43 Brouns SJJ, Jore MM, Lundgren M *et al.* Small Crispr RNAs guide antiviral defense in prokaryotes. *Science.* 2008; 321:960–964.

44 Lander. The heroes of Crispr.

45 Makarova *et al.* A putative RNA-interference-based immune system in prokaryotes.

46 In short, self-splicing occurs through the breaking of electron bonds in the phosphate groups that binds a string of nucleic acids into a molecular sequence. RNA is subtly different from DNA in that it has an extra hydroxyl group, an OH, and the hydrogen proton from this hydroxyl group can free itself from the molecule, "deprotonate," resulting in an oxygen with a negative charge, or it can acquire a free hydroxyl with a

negative charge, which can go on the attack to steal an electron bond from a phosphate group, breaking the phosphate backbone.

47 Marraffini LA, Sontheimer EJ. Crispr interference limits horizontal gene transfer in staphylococci by targeting DNA. Science. 2008; 322:1843–1845.

48 Horvath P, Romero DA, Coûté-Monvoisin AC *et al.* Diversity, activity, and evolution of Crispr loci in *Streptococcus thermophilus. Bacteriol.* 2008; 190:1401–1412.

49 Deveau H, Barrangou R, Garneau JE *et al.* Phage response to Crispr-encoded resistance in *Streptococcus thermophilus.Bacteriol.* 2008; 190:1390–1400.

50 Sternberg SH, Redding S, Jinek M, Greene EC, Doudna JA. DNA interrogation by the Crispr RNA-guided endonuclease Cas9. *Nature.* 2014; 507:62–67. doi: 10.1038/nature13011; pmid: 24476820.

51 Maxmen. The Genesis Engine.

52 Mangold M, Siller M, Roppenser B *et al.* Synthesis of group A streptococcal virulence factors is controlled by a regulatory RNA molecule. *Mol. Microbiol.* 2004; 53:1515–1527.

53 Deltcheva E, Chylinski K, Sharma CM *et al.* Crispr RNA maturation by trans-encoded small RNA and host factor RNase III. *Nature.* 2011; 471:602–607.

54 Charpentier, now operating out of the Max Planck Institute for Infection Biology, told me there are at least six types of Crispr-Cas systems. "Type I" is complex and involves a "cascade" of a number of Cas proteins which must act together in tight coordination, while the "type II" system is the one that includes a neighboring tracrRNA molecule and consists of one protein with a dual-tracrRNA-CRISPR-RNA. Among those microbes that include type II systems include *S. pyogenes, S. mutans, L. innocua, N. meningitidis* and *S. thermophilus.* Cas9 is now one of the few microbial enzymes that is a household name, but it gained its popularity for accidental reasons, mainly it is one of the largest such Cas nucleases. In fact, there are numerous Cas endonucleases in the neighborhood of tracrRNA including Csn1 (Cas9), but also a Csn2…which constitute an "operon," meaning several genes which are expressed together under a single regulatory control. Those additional genes in the operon are responsible for the memorization step of the immune system, but in type I systems, for instance, several Cas proteins must bundle together into a larger unit to get the job done. What's so special about Cas9? It can work all by itself without any "supporting cas(t) just with the dual-tracrRNA-CRISPR-RNA." The best technical review paper of the six types of Crispr-Cas system in the wild is: Wright AV, Doudna JA. Biology and applications of Crispr systems: harnessing nature's toolbox for genome engineering. *Cell.* 2016; 164(1):29–44.

55 Maxmen. The Genesis Engine.

56 Jinek M, Jiang F, Taylor D *et al.* Structures of Cas9 endonucleases reveal RNA-mediated conformational activation. *Science.* 2014; 343:1247997. doi: 10.1126/science.1247997; pmid: 24505130.

57 Nishimasu H, Ran FA, Hsu PD *et al.* Crystal structure of Cas9 in complex with guide RNA and target DNA. *Cell.* 2014; 156:935–949. doi: 10.1016/j.cell.2014.02.001; pmid: 24529477.

58 "Molecular structures of Cas9 determined by electron microscopy and x-ray crystallography show that the protein undergoes large conformational rearrangement upon binding to the guide RNA, with a further change upon association with a target double-stranded DNA (dsDNA). This change creates a channel, running between the two structural lobes of the protein that binds to the RNA-DNA hybrid as well as to the coaxially stacked dual-RNA structure of the guide corresponding to the crRNA repeat–tracrRNA anti-repeat interaction." Doudna JA, Charpentier E. Genome editing. The new frontier of genome engineering with Crispr-Cas9. *Science.* 2014 Nov 28; 346(6213):1258096. doi: 10.1126/science.1258096.

59 Sapranauskas R, Gasiunas G, Fremaux C *et al.* The *Streptococcus thermophilus* Crispr/Cas system provides immunity in *Escherichia coli. Nucleic Acids Res.* 2011; 39:9275–9282.

60 Karvelis *et al. RNA Biology,* 10(5):841–851.

61 Doudna and Charpentier. Genome Editing. The new frontier of genome engineering with Crispr-Cas9 Science. 2014 Nov 28;346(6213):1258096. Doi: 10.1126/science. 1258096d.

62 HNH and RuvC-like domains are just parts of a Cas protein, and the only reason this is important is because each of them cuts one strand of the double-stranded DNA helix.

63 Jinek M, Chylinski K, Fonfara I *et al.* A programmable dual-RNA-guided DNA endonuclease in adaptive bacterial immunity. *Science.* 2012; 337:816–821.

64 Doudna and Charpentier. Genome Editing. The new frontier of genome engineering with Crispr-Cas9 Science. 2014 Nov 28;346(6213):1258096. Doi: 10.1126/science. 1258096d.

65 Maxmen. The Genesis Engine.

66 In 2012, Siksnys, Barrangou and Horvath also showed Crispr-Cas9 could cut DNA in a test tube.

67 Lander. The heroes of Crispr.

68 Lander. The heroes of Crispr.

69 Mali P, Yang L, Esvelt KM *et al.* RNA-guided human genome engineering via Cas9. *Science.* 2013; 339:823–826.

70 Cong L, Ran FA, Cox D *et al.* Multiplex genome engineering using Crispr/Cas systems. *Science.* 2013; 339:819–823.

71 Mali *et al.* RNA-guided human genome engineering via Cas9. *Science.* 2013; 339:823–826.

72 Hwang WY, Fu Y, Reyon D *et al.* Efficient genome editing in zebrafish using a Crispr-Cas system. *Nat. Biotechnol.* 2013; 31:227–229.

73 Cho SW, Kim S, Kim JM, Kim J-S. Targeted genome engineering in human cells with the Cas9 RNA-guided endonuclease. *Nat. Biotechnol.* 2013; 31:230–232.

74 Jinek M, East A, Cheng A *et al.* RNA-programmed genome editing in human cells. *eLife.* 2013; 2:e00471.

75 Lander. The heroes of Crispr.

76 Begley S. Controversial Crispr history sets off an online firestorm. *STAT News.* January 19, 2016.

77 Vence T. "Heroes of Crispr" disputed. *The Scientist.* January 19, 2016.

78 Comfort N. A Whig history of Crispr. January 18, 2016. http://genotopia .scienceblog.com/573/a-whig-history-of-Crispr/ (accessed June 2016).

79 Regalado A. A scientist's contested history of Crispr. *Technol. Rev.* January 19, 2016.

80 Comfort. Genes are overrated.

81 The Rockefeller Institute's Phoebus Levene thought the "comically plain" structure of DNA "disqualified it as a carrier of genetic information"; he even called DNA, Mukherjee reports, a "stupid molecule." Instead, "Nobel Prizes were awarded three times for elucidating aspects of it: in 1910 (Albrecht Kossel), 1957 (Alexander Todd), and 1962 (Watson, Crick, and Wilkins). There's no evidence that Phoebus Levene – Kossel's student – called it a "stupid molecule," as Mukherjee claims. Max Delbrück did, in the mid-1940s, after Oswald Avery and colleagues had shown it to be the molecule of heredity in pneumococcus. Delbrück, Watson's most important mentor, used such blunt skepticism to spur scientific rigor among his followers. The "stupid molecule" remark, then, is best understood as prologue to the solution of the double helix in 1953, rather than as an obstacle to its having been solved sooner. Comfort. Genes are overrated.

82 Comfort. A Whig history of Crispr.

83 Doudna and Charpentier. Genome editing.

84 Wright and Doudna. Biology and applications of Crispr systems.

85 Franklin was a colleague of Maurice Wilkins, who shared the Nobel with Crick and Watson, working at the MRC Laboratory of Molecular Biology in Cambridge.

86 Kaufman R. It doesn't add up. *Science*. December 16, 2011. doi: 10.1126/science.caredit.a1100139.

87 Kaufman. It doesn't add up.

88 Berg P, Mertz JE. Personal reflections on the origins and emergence of recombinant DNA technology. *Genetics*. January 2010; 184(1):9-17. doi: 10.1534/genetics.109.112144.

89 Shapin S. The desire to know: Scientific virtue is worth saving. *The Boston Review*. January and February 2015: 32.

90 For Chomsky, institutions do not simply exist to exert power for those within them, at the expense of those outside of them, as Foucault had stated. He argued, instead, and rather effectively over the years, that institutions manifest our basic desire for some justice which is unbiased to private interests. "I think it's too hasty to characterize our existing systems of justice as merely systems of class oppression; I don't think that they are that. I think that they embody systems of class oppression, but they also embody a kind of groping towards the true humanly valuable concepts of justice and decency and love and kindness and sympathy, which I think are real." – Chomsky vs. Foucault debate. Human Nature: Justice vs. Power (1971).

91 Molecular evolution, too, is a series of blind contingencies, doors opening unexpectedly in pathways – usually with catastrophic outcomes. It happens on boring, sunny days for no particular reason. And when geneticists look at that, it's staggering, really, not just because it exposes the daunting risks of life, not just because they know that molecular door can pop open or closed in a pathway and wreck everything in an instant, but because they can open doors, too. Evolution is the most dangerous idea out there and still is.

92 Keats said famously: "I had not a dispute but a disquisition with Dilke, upon various subjects; several things dove-tailed in my mind, and at once it struck me what quality went to form a Man of Achievement, especially in Literature, and which Shakespeare possessed so enormously – I mean Negative Capability, that is, when a man is capable of being in uncertainties, mysteries, doubts, without any irritable reaching after fact and reason – Coleridge, for instance, would let go by a fine isolated verisimilitude caught from the Penetralium of mystery, from being incapable of remaining content with half-knowledge. This pursued through volumes would perhaps take us no further than this, that with a great poet the sense of Beauty overcomes every other consideration, or rather obliterates all consideration."

93 Sherkow J. The Crispr patent interference showdown is on: How did we get here and what comes next? Stanford Center for Law and Biosciences Blog. December 29, 2015.

94 In March 2016, Harvard's Alpert Prize was issued for Crispr and awarded to five scientists: Rodolphe Barrangou, associate professor in the Department of Food, Bioprocessing and Nutrition Sciences and the Todd R. Klaenhammer Distinguished Scholar in Probiotics Research at North Carolina State University; Philippe Horvath, senior scientist at DuPont in Dangé-Saint-Romain, France; Jennifer Doudna, the Li Ka Shing Chancellor's Chair in Biomedical and Health Sciences and professor of molecular and cell biology and of chemistry at the University of California, Berkeley; Emmanuelle Charpentier, scientific member and director at the Max Planck Institute for Infection Biology in Berlin and professor at Umeå University in Sweden; Virginijus Siksnys, professor, chief scientist and department head at the Institute of Biotechnology at Vilnius University in Lithuania.

95 The initial proof of Crispr adaptive interference was made by Barrangou and Horvath in the 2007 *Science* paper. Sontheimer argues this paper provided the Crispr field's "Fire and Mello moment" (i.e. when the pathway was revealed), drawing an analogy to a mechanism called RNA interference, or RNAi, which was revealed as a means that a cell has to use RNA molecules to interfere with the translation of other RNA molecules into proteins, thereby regulating the expression of genes. Andrew Fire and Craig Mello uncovered the RNAi pathway in 1998. "To continue the RNAi analogy, the contributions of Doudna, Charpentier, Siksnys, Zhang, Church, Joung, and Kim in their 2012/2013 papers are more analogous to the RNAi field's 'Tuschl moment,' which was when the primary reduction-to-practice advance was provided," alluding to Thomas Tuschl who made the RNAi technology applicable to human cells in 2001.

96 Regalado A. Engineering the perfect baby. *Technol. Rev.* March 5, 2015.

97 Regalado. Engineering the perfect baby.

98 Kahn J. The Crispr quandry. *The New York Times Magazine.* November 9, 2015.

99 Huebbe P, Nebel A, Siegert S *et al.* APOE e4 is associated with higher vitamin D levels in targeted replacement mice and humans. *FASEB J.* September 2011; 25(9):3262–3270. doi: 10.1096/fj.11-180935. PMID 21659554.

100 The gene *PCSK9* has a role in hypercholesterolemia and ischemic stroke. An inhibitor shows an ability to reduce LDL-C levels, which we tend to want to keep low for cardiovascular health. Although the findings have been controversial, and appear to be subject to the genetic background, evidence suggests that this gene can affect risk to stroke. In a meta-analysis, one single nucleotide polymorphism (rs505151) in which a person has two copies of a guanine nucleotide at that site associates with risk for ischemic stroke patients. People who have two copies of adenine, or are heterozygous, meaning they have one copy of adenine and one copy of guanine, have levels of LDL-C which are twice as high as the normal control subjects, and this may indicate the risk of ischemic stroke is "mediated by increased levels of LDL-C." Au A, Griffiths LR, Cheng KK *et al.* The influence of OLR1 and PCSK9 gene polymorphisms on ischemic stroke: Evidence from a meta-analysis. *Sci Rep.* 2015; 15(5):18224.

101 A pair of papers dropped in 2012 characterizing rates of germline mutations in humans to much sensation. Men average two new mutations per year in each germline cell, and by the age of 40, most fathers pass on as many as 80 new mutations to their offspring. The implication was that paternal age contributes to the rates of autism and schizophrenia, since more mutations are tossed into the mix. Kong A, Frigge ML, Masson G, *et al.* Rate of *de novo* mutations and the importance of father's age to disease risk. *Nature.* August 23 2012; 488:471–475. doi: 10.1038/nature11396. Michaelson JJ. Whole-genome sequencing in autism identifies hot spots for de novo germline mutation. *Cell.* December 21 2012; 151(7):1431–1442. doi: 10.1016/j.cell.2012.11.019.

102 Madabhushi R, Gao F, Pfenning AR *et al.* Activity-induced DNA breaks govern the expression of neuronal early-response genes. *Cell.* June 18, 2015; 161:1592–1605.

103 Regalado. Engineering the perfect baby.

104 Skerrett P. Experts debate: Are we playing with fire when we edit human genes? *STAT News.* November 17, 2015.

105 Müller-Hill B. *The lac Operon: A Short History of a Genetic Paradigm.* Walter de Gruyter. 1996.

106 Harrison RP. *Juvenescence: A Cultural History of our Age.* University of Chicago Press. 2014.

107 Berg and Mertz. Personal reflections.

108 Moreno J. *The Body Politic.* Bellevue Literary Press. 2011.

CHAPTER 2

109 Lederberg J. Interview with Prof. Lederberg, Winner of the 1958 Nobel Prize in Physiology and Medicine. Conducted by Lev Pevzner, 20 March 1996.

110 Massachusetts Institute of Technology Oral History Program. *Oral History Collection on the Recombinant DNA Controversy, 1966–1978*, 1988. MC.0100.

111 Tucker A. Obituary: ES Anderson. *The Guardian.* Tuesday 21 March 2006.

112 Kala-azar is the second-largest parasitic killer in the world after malaria. Protozoa are single-cell eukaryotic cells, which are in the broad domain that include mammals, including humans, in contrast to prokaryotic cells, which consist mainly of single-celled bacteria and Archaea. A vector refers to a small organism such as a mosquito or tick, which can carry protozoan from animal to person. A reservoir is a long-term host, in which a pathogen may reside at a subclinical level, including birds, livestock, pigs and dogs. Once the protozoan infects a human, it causes Leishmania or dumdum fever.

113 Friedberg EC. Master molecule, heal thyself. *J. Biol. Chem.* 2014 May 16; 289(20):13691–13700. Published online April 72014. doi: 10.1074/jbc.X114.572115.

114 Beadle and Tatum were studying genetic mutations in *Neurospora crassa*, a simple bread mold. It could be cultured in a bath of sugar, inorganic salts and the vitamin biotin. They used radiation on large numbers of the mold to produce some organisms with mutant genes. They showed that some of these mutant spores would not replicate, again, without the addition of a specific amino acid – arginine. This showed that the mutation compromised a discrete gene, which builds a specific protein, or enzyme, that is needed for the mold to produce arginine on its own. In fact, there are many amino acids that an organism can produce on its own, but some so-called "essential amino acids" are those that must come from nutritional sources. Arginine was one that the mold could produce on its own, but not after the mutation. And so, without adding arginine, the mold would simply not grow. This showed that a mutation affected a specific gene.

115 In fact, the idea of discrete particles of inheritance had been around a while. Mendel's original pea plant experiments suggested particulate units of inheritance. The implication was that particular traits must be

traceable to particulate molecules. When Hugo De Vries replicated Mendel's experiments, the basic mathematics of the laws of inheritance became widely accepted. De Vries began to champion the idea that there must be "tiny packets" of some sort of material, most likely related to these newfound chromosomes, which carried inherited traits across cell boundaries. August Weismann advanced his "germ plasm theory," splitting these packets into "germ cells" and "somatic cells."

116 As Stephen Jay Gould has noted, the notion of a "master template" of heredity traces back at least to the Renaissance, as he explained it in his masterpiece *The Structure of Evolutionary Theory*. The Renaissance Man has always been looked upon with skepticism by the experts of a field who have devoted decades to their discipline. In fact, he has been chastened at least since the fourth century BC, long before there was a Renaissance. At that time, the motto appeared: "a cobbler should stick to his last," where "a last" was a shoemaker's model foot. In other words, cobblers: mind your own business and stick to building shoes, please. No need to throw around your advice. But a polymath with a liberal arts background can often toss surprising insights into the mix, garnering an advantage of new perspective, what we might call beginner's luck. This was the case in the eighteenth century, when the poet J. W. von Goethe dared to suggest some ideas for the biologists, both drawing rebuke and shaking up their field. (The aphorism of the cobbler can be traced to Pliny the Elder, in the original Latin, *ne supra crepidam sutor indicaret*.) Biology had been stuck on the problem of "Paley's watch," which was conceived by the Reverend William Paley. If any of us came upon a watch, Paley suggested, we must imagine a watchmaker; in his words: "there cannot be design without designer; contrivance without a contriver; arrangement, without anything capable of arranging." But Goethe had a moment of insight, or "Einfalle," a German word for "idea," which translates something close to "facts that fall into the head." He came up with his "theory of archetypes" while pondering a leaf. Goethe saw patterns in nature all around him, but his intuition told him that these patterns and models weren't as static as Paley had suggested. Goethe observed that leaves are constrained by a pattern that is modifiable. "The plant forms which surround us were not all created at some given point in time and then locked into the given form, they have been given... a felicitous mobility and plasticity that allows them to grow and adapt themselves to many different conditions in many different places." Goethe was alive to the insight that there are deep patterns in nature, patterns that we've all stuck by, like blueprints –

whale fins, bat wings and human hands are built on pretty much the same plan, tinkered to degrees. Call the blueprint a "Baupläne," if you like, German for "blueprint" or "body plan." In 1978, E. B. Lewis was studying gene dosage in flies and became interested in a duplicated *Hox* gene, called BX-C. Lewis explained that the dosage of this gene (0, 1, 2 or any number of copies of the gene on a single chromosome) controlled a gradient of development up and down the fly. Adding dosage, or "gain-of-function," gene variants would strengthen the gradient and enable posterior structure to develop in more anterior positions, while "loss-of-function," or reduced dosage, would weaken the gradient and allow anterior structures to develop in more posterior positions (added legs). *Hox* genes were identified as a family of genes responsible for the regulation of the body plan, and bilateral development, the segmentation of teeth and fingers, the symmetrical body patterning. It was the underlying genetics for William Bateson's early discovery of "homeotic" transformations or examples of "fast evolution" in insects and plants, and the duplicated thoraxes in insects that Thomas Hunt Morgan had spotted in 1915. Biologists were hitting on the genes responsible for the "Baupläne" that Goethe had anticipated two centuries before.

117 Müller-Hill. *The lac Operon.*

118 Moreno. *The Body Politic.*

119 Shapin. The desire to know.

120 Shapin. The desire to know.

121 Müller-Hill. *The lac Operon.*

122 Müller-Hill. *The lac Operon.*

123 Avery's group was able to isolate DNA by using a battery of tests, including the use of trypsin and ribonuclease, enzymes that break down proteins and RNA, leaving only the DNA intact. They then used techniques for destroying the protein in virulent strains of bacteria while leaving its DNA unharmed, and for destroying the DNA in others while leaving the protein unharmed. Thus, the physicians reaffirmed Frederick Griffith's famous declaration that a "transforming principle" was conveyed through the DNA.

124 Fredrickson DS. *The Recombinant DNA Controversy: A Memoir. Science, Politics, and the Public Interest 1974–1981.* ASM Press, 2001.

125 Friedberg. Master molecule, heal thyself.

126 Friedberg. Master molecule, heal thyself.

127 Shapin. The desire to know.

128 Shapin. The desire to know.

129 Typhoid is a type of *Salmonella* bacteria that can give rise to typhoid fever.

130 Typhus is a number of similar diseases caused by *Rickettsia* bacteria, which killed more than 3 million people in WWI; typhus is not to be confused with typhoid-type *Salmonella*, which has an alias as typhoid bacillus or *Salmonella enteric typhi*, which uses humans as a host, or *Salmonella typhimurium*, which uses cattle and pigs as its host, or its associated typhoid fever.

131 An antigen is a molecular structure, usually a protein, which is the target for an adaptive immune response. For instance, an antigen on a virus or bacterial cell is the target for an antibody made by a human immune cell.

132 Before transferring a plasmid, it is usually replicated, or copied, by a means of "rolling circle amplification," where the plasmid is nicked by an enzyme unimaginatively called a "nickase" and then the genetic material is copied and then fixed again into a new circular plasmid.

133 Lederberg J. Cell genetics and hereditary symbiosis. *Physiol. Rev.* 1952; 32(4):403–430.

134 Lederberg J, Cavalli LL, Lederberg EM. Sex compatibility in *Escherichia coli. Genetics* November 1952; 37(6):720–730.

135 Zinder ND, Lederberg J. Genetic exchange in *Salmonella. J. Bacteriol.* 1952; 64(5):679–699.

136 Berg and Mertz. Personal reflections.

137 Lysogenize means to infect. This means that he wants to try to infect the *Salmonella* type F1 with a phage that only infects the type F2. As his hypothesis goes, he would expect the F2 type *Salmonella* to transform the phage, transferring to it new code that would allow it to convey F2 type properties. Now when the phage entered an F1 microbe, it would convey its F2 properties, and transform F1 type into F2 type.

138 In 2003 it became known as the Health Protection Agency in Britain.

139 Berg P. Moments of discovery: My favorite experiments. *JBC.* July 31, 2003; 278:40417–40424. doi: 10.1074/jbc.X300004200.

140 In 1947, Alfred Mirsky and Hans Ris published a report on the chemical composition of a chromosome, showing that 90 percent of it is composed of nucleohistone (mostly protein), while the remainder was a "coiled thread containing some 12 to 14 percent of ribose nucleic and about one-fifth as much desoxyribose [sic] nucleic acid." The authors deduced "The form of the chromosome is due primarily to the protein thread of the residual chromosome... (This) provides evidence for considering the residual chromosome to be the basis of the linear order of

the genes." It would take a decade before Watson and Crick unveiled its exact structure.

141 By the end of the 1950s, Matthew Meselson and Franklin Stahl showed the mechanism of inheritance was "semi-conservative," in other words, when a cell divides, the double-stranded DNA splits and each original strand remains intact and serves as a template while synthesizing a new additional strand. Thus one half of each double-stranded helix that emerges in a cell division is conserved from the former cell, and one half is newly minted.

142 Berg. Moments of discovery.

143 Protein is made of small units of amino acids of which there are 20 essential types that are native to the body, which each have one type of molecule at one end, a carboxyl group, designated as the C-terminus, and at the other end a molecule called an amine group, or N-terminus.

144 The other lab that co-discovered tRNA was Hoagland and Zamecnik at Harvard.

145 Jim Offengand, a graduate student, and Jack Preiss, a postdoctoral fellow, in the Berg lab, went on to describe the mechanism, showing the reaction was carried out by a highly specific enzyme.

146 Berg. Moments of discovery.

147 There are 20 amino acids and each one matches a specific three-base nucleotide code, a triplet of nucleotides, which is called a codon.

148 Elliot Volkin and Lazarus Astrachan in 1956 declared the composition of RNA closely resembled that of DNA. Crick, along with Jacques Monod, Francois Jacob, Sydney Benner and Arthur Beck Pardee, began conducting experiments which involved phages and would provide a full explanatory force of the dogma.

149 Szilard helped write the letter Albert Einstein sent to US President Roosevelt in favor of constructing the atom bomb. He tried to stop the bomb being dropped on civilians, and left physics after the bombing of Hiroshima and Nagasaki. "He published science fiction. In one story, an extra-terrestrial expedition of scientists excavates Central Station in New York City after an atomic war has destroyed all human life on earth. The pay toilets with their coin deposit start a controversy. The older, established scientists believe that the coins were deposited as part of a religious cult. A young iconoclast scientist proposes the hypothesis that the economic system of Terra demanded payments for everything, even for toilet use, and that this extreme form of capitalism ruined the civilization of Terra. The young man is ridiculed by

his elders for proposing a clever but absurd idea." Müller-Hill. *The lac Operon.*

150 The experiment is named for the trio of Arthur Beck Pardee, Francois Jacob and Jacques Monod.

151 Müller-Hill. *The lac Operon.*

152 Messenger RNA, or mRNA, was officially reported by Jacob, Sydney Brenner and Matthew Meselson at the California Institute of Technology in 1961.

153 Crow JF, Dove WF (eds). *Perspectives: Anecdotal, Historical and Critical Commentaries on Genetics.* The Genetics Society of America. 1995.

154 Datta N, Pridie RB, Anderson ES. An outbreak of infection with *Salmonella typhimurium* in a general hospital. *J. Hygiene.* 14 May 2009; 58(02): 229. doi: 10.1017/S0022172400038316.

155 Datta N. Transmissible drug resistance in an epidemic strain of *Salmonella typhimurium. J. Hygiene.* September 1962; 60(3): 301–310. doi: 10.1017/s0022172400020416.PMC2134509.PMID14025218.

156 Antibiotics.

157 A resistance transfer factor (R-factoror RTF) is an old name for a plasmid that codes for antibiotic resistance.

158 Tucker. Obituary: ES Anderson.

159 Cohen SN. DNA cloning: A personal view after 40 years. *Proc. Natl. Acad. Sci. USA.* 2013; 110(39):15521–15529. doi: 10.1073/pnas.1313397110.

160 Lederberg *et al.* Sex compatibility in *Escherichia coli.*

161 Harada K, Kameda M, Suzuki M, Mitsuhashi S. Drug resistance of enteric bacteria. 3. Acquisition of transferability of nontransmissible R(Tc) factor in cooperation with F factor and formation of Fr(Tc). *J. Bacteriol.* 1964; 88:1257–1265.

162 Watanabe T, Ogata C, Sato S. Episome-mediated transfer of drug resistance in Enterobacteriaceae. 8. Six-drug-resistance R factor. *J. Bacteriol.* 1964; 88:922–928.

163 Watanabe T, Fukasawa T. Episome-mediated transfer of drug resistance in Enterobacteriaceae. I. Transfer of resistance factors by conjugation. *J. Bacteriol.* 1961; 81:669–678.

164 Campbell AM. Episomes. *Adv. Genet.* 1963; 11:101–145.

165 Jacob F, Brenner S, Cuzin F. On the regulation of DNA replication in bacteria. Cold Spring Harb. Symp. Quant. Biol. 1963; 28:329–348.

166 Cohen. DNA cloning.

167 Cohen. DNA cloning.

168 Cohen. DNA cloning.

169 Ssu was the name of one of Anderson's plasmids and pSC101 was one of Cohen's plasmids (pSC stands for plasmid of Stanley Cohen). EcoRI is a restriction enzyme that works as a pair of tiny scissors to cut and paste the plasmids into his own recombination and hybrid plasmids. Restriction enzymes are explained in the next chapter.

170 Shapin. The desire to know.

171 Some have quipped that science today is so dogmatic we currently live in an age of the "conference industrial complex."

172 Shapin. The desire to know.

173 Shapin. The desire to know.

174 I can find no better example of the triumphant mode of data-driven decision-making over gut instinct than the Associated Press story of the Discovery shuttle. NASA chief Michael Griffin, was exulted by the *Associated Press* for making an "emotion-free logical decision based on hard numbers" that saved a mission. "And he's so cool under pressure," a reporter gushed. After Discovery's successful July 4th launch, Griffin, when asked to comment on his mood at the time of events, reportedly said: "I'll have time for feelings after I'm dead." Borenstein S. NASA chief's gamble – or calculated decision – that paid off, big time. *Associated Press.* July 17, 2006.

175 The scientific method is only one way to make decisions, and you can reach this conclusion through the ostensive realization that your gut instincts, intuitions and common sense logic continue to persist even at times when you are not following the scientific method. It is an obnoxious and persistent reaction that emotions or activities don't "count," unless they are particularized, and evaluated under a rubric of consequential ethics, whereby everything must somehow be evaluated through its length and quality metrics to determine if it was worth doing; this girds against virtue ethics, which means I could do something based on the intent. I have to remind myself, what I *must* do is not science, but survive.

176 Nitrogen fixation is a mechanism by which a microbe generates the large amounts of ATP needed to transform nitrogen found in the soil or atmosphere into nitrogen dioxide, ammonia, which a plant can then use to make nucleotides, its basic building blocks. This can be an example of symbiosis, or mutualism, between a microbe and plant with its roots in the ground. For example, a *Rhizobium* microbe can fix nitrogen for a legume plant which provides a niche in the soil with the precise oxygen content the microbe needs.

177 Berg P, Baltimore D, Boyer HW *et al.* Potential biohazards of recombinant DNA molecules. *Science* 1974; 185:303.

178 Signers of the letter included Paul Berg, David Baltimore, Herbert Boyer, Stanley Cohen, Ronald Davis, David Hogness, Daniel Nathans, Richard Roblin, James Watson, Sherman Weissman and Norton Zinder.

CHAPTER 3

179 Crichton M. *Jurassic Park*. Century Books. 1991.

180 In 2006, I went on a family trip to Poland to meet with our relatives in the Old World. I was 30, my father, 60, my grandmother, 90, and we all went, but I took a later, separate flight. My family had touched down in Krakow. I arrived at the airport late, missing my flight by mere moments. I told the flight desk that I was going to Poland, and took the next flight, but the attendant never told me that flight was heading to Warsaw, where I ended up, 183 miles away from Krakow. I called my father and said I was on Powisle Street at the correct meeting address, and he said, no, he was at the address and I wasn't there. Confused, we agreed to meet at the Sheraton. I called him again, protesting that I was in the lobby. Indeed, we were both at the Sheraton, but I was at Sheraton Warsaw and he was at Sheraton Krakow. I'd like to blame Lufthansa Airlines. But isn't that the stereotypical story of a family trip to Poland? It's also the perfect story to explain "off-target effects": incidentally hitting multiple sites in the genome that are precisely the same address, but which occur in different neighborhoods, regions or chromosomes.

181 "It is possible that a given 20 base, or bp (base pair), sequence occurs more than once in the genome but (this is) relatively rare. What do occur more frequently are closely related sites that differ at one or more positions within the 20 bp sequence. The more mismatches that one allows for, the higher number of sites one can find in the genome. For example, sites with 1 or 2 mismatches are still relatively infrequent but sites with 5 or 6 mismatches can occurs thousands or tens of thousands of times in the genome." Keith Joung, personal correspondence.

182 *Streptococcus pyogenes*, *Staphylococcus aureus* and *Streptococcus thermophiles* are among the microbes that contain the Crispr-Cas9 immune defense system. I asked George Church whether he thought nature might have targeted defense system tricks in store for us that are even more applicable for gene engineering. "Almost certainly yes," he told me.

183 Crispr-Cas9 can be designed to target virtually any 20-nucleotide sequence in the human genome, with one caveat: the target must end with a three-base sequence, a "protospacer adjuster motif," or PAM, in which any nucleotide is followed by two guanine DNA bases. Joung evolved Cas9 in the lab, using bacterial-based genetic selection systems to identify rare mutants. By doing so, they've been able to identify new systems that can target sequences that do not end with a traditional PAM, and that are less likely to induce an "off-target" effect.

184 Regaldo. Engineering the perfect baby.

185 Regaldo. Engineering the perfect baby.

186 Maxmen. The Genesis Engine.

187 Greely H. On Science, Crispr-Cas9, and Asilomar. Law and Biosciences Blog. *Stanford Law Rev.* April 4, 2015.

188 Baltimore D, Berg P, Botchan M *et al.* Biotechnology: A prudent path forward for genomic engineering and germline gene modification. *Science.* April 3, 2015;348(6230):36–38. doi: 10.1126/science.aab1028. Epub March 19 2015.

189 Regaldo. Engineering the perfect baby.

190 "Enhancement purposes" would be adding a non-medically necessary gene or gene edit that provides a boost for cognitive or athletic advantage, while "disease prevention purposes" would mean making an edit to a gene *in vitro*, post-fertilization and prior to implantation of a pregnancy to intervene on a genetic abnormality before a baby is actually born. Furthermore, "human embryonic cell lines (hESCs)" are cells that are derived from an embryo resulting in the destruction of the embryo for the sake of creation of a useful cell line of embryonic stem cells which can be used for research or therapeutic purposes since they can give rise to virtually any type of cell, while "human induced pluripotent cell lines" (hiPSCs) are the same type of general-purpose, highly useful cells, which can be engendered without the destruction of an embryo. The important distinction here is that some types of genetic engineering mentioned here give rise *to* living beings, and some are derived *from* living beings. Greely H. On Science, Crispr-Cas9, and Asilomar.

191 Between 1856 and 1863 the monk Gregor Mendel had cultivated and tested 29000 peaplants, demonstrating that traits were inherited independently. For instance, a trait for the roundness of a pea was inherited separately from a trait for the greenness of a pea. Moreover, some traits appeared to be "dominant," while some were "recessive." He showed when yellow and green peas were bred together, the result was always a

yellow pea, but in the next generation one third of the peas were again green. But, William Bateson and Reginald Punnett had been critical of Mendel's experiments and reported that certain traits were co-inherited, or "linked." Thomas Hunt Morgan then countered with an observation that these supposed linked traits were also, sometimes, inherited independently. How could this happen? Morgan suggested "cross-overs," in which a form of a gene, or allele, from one chromosome is swapped for a different version of the gene on its paired chromosome. In 1931, a budding young scientist named Barbara McClintock made use of a new invention, the electron microscope, and showed Morgan's cross-overs did indeed happen each time an embryonic, or germ, cell divides. These recombination events became known as "crossing over." McClintock suggested that a purpose of this mechanism of crossing over was to shuffle the deck, so that the same versions of genes did not remain clustered together on the same chromosome and become passed down together through the generations. In other words, it was a means for chromosomes to "unlink" versions of genes, and introduce a healthy mix of genetic variation in the code that would be passed forth. It happens by homologous recombination.

192 Bianconi E. An estimation of the number of cells in the human body. *Ann. Hum. Biol.* Nov–Dec 2013; 40(6):463–471.

193 "My mother is one of the last disciples of Gestalt psychology. I mean, Kohler is her God." Massachusetts Institute of Technology Oral History Program. *Recombinant DNA Controversy.*

194 Massachusetts Institute of Technology Oral History Program. *Recombinant DNA Controversy.*

195 Massachusetts Institute of Technology Oral History Program. *Recombinant DNA Controversy.*

196 I took a class with Philip I. Marcus in virology before he died. He taught into his 90s, wore a white lab coat even while lecturing and he was an old-school grader: he thought a C was a good grade. He taught virology as if it was a mystery novel unfolding, showing us shadows of icosahedra and how scientists used those shadows to deduce its shape, or regaling us with stories of tobacco mosaic virus, which assembles from several disparate molecules. He once read a prepared statement on the journalist Rebecca Skloot, excoriating her for not contacting him and reporting more in depth on the scientists' point of view for her book on HeLa cells. Then he passed out autographed copies of the journal *Emerging Infectious Diseases.* Why is any of this important? If we couldn't culture HeLa cells, or T-cells, or other types of human cells, we could

never engineer them. So, despite how out-of-the-blue genome engineering is, its technology really depends on a gradual pitch of science, figuring out how to culture cells in a laboratory, and other small advances.

197 Massachusetts Institute of Technology Oral History Program. *Recombinant DNA Controversy.*

198 "Detlev Bronk accepted me and it was only because some guy had dropped out to study cello." Massachusetts Institute of Technology Oral History Program. *Recombinant DNA Controversy.*

199 Massachusetts Institute of Technology Oral History Program. *Recombinant DNA Controversy.*

200 Massachusetts Institute of Technology Oral History Program. *Recombinant DNA Controversy.*

201 Massachusetts Institute of Technology Oral History Program. *Recombinant DNA Controversy.*

202 Massachusetts Institute of Technology Oral History Program. *Recombinant DNA Controversy.*

203 Massachusetts Institute of Technology Oral History Program. *Recombinant DNA Controversy.*

204 Berg and Mertz. Personal reflections.

205 Berg and Mertz. Personal reflections.

206 Mertz and Davis. Cleavage of DNA by R 1 restriction.

207 Massachusetts Institute of Technology Oral History Program. *Recombinant DNA Controversy.*

208 Berg and Mertz. Personal reflections.

209 Berg and Mertz. Personal reflections.

210 Berg and Mertz. Personal reflections.

211 "These molecules would not have replicated in *E. coli* because a gene in the plasmid cloning vector, the lambda *O* gene, had been disrupted by insertion of the SV40 sequences," said Janet Mertz. However, some of the molecules she created in June of 1972, using a far more efficient method, retained this gene in an intact form, meaning that genetically recombined molecules had been created that could have been spread through replication in *E coli.*

212 Arber W. Host-controlled modification of bacteriophage. *Annu. Rev. Microbiol.* 1965; 19:365–378.

213 Odelberg W (ed). *Les Prix Nobel: The Nobel Prizes 1978.* Nobel Foundation. 1979.

214 Kelly TJ Jr, Smith HO. A restriction enzyme from *Hemophilus influenzae. J. Mol. Biol.* July 28, 1970; 51(2):393–409.

215 Boyer's lab at University of California San Francisco did not publish their findings with EcoRI until late 1972, yet had already generously provided this enzyme to John Morrow and Janet Mertz, members of Berg's lab, in the summer of 1971 so they could perform their experiments with SV40. This was before a modern biotech apparatus would emerge whereby companies such as AddGene and New England Biolabs supply "reagents" and molecular recipes to anyone.

216 Massachusetts Institute of Technology Oral History Program. *Recombinant DNA Controversy.*

217 "Meselson and Yuan had purified a restriction enzyme which was completely different from the one the Japanese workers had reported on. It turned out to have such bizarre properties... these crazy co-factor requirements; they required S-adenosyl-L-methionine (which adds the methyl groups) and ATP (a molecular fuel) for activity. And once that clue was available we picked up this and proceeded to purify what is now called the *EcoB* restriction endonucleolytic activity." But it turns out that *EcoB* and *EcoK* restriction enzymes (the B and K refer to strains of *E. coli*) had "a number of properties about them which make them unsuitable for DNA manipulation. I later referred to these as Type I restriction enzymes." In fact, these types of restriction enzymes were complicated to use because they required these additional molecules, or co-factors, and did not cleave DNA at precise and reliable locations. "I guess it was about 1968, we went back and had a look at the literature. And the Japanese group had reported that their activity didn't require S-adenosyl-L-methionine and ATP. And that sort of bothered me. Bob Yoshimori, a postdoc, scoured a number of microbes and we found one that was different, and that's the *EcoRI* activity. Then it went fairly well after that."

218 Mertz and Davis. Cleavage of DNA by R 1 restriction endonuclease.

219 Berg P. *A Stanford Professor's Career in Biochemistry, Science Politics, and the Biotechnology Industry* (typescript of an oral history conducted in 1997 by Sally Smith Hughes). Regional Oral History Office, University of California. 2000.

220 Hedgpeth J, Goodman HM, Boyer HW. DNA nucleotide sequence restricted by the RI endonuclease. *Proc. Natl. Acad. Sci. USA.* November 1972; 69(11):3448–3452.

221 Morrow JF, Berg P, Kelly TJ Jr, Lewis AM Jr. Mapping of simian virus 40 early functions on the viral chromosome. *J. Virol.* September 1973; 12(3):653–658.

222 Mertz and Davis. Cleavage of DNA by R 1 restriction endonuclease.

223 Massachusetts Institute of Technology Oral History Program. *Recombinant DNA Controversy.*

224 Hedgpeth *et al.* DNA nucleotide sequence.

225 Boyer HW. *Recombinant DNA Research at UCSF and Commercial Application at Genentech.* Interviews Conducted by Sally Smith Hughes. The UCSF Oral History Program and the Program in the History of the Biological Sciences and Biotechnology. 1994. http://content.cdlib.org/ark:/13030/kt5d5nb0zs/.

226 Sgaramella V. Enzymatic oligomerization of bacteriophage P22 DNA and of linear Simian virus 40 DNA. *Proc. Natl. Acad. Sci. USA.* November 1972; 69(11):3389–3393.

227 Sgaramella showed that he could ligate together the ends of phage P22 DNA with a different DNA ligase, one encoded by the phage T4, as well as SV40 ends generated by cutting with EcoRI enzyme, but he was unable to make P22-SV40 recombinant DNAs by incubating them together with DNA ligase. The ends of phage P22 DNA were known to be blunt. Thus, Sgaramella had made the important discovery that blunt-ended DNAs can be joined together using T4 DNA ligase, albeit at much lower efficiency than can EcoRI-generated DNA ends. However, his failure to make recombinant DNAs simply indicated that the EcoRI-generated ends were *different* in some way from the P22 naturally blunt ends. In fact, they were cohesive. But, Mertz argues, his data didn't indicate how they were different. Mertz says, "My lab notebooks (available within the Berg archive held at Stanford) show that I already knew EcoRI-cleaved SV40 DNA was infectious in August 1971 suggesting the ends might be cohesive, before Sgaramella arrived at Stanford that fall. After learning about the Berg lab findings, Sgaramella obtained EcoRI-cut DNA from Morrow. P22 DNA from Lobban, and *E. coli* DNA ligase from Modrich. It is these DNAs that he used to show that he could not make P22-SV40 DNA recombinants. His findings only indicated the ends of the 2 DNAs were different. He never determined how they differed; nor did he make any recombinant DNAs. Davis and I proved the EcoRI-generated ends were cohesive, with Boyer's lab then sequencing them after learning this fact from me."

228 Cohen. DNA cloning.

229 Cohen. DNA cloning.

230 Cohen SN, Chang AC, Hsu L. Nonchromosomal antibiotic resistance in bacteria: Genetic transformation of *Escherichia coli* by R-factor DNA. *Proc. Natl. Acad. Sci. USA.* 1972; 69(8):2110–2114.doi:10.1073/pnas.69.8.2110.PMC426879.PMID4559594.

231 Cohen S, Chang A, Boyer H, Helling R. Construction of biologically func tional bacterial plasmids *in vitro*. *Proc. Natl. Acad. Sci. USA*. 1973; 70(11): 3240–3244.doi:10.1073/pnas.70.11.3240.PMC427208.PMID4594039.

232 Berg and Mertz. Personal reflections.

233 Cohen. DNA cloning.

234 Chang ACY, Cohen SN. Genome construction between bacterial species *in vitro*: Replication and expression of *Staphylococcus* plasmid genes in *Escherichia coli*. *Proc. Natl. Acad. Sci. USA*. 1974; 71(4):1030–1034.

235 Berg and Mertz. Personal reflections.

236 Massachusetts Institute of Technology Oral History Program. *Recombinant DNA Controversy*.

237 Morrow JF, Cohen SN, Chang AC, *et al*. Replication and transcription of eukaryotic DNA in *Escherichia coli*. *Proc. Natl. Acad. Sci. USA*. May 1974;71(5):1743–1747.

238 Cohen. DNA cloning.

239 Morrow *et al*. Replication and transcription.

240 Berg and Mertz. Personal reflections.

241 Fredrickson.*The Recombinant DNA Controversy*.

242 By another account, he said, "Well, now we can put together any DNAs we want to." Lear J. *Recombinant DNA: The Untold Story*. Crown Publishers. 1978.

243 Fredrickson. *The Recombinant DNA Controversy*.

244 Berg P. Meetings that changed the world: Asilomar 1975: DNA modification secured. *Nature*. 2008; 455(7211):290–291.

245 Berg *et al*. Potential biohazards. Also NAS ban on plasmid engineering. *Nature* 19 July 1974; **250**:175.

246 A prior conference had also been held at Asilomar in 1973, but focused on containment of genetically modified organisms in the context of biological warfare and biohazard. But, tensions around bio-warfare were already easing after Nixon unexpectedly called for an end to the Biological Weapons Program in 1969. In fact, this led to an international Biological Weapons Convention, which opened for signing in April 1972 and drew signatures from 22 states, the UK, US and Soviet Union, taking effect in March 1975.

247 It is easy to dismiss bio-warfare as a piece of science fiction drummed up by Michael Crighton or Richard Preston. In November 2015, a local source in Nineveh province said that ISIS had executed the head of the Department of Physics at the University of Mosul because of his refusal to develop biological weapons. The source said: "Militants belonging to

ISIS executed the president of the Department of Physics at the Faculty of Science in the University of Mosul," adding that, "The execution came on the back of his rejection to cooperate with the organization in the development of biological weapons, which ISIS is seeking to possess and use in the fighting against government forces." The source, who requested to remain anonymous, noted: "The execution took place in a public square in the center of Nineveh," pointing out that, "the organization has handed over the body to the forensic medicine department." Stanford ethicist Hank Greely explained the problem to me: Crispr-Cas9 can be used to edit virtually any gene with incredible precision and it can be used to alter microbes and turn them into highly infectious and pathogenic strains. And if Crispr becomes easy enough to use, then it's just a step away from building a weapon, since microbes can be found under any toilet seat. You may not be able to get enriched uranium, but you can get microbes and a Crispr-Cas9 kit.

248 Maxmen. The Genesis Engine.

249 Berg. Meetings that changed the world.

250 Fredrickson. *The Recombinant DNA Controversy.*

251 Fredrickson. *The Recombinant DNA Controversy.*

252 Fredrickson. *The Recombinant DNA Controversy.*

253 Berg. Meetings that changed the world.

254 Maxmen. The Genesis Engine.

255 Berg. Meetings that changed the world.

256 Fredrickson. *The Recombinant DNA Controversy.*

257 In 1916, Nocolae Paulescu used a pancreatic extract from a fish to treat his sick dog, but it's composition was unclear. Then, in 1921, J. J. R. Macleod and Frederick Banting isolated insulin from an actual dog, showing they could alter glucose levels in the animal with the insulin. The first successful clinical trial was conducted the following year. Eli Lilly & Co. went into mass production of insulin in 1923, and the drug caught on like wildfire, since it seemed to raise some sick children from their deathbeds. Eli's patent was soon transferred to the British Medical Research Council to prevent exploitation. In 1926, it was discovered that proteins could act as enzymes, catalyzing the body's metabolic processes. That same year, researchers figured out how to crystalize proteins, hardening them into a rigid form so that their structures could be studied. Insulin was so important that it became one of the first proteins to be crystalized in pure from. Proteins were found to be wildly complex, composed of crazy swirling ribbon-like strings of all sorts of amino acids.

258 Cohen. DNA cloning.

259 Mulligan RC, Howard BH, Berg P. Synthesis of rabbit β-globin in cultured monkey kidney cells following infection with a SV40 β-globin recombinant genome. *Nature.* 11 January 1979; 277:108–114. doi:10.1038/277108a0.

260 Berg and Mertz. Personal reflections.

CHAPTER 4

261 Mulligan RC. Development of gene transfer technology. *Hum. Gene Ther.* December 2014; 25:995–1002. doi: 10.1089/hum.2014.2543.

262 Mulligan. Development of gene transfer technology.

263 Mulligan. Development of gene transfer technology.

264 Matfield M. New vectors for gene therapy. *New Sci.* January 23, 1986: 32.

265 Kang EM, MalechHL. *Methods in Ezymology, 1st edn.* Volume 507, Gene transfer vectors for clinical application.

266 Matfield. New vectors for gene therapy.

267 Matfield. New vectors for gene therapy.

268 Friedberg. Master molecule, heal thyself.

269 Friedberg EC, Goldthwait DA. Endonuclease II of *E. coli. Cold Spring Harbor Symp. Quant. Biol.* 1969; 33:271–275.

270 Friedberg EC, Goldthwait DA. Endonuclease II of *E. coli.* I. Isolation and purification. *Proc. Natl. Acad. Sci. USA.* 1969; 62:934–940.

271 Friedberg EC, Hadi SM, Goldthwait DA. Endonuclease II of *E. coli.* II. Enzyme properties and studies on the degradation of alkylated and native deoxyribonucleic acid. *J. Biol. Chem.* 1969; 244:5879–5889.

272 Feaver WJ, Svejstrup JQ, Bardwell L *et al.* Dual roles of a multiprotein complex from *Saccharomyces cerevisiae* in transcription and DNA repair. *Cell.* 1993; 75:1379–1387.

273 Wang Z, Svejstrup JQ, Feaver WJ *et al.* Requirement for RNA polymerase II transcription factor b (TFIIH) during nucleotide excision repair in the yeast *Saccharomyces cerevisiae. Nature.* 1994; 368:74–76.

274 Bardwell AJ, Bardwell L, Iyer N *et al.* Yeast nucleotide excision repair proteins Rad2 and Rad4 interact with RNA polymerase II basal transcription factor b. *Mol. Cell. Biol.* 1994; 14:3569–3576.

275 Bardwell L, Bardwell AJ, Feaver WJ *et al.* Yeast Rad3 protein binds directly to both Ssl2 and Ssl1 proteins: implications for the structure

and function of transcription/repair Factor b. *Proc. Natl. Acad. Sci. USA*. 1994; 91:3926–3930.

276 Bardwell AJ, Bardwell L, Wang Z *et al*. Recent insights on DNA repair: the mechanism of damaged nucleotide excision in eukaryotes and its relationship to other cellular processes. *Ann. N.Y. Acad. Sci*. 1994; **726**:281–291.

277 Friedberg EC, Bardwell AJ, Bardwell L *et al*. Nucleotide excision repair in the yeast *Saccharomyces cerevisiae*: its relationship to specialized mitotic recombination and RNA polymerase II basal transcription. *Philos. Trans. R. Soc. Lond. B Biol. Sci*. 1995; 347:63–68.

278 Friedberg EC. Xeroderma pigmentosum, Cockayne syndrome, essential genes, helicases and DNA repair: what's the relationship? *Cell*. 1992; 71:887–889.

279 The 2015 Nobel Prize in Chemistry was awarded toTomas Lindahl, Paul Modrich and Aziz Sancar for their work on the molecular mechanisms of DNA repair processes.

280 Botchan M, Stringer J, Mitchison T, Sambrook J. Integration and excision of SV40 DNA from the chromosome of a transformed cell. *Cell*. 1980; 20:143–152.

281 Wilson JH, Berget PB, Pipas JM. Somatic cells efficiently join unrelated DNA segments end-to-end. *Mol. Cell Biol*. 1982; 2:1258–1269.

282 Winocour E, Keshet I. Indiscriminate recombination in simian virus 40-infected monkey cells. *Proc. Natl. Acad. Sci. USA*. 1980; 77:4861–4865.

283 Capecchi later explained the thrust of the mechanism in a 2008 interview. "The reason that somatic cells use homologous recombination is that every day each of your cells receives about 10,000 insults to its DNA. The insults arise from oxygen radicals produced in the cells, or from sunlight, or from everything else that's happening to your poor cells. Often, a DNA strand gets broken. When it breaks, you not only lose the gene at the breakage point, but upon cell division you lose all the genes that are no longer associated with a centromere. The first thing a cell wants to do is stick those two pieces of DNA back together so that, rather than losing a thousand genes, it just loses one gene. Once that is done, the damaged DNA at the junction is tagged and the cell can use the copy of the gene from the other homologous chromosome to repair it. For example, if the maternal copy is broken, then the paternal copy can be used to repair the damaged gene. Homologous recombination is the machinery that mediates this repair."

284 By gene swapping between paired chromosomes during meosis or "crossing over" when male and female germ cells first meet and fuse.

285 Mulligan. Development of gene transfer technology.

286 IL-2 alpha receptor is on chromosome 10 and IL-2 beta receptor is on chromosome 22. So what's so special about IL-2 gamma? Men have only one X chromosome, so if there is a defective copy of only one gene, they don't have a backup. While if there is a defective copy of the alpha or beta receptors, there is a second backup copy, since we all have two copies of each of the 22 "autosomal" chromosomes.

CHAPTER 5

287 Moreno. *The Body Politic.*

288 Hypertrophy is an enlarged cell, in this case giving rise to larger muscle. Ski is the name of a gene, the "v" in v-ski means it is a component of a virus, and in short, the "c" in c-ski means that it's a cancer-related, or oncogene, now incorporated into the cattle's genome.

289 Gordon JW. Genetic enhancement in humans. *Science* March 26, 1999; 283(5410):2023–2024. doi:10.1126/science.283.5410.2023.

290 Chen C. These superhumans are real and their DNA could be worth billions. *Bloomberg.* July 22, 2015.

291 Chen. These superhumans are real.

292 To be sure, beneficial mutations are rare. Mutations when randomly inserted, in vast cases, cause harm to complex systems. I suggest the exhilarating experiment: open the hood of your automobile and make a small random alteration to one of the systems, then drive. Did it improve or harm the function? (As an amateur auto mechanic, and an obstinate American male, I know the painful answer.) In one study on RNA viruses, it was shown that 39.6% of mutations were lethal, 31.2% were non-lethal but harmful and 27.1% were neutral, with a modest 2% of the changes being actually beneficial. It's why Stephen Jay Gould noted "a good bookkeeper wants an unimpeachable record." It's also why we obtain human diseases much more frequently than we evolve useful new biological properties.

293 How does this happen? Susumu Ohno was prescient when writing in *Evolution by Gene Duplication* in 1970 that "the creation of a new gene from a redundant copy of an old gene is the most important role that gene duplication played in evolution." Soon, the literature was loaded with instances of genes evolving from other genes. That includes crystallins, a group of proteins found in eye lenses that account for their transparency, which have similar sequences as antioxidants and heat

shock proteins, molecular chaperones that assist proteins in maintaining folding structures under stressful conditions. Evolution was taking a second superfluous copy of a gene, a "paralogue," and re-engineering it for a new purpose, a new concept in evolutionary biology called "exaptation." If adaptation was slow tinkering and development of a new gene, then exaptation was the repurposing of an existing gene, which could lead to fast evolution. Sometimes a gene can lose its old function, and take on a new function; and sometimes a gene can acquire mutations that enable it to add a second or third role, keeping the first.

294 The fourteenth century medieval philosopher William of Ockham was a nominalist, a thinker who believed that there are no universals, but rather that universals are just formed as categories of the mind. In fact, all that exists are particulates, he thought. Intriguingly, particle physics and the particulate nature of biology has made nominalism a dominant mode of science, albeit, now a special form of the classification, "trope nominalism."

295 Or, sometimes nothing at all. When scientists first saw that much of the genome was transcribed into RNA, but did not become protein, so called "non-coding RNA," the explanation was that it had minimal function, or more likely, that it had no function at all, existing as mere "junk DNA." Ask a scientist what an undescribed molecule does, and usually their first response is probably just one thing, or more likely, nothing at all. But a group called ENCODE later came to publish results suggesting that while only 2 percent of the genome is involved with the construction of proteins, hence official "genes," about 80 percent of it is biochemically functional.

296 Genes associated with pigmentation also include *SLC24A5, SLC45A2, TYR* and *HERC2/OCA2*.

297 Roman soldiers overpowered a Jewish resistance, and by 75 AD, the insurrection was in retrenchment. Having sustained severe casualties, the resistance was limited to a weakened existence outside the empire. The colonies resurged, but by 1000 AD, a population size that hourglassed back into the millions was now reduced back in size to 400 wandering families. Further expulsions during the Crusades pushed the Diaspora into Lithuania and Poland between 1100 and 1400 AD. Thus, we got the concept of the "wandering Jew"; an ethnic group whose populations peaked and plummeted. Imagine what it did to their genes.

298 A long stretch of DNA that is similar in many people in a subpopulation is called "extended haplotype homozygosity."

299 "Give me a fruitful error anytime, full of seeds, bursting with its own corrections. You can keep your sterile truth for yourself," wrote the Italian economist Vilfredo Pareto. Mutations aren't flaws that sometimes occur in a perfect system. Instead the whole system is a bundle of flaws, beat out over time. Simply put, we are the best of flaws. As Pareto foretold in his writing, errors that occur in systems are often the basis of innovation – indeed, spontaneous mutations, in effect, molecular typos, initiate the start of all evolutionary processes. Indeed, it's apt to be flukes in multiple genes such as the speech-related gene *FOXP2* that forged a separation of *Homo sapiens* from *erectus*. While *Homo sapiens* enjoyed an abrupt cultural expansion, burying symbolic artifacts with its dead and using intricate tools, the linguist Derek Bickerton noted *Homo erectus* "sat for 0.3 million years in the drafty, smoky caves of Zhoukoudian, cooking bats over smoldering embers and waiting for the cave to fill up with their own garbage." Flukes in ASPM, a brain size gene, arose 5800 years ago and were oddly correlated with the emergence of written language, arts and religion in the Axial Period – and certainly were promulgated through the mechanisms of selective sweep. The changes in brain expansion genes highlight the profound implication of evolution, and why it has such an unsettling effect – it is its insistence on oblivion, the very fact that history and meaning must be lost for growth and change to occur. Pareto had it right. Flukes and accidents made us human.

300 East EM. Studies on size inheritance in nicotiana. *Genetics*. January 6, 1916; 1:164–176.

301 Fosse R, Joseph J, Richardson K. A critical assessment of the equal-environment assumption of the twin method for schizophrenia. *Front. Psychiatry*. 2015; 6:62. doi:10.3389/fpsyt.2015.00062.

302 Tavernise S. US suicide rate surges to a 30-year high. *The New York Times* April 22, 2016.

303 Thompson *et al.* Genetics of the connectome.

304 Rope AF, Wang K, Evjenth R *et al.* Using VAAST to identify an X-linked disorder resulting in lethality in male infants due to N-terminal acetyl transferase deficiency. *Am. J. Hum. Genet.* July 15, 2011; 89(1):28–43.

305 Farrer LA, Cupples LA, Haines JL *et al.* Effects of age, sex, and ethnicity on the association between apolipoprotein E genotype and Alzheimer disease: A meta-analysis. *APOE* and Alzheimer Disease Meta Analysis Consortium. *JAMA*. 1997; 278:1349–1356.

306 Jahanshad N, Rajagopalan P, Thompson PM. Neuroimaging, nutrition, and iron-related genes. *Cell. Molec. Life Sci.* 2013; 70(23):4449–4461. doi: 10.1007/s00018-013-1369-2.

307 Yang J, Benyamin B, McEvoy BP *et al.* Common SNPs explain a large proportion of the heritability for human height. *Nat. Genet.* 2010; 42:565–569.

308 Thompson *et al.* Genetics of the connectome.

309 Carey B. Scientists move closer to understanding schizophrenia's cause. *The New York Times.* January 27, 2016.

310 Sekar A. Schizophrenia risk from complex variation of complement component 4. *Nature.* February 11, 2016; 530(7589):177–183. doi: 10.1038/nature16549.

311 As I previously wrote in *The Atlantic*, "RNA is tailored by seamstresses in our cells, leading to many species or 'isoforms' of RNA and protein. I like to think of these isoforms as tiny dresses. A single gene can be patterned to build many styles of a dress. And some RNA can regulate other RNA, tuning its expression 'up' or 'down,' deciding how many dresses are made. Furthermore, a series of 'epigenetic' molecules attaches to the structure of the genome and switches genes 'on' or 'off.' Thus, our genes are regulated by disparate forces, which decide when, which, and how many of these dresses are sewn in the cellular factory." Kozubek J. Why can't we prevent Alzheimer's? *The Atlantic.* January 30, 2016.

312 The scientists evaluated 28799 schizophrenia cases and 35986 controls from 22 countries to study the association of 7751 SNP markers across the MHC locus to predict the structure of *C4* structural alleles, and then used the versions or alleles to predict the expression.

313 Carey. Scientists move closer.

314 O'Rourke M. *Infectious Madness* by Harriet A. Washington. Book Review. *The New York Times.* December 31, 2015.

315 Huttlin EL, Ting L, Bruckner RJ *et al.* The BioPlex Network: A systematic exploration of the human interactome. *Cell.* July 16, 2015; 162(2):425–440. doi:10.1016/j.cell.2015.06.043.

316 Ashton CH. Anything for a quiet life? www.benzo.org.uk/afaql2.htm.

317 Shenk JW. The end of "genius." *The New York Times.* July 19, 2014.

318 Abraham A. Is there an inverted-U relationship between creativity and psychopathology? *Front. Psychol.* 2014; 5:750.

319 Kaufman JC (ed). *Creativity and Mental Illness.* Cambridge University Press. 2014.

320 Thompson *et al.* Genetics of the connectome.

321 Thompson *et al.* Genetics of the connectome.

322 Thompson *et al.* Genetics of the connectome.

323 Anticevic A, Van Snellenberg JX, Barch DM. Neurobiology of emotional dysfunction in schizophrenia: new directions revealed through meta-analyses. *BP*. 2012; 71:e23–e24. author reply e25.

324 Whitfield-Gabrieli S, Thermenos HW, Milanovic S *et al*. Hyperactivity and hyperconnectivity of the default network in schizophrenia and in first-degree relatives of persons with schizophrenia. *Proc. Natl. Acad. Sci. USA*. 2009; 106:1279–1284.

325 Thompson *et al*. Genetics of the connectome.

326 Zalocusky KA, Ramakrishnan C, Lerner TN *et al*. Nucleus accumbens D2R cells signal prior outcomes and control risky decision-making. *Nature*. 2016; 531(7596):642–646. doi:10.1038/nature17400.

327 Chiang MC, Barysheva M, Shattuck DW *et al*. Genetics of brain fiber architecture and intellectual performance. *J. Neurosci*. 2009; 29:2212–2224.

328 Kochunov P, Glahn DC, Lancaster JL *et al*. Genetics of microstructure of cerebral white matter using diffusion tensor imaging. *Neuroimage*. 2010; 53:1109–1116.

329 Thompson *et al*. Genetics of the connectome.

330 Egan MF, Kojima M, Callicott JH *et al*. The *BDNF* val66met polymorphism affects activity-dependent secretion of BDNF and human memory and hippocampal function. *Cell*. 2003; 112:257–269.

331 Chiang MC, Barysheva M, Toga AW *et al*. *BDNF* gene effects on brain circuitry replicated in 455 twins. *Neuroimage*. 2011; 55:448–454.

332 Braskie MN, Jahanshad N, Stein JL *et al*. Relationship of a variant in the *NTRK1* gene to white matter microstructure in young adults. *J. Neurosci*. 2012; 32:5964–5972.

333 Jahanshad N, Kohannim O, Hibar D *et al*. Brain structure in healthy adults is related to serum transferrin and the H63D polymorphism in the *HFE* gene. *Proc. Natl. Acad. Sci. USA*. 2012;109: E851–E859.

334 Matsumoto M, Weickert CS, Akil M *et al*. Catechol O-methyltransferase mRNA expression in human and rat brain: evidence for a role in cortical neuronal function. *Neuroscience*. 2003; 116:127–137.

335 Tunbridge EM, Harrison PJ, Weinberger DR. Catechol-o-methyltransferase, cognition, and psychosis: Val158Met and beyond. *BP*. 2006; 60:141–151.

336 Chen J, Lipska BK, Halim N *et al*. Functional analysis of genetic variation in catechol-O-methyltransferase (*COMT*): effects on mRNA, protein, and enzyme activity in postmortem human brain. *Am. J. Hum. Genet*. 2004; 75:807–821.

337 Liu B, Song M, Li J et al. Prefrontal-related functional connectivities within the default network are modulated by *COMT* val158met in healthy young adults. *J. Neurosci.* 2010; 30:64–69.

338 Dennis EL, Jahanshad N, Rudie JD et al. Altered structural brain connectivity in healthy carriers of the autism risk gene, CNTNAP2. *Brain Connect.* 2011; 1:447–459.

339 Kohannim O, Jahanshad N, Braskie MN et al. Predicting white matter integrity from multiple common genetic variants. *Neuropsychopharmacol.* 2012; 37(9):2012–2019.

340 Wray H. On the trail of the Orchid Child. *Sci. Am. Mind.* November 1, 2011.

341 Gottschall J. *The Storytelling Animal: How Stories Make Us Human.* Houghton Mifflin Harcourt. 2012.

342 One of the hardest lessons of my life was accepting that there are not huge variations in intelligence between people. Any penetrating insight or profound experience I've ever had that leads me to put something down in ink is not something that at least someone else could not experience, or comprehend or at least partially express. That's why things are so competitive. Darwin had it right. It really is only small variations in biology that distinguish us. As unique as any of us is, we are really not *that* different.

343 Mackinnon DW, Nielson G. (eds) The personality correlates of creativity: A study of American architects. Proceedings of the XIV International Congress of Applied Psychology. Volume 2, Personality Research. Munksgaard. 1962: 11–39.

344 Ernest Hemmingway wrote of the dead leopard at the top of the peak in the Snows of Kilimanjaro; it is a sense that intelligence is not something calculated and achieved, but something punishing and surpassing even itself.

345 Zizek S. *The Puppet and the Dwarf: The Perverse Core of Christianity.* The MIT Press. 2003.

346 Makari G. Notes from psychiatry's battle lines. *The New York Times.* February 23, 2016.

347 I owe the connection between Foucault and Sapolsky in this context, and its basic presentation here, to Daniel Lord Smail's fascinating 2009 book, *On Deep History and the Brain.*

348 Sapolsky RM. Stress and the brain: individual variability and the inverted-U. *Nat. Neurosci.* October 2015; 18(10):1344–1346. doi: 10.1038/nn.4109.

349 Cheng MY, Sun G, Jin M et al. Blocking glucocorticoid and enhancing estrogenic genomic signaling protects against cerebral ischemia. *J. Cereb. Blood Flow Metab.* 2009; 29(1):130–136.

350 Cheng MY, Lee IP, Jin M *et al.* An insult-inducible vector system activated by hypoxia and oxidative stress for neuronal gene therapy. *Transl Stroke Res.* 2011; 2(1):92–100.

351 Beck T. A vaccine for depression? *Nautilus.* December 17, 2015.

352 Beck. A vaccine for depression?

353 Sapolsky. Stress and the brain.

354 Benyamin B, Pourcain BS, Davis OS *et al.* Childhood intelligence is heritable, highly polygenic and associated with FNBP1L. *Mol Psychiatry.* February 2014; 19(2):253–258. doi: 10.1038/mp.2012.184.

355 Pinker S. Steven Pinker on new advances in behavioral genetics. *The Washington Post.* December 31, 2015.

356 Fitch WT, Hauser MD, Chomsky N. The evolution of the language faculty: clarifications and implications. *Cognition* 2005; 97(2):179–210.

357 Steven Pinker and Ray Jackendoff responded with an article in *Cognition* (March 2005; 95(2):201–236) entitled "The faculty of language: what's special about it?"

358 Pinker S, Jackendoff R. The nature of the language faculty and its implications for evolution of language. *Cognition* 2005; 97:211–225.

359 Gordon. Genetic enhancement in humans.

360 Specter M. The Gene Hackers: A powerful new technology enables us to manipulate our DNA more easily than ever before. *The New Yorker.* November 16, 2015.

361 Boeke JD, Church G, Hessel A *et al.* The Genome Project – Write. *Science.* June 2, 2016. doi:10.1126/science.aaf6850.

362 Pollack A. Scientists talk privately about creating a synthetic human genome. *The New York Times.* May 13, 2016.

363 Wang H, Isaacs F, Carr P *et al.* Programming cells by multiplex genome engineering and accelerated evolution. *Nature.* 2009; 460 (7257):894–898.

364 Bessen J. What does it mean for researchers, journalists and the public when secrecy surrounds science? theconversation.com May 24, 2016.

365 Gibson DG, Glass JI, Lartigue C *et al.* Creation of a bacterial cell controlled by a chemically synthesized genome. *Science.* May 20, 2010; 329:52–56. doi: 10.1126/science.1190719.

366 Hutchison CA 3rd, Chuang RY, Noskov VN *et al.* Design and synthesis of a minimal bacterial genome. *Science.* March 25, 2016; 351:1414. doi: 10.1126/science.aad6253.

367 A Canadian poet named Christian Bök created the Xenotext project, which included among its feats, an inscription of poetry into DNA of a harmless bacterium, *Deinococcus radiodurans*, which translates into a chain of peptides that spits back an answer. In Bök's words, "It's a very

short poem; a very masculine assertion about the aesthetic creation of life. The organism reads the poem, and writes in response a very melancholy, feminine – almost surreal – poem about the aesthetic of the loss of life. They're in dialogue with each other."

Bök coded a line into the DNA sequence of the bacteria that read: *Any style of life / is prim.*

The bacteria (which emits a red luminescence) always writes back in peptide code: *The faery is rosy / of glow.*

368 Endy D, Zoloth L. Should we synthesis a human genome? May 10, 2016. https://dspace.mit.edu/bitstream/handle/1721.1/102449/ShouldWe Genome.pdf?sequence=1.

CHAPTER 6

369 The Hinxton Group. *An International Consortium on Stem Cells, Ethics and Law.* Consensus Statement. February 24, 2006.

370 Havel uses the smokestack as a brilliant metaphor for contrasting the delineations of science and technology from the noumenon of raw nature. "To me, personally, the smokestack soiling the heavens is not just a regrettable lapse of a technology that failed to include 'the ecological factor' in its calculation, one which can be easily corrected with the appropriate filter. To me it is more, the symbol of an age which seeks to transcend the boundaries of the natural world and its norms and to make it into a merely private concern, a matter of subjective preference and private feeling, of the illusions, prejudices, and whims of a 'mere' individual. It is a symbol of an epoch which denies the binding importance of personal experience including the experience of mystery and of the absolute and displaces the personally experienced absolute as the measure of the world with a new, man-made absolute, devoid of mystery, free of the 'whims' of subjectivity and, as such, impersonal and inhuman. It is the absolute of so-called objectivity: the objective, rational cognition of the scientific model of the world. Modern science, constructing its universally valid image of the world, thus crashes through the bounds of the natural world, which it can understand only as a prison of prejudices from which we must break out into the light of objectively verified truth. The natural world appears to it as no more than an unfortunate leftover from our backward ancestors, a fantasy of their childish immaturity. With that, of course, it abolishes as mere Fiction even the innermost foundation of our natural world; it kills God

and takes his place on the vacant throne so that henceforth it would be science which would hold the order of being in its hand as its sole legitimate guardian and be the sole legitimate arbiter of all relevant truth. For, after all, it is only science that rises above all individual subjective truths and replaces them with a superior, suprasubjective, suprapersonal truth, which is truly objective and universal."

371 Doudna J. Genome-editing revolution: My whirlwind year with Crispr. *Nature.* December 24, 2015; 528(7583):469–471. doi: 10.1038/528469a.

372 Sherman Elias, a thoughtful man, died a year after I met him from autoimmune hepatitis.

373 Knight H. A metabolic master switch underlying human obesity. *MIT News.* August 19, 2015.

374 Cyranoski D. Scientists sound alarm over DNA editing of human embryos: Experts call for halt in research to work out safety and ethics issues. *Nature News.* March 12, 2015. doi: 10.1038/nature.2015.17110.

375 Cyranoski. Scientists sound alarm.

376 Lander ES. Brave new genome. *N. Engl. J. Med.* July 2, 2015; 373:5–8. doi: 10.1056/NEJMp1506446.

CHAPTER 8

377 Liu X, Jiang S, Fang C *et al.* Affinity-tuned ErbB2 or EGFR chimeric antigen receptor T cells exhibit an increased therapeutic index against tumors in mice. *Cancer Res.* September 1, 2015; 75:3596. doi: 10.1158/0008-5472.CAN-15-0159.

378 Grady D. An immune system trained to kill cancer. *The New York Times.* September 12, 2011: D1.

379 Ehrlich's work specifically focused on an antiserum for diphtheria, and was only later extrapolated to a broad therapeutic potential.

380 Epitopes are structural properties on the surface of antibodies which are not only due to the composition of the antibody, but additional molecules added in a process called glycosylation. Titers refer to the load of antibodies in the circulatory system, particularly the blood circulation.

381 Edelman G. *Second Nature: Brain Science and Human Knowledge.* Yale University Press. 2006.

382 The differences in antibody or receptor epitopes relate to their specificity and affinity for antigens, notably variable (V) and diverse (D) regions, while categories or classes of antibodies, or immunoglobulins, specify they be dispatched for general roles. "Class switching" is a mechanism

by which the constant (C) region portion of the antibody heavy chain is swapped out, while the variable region (V) stays the same. Antibodies come in classes (IgA, IgD, IgE, IgG, IgM) and can switch classes to better tune to allergen, pollen or specific pathogenic elements.

383 In the winter of 1944, Barbara McClintock was investigating self-pollinating corn plants, which were inbred and recessive due to their self-pollinating abilities. The corn she was experimenting with had unusual color patterns and blotches on its leaves, and she began to believe chromosomal regions in the corn had undergone a loss of genetic material, while other regions had picked up parts of chromosomes. What she then found was more than strange. Some genes appeared to be "hopping." Her experiments would question the orthodoxy that genes were absolutely fixed in their address on a chromosome. These regions of hopping code would later be given a host of names, such as "transposable elements," "transposons," "mobile elements" or "jumping genes."

384 Oettinger MA, Schwatz DG, Gorka C, Baltimore D. RAG1 and RAG2, adjacent genes that synergistically activate V(D)J recombination. *Science.* 1990; 248:1517–1523.

385 The homology between RAG and transposase suggests evolution generated a highly adaptive immune system from chaotic elements that perpetrated havoc upon it, by random error.

386 In fact, the concept was established two years prior. Kuwana Y, Asakura Y, Utsunomiya N *et al.* Expression of chimeric receptor composed of immunoglobulin-derived V regions and T-cell receptor-derived C regions. *Biochem. Biophys. Res. Commun.* December 31, 1987;149 (3):960–968.

387 Walker RE, Bechtel CM, Natarajan V *et al.* Long-term in vivo survival of receptor-modified syngeneic T cells in patients with human immuno deficiency virus infection. *Blood.* July 15, 2000; 96(2):467–474.

388 Mitsuyasu RT. Prolonged survival and tissue trafficking following adoptive transfer of CD4zeta gene-modified autologous CD4(+) and CD8(+) T cells in human immunodeficiency virus-infected subjects. *Blood.* August 1, 2000; 96(3):785–793.

389 Kim YJ, Mantel PL, June CH, Kim SH, Kwon BS. 4-1BB costimulation promotes human T cell adhesion to fibronectin. *Cell Immunol.* February 25, 1999;192(1):13–23.

390 Grady. An immune system trained to kill cancer.

391 A second patient also had a complete response by October 2010.

392 Avery Walker of Redmond, Oregon and Madison Gorman of Maryland subsequently relapsed and died. Emily Whitehead lives and is cancer

free at time of this writing. The technology is not a silver bullet, and there have been let downs and deaths, but 90 percent of patients with one form of acute lymphoid leukemia are in complete remission.

393 Liu *et al.* Affinity-tuned ErbB2 or EGFR.

394 Begley and Ellis. Drug development.

395 Tomlinson I. How many mutations in a cancer? *Am. J. Pathol.* March 2002; 160(3):755–758. doi: 10.1016/S0002-9440(10)64896-1.

396 Knudson A. Mutation and cancer: statistical study of retinoblastoma. *Proc. Natl. Acad. Sci. USA.* 1971; 68(4):820–823.

397 Cancer stem cells: The root of all evil? *The Economist.* September 11, 2008.

398 Apple S. An old idea revived: Starve cancer to death. *The New York Times.* May 12, 2016.

399 Apple. An old idea revived.

400 Apple. An old idea revived.

401 Flavahan WA, Drier Y, Liau BB *et al.* Insulator dysfunction and oncogene activation in IDH mutant gliomas. *Nature.* January 7, 2016; 529:10–114. doi: 10.1038/nature16490.

402 Kolata G. Scientists discover reason brain tumors grow fast. *The New York Times.* December 24, 2015.

403 Apple. An old idea revived.

404 Wilson J. Oxidants, antioxidants and the current incurability of metastatic cancers. *Open Biol.* January 8, 2013; 3(1):120144. doi: 10.1098/rsob.120144.

405 Breivikmay J. Obama's pointless cancer "moonshot." *The New York Times.* May 27, 2016.

406 Gromeier M, Lachmann S, Rosenfeld MR, Gutin PH, Wimmer E. Intergeneric poliovirus recombinants for the treatment of malignant glioma. *Proc. Natl. Acad. Sci. USA.* 2000; 97:6803–6808.

407 Merrill MK, Bernhardt G, Sampson JH *et al.* Poliovirus receptor CD155-targeted oncolysis of glioma. *Neuro-oncol.* 2004; 6:208–217.

408 Dobrikova EY, Broadt T, Poiley-Nelson J *et al.* Recombinant oncolytic poliovirus eliminates glioma in vivo without genetic adaptation to a pathogenic phenotype. *Mol Ther.* 2008; 16:1865–1872.

409 Pelley S. Transcript from "Breakthrough Status" which aired on May 15, 2016 on CBS News. Denise Schrier Cetta and Michael Radutzky producers.

410 Pelley. Transcript from "Breakthrough Status."

CHAPTER 9

411 Pollack A. A biotech evangelist seeks a Zika dividend. *The New York Times Magazine*. March 5, 2016.

412 Most of this interview previously appears in: Kozubek J. An ON/OFF switch for genes. *Sci. Am.* 2016; 314:52–57. doi: 10.1038/scientificamerican0116-52.

413 The immune system is designed to mobilize based on the flagging of foreign molecules, or "non-self" antigens, on microbes or viruses that do not have a hall pass to be circulating in the body. Just how does it pick up on the train of cancer cells, which carry "self" badges? In the 1960s, a non-conformist French scientist named Polly Matzinger suggested the immune system could not only target "non-self" markers on foreign microbes and viruses, but also "self" markers on its own cells. Matzinger called it the "danger signal" and she suggested the immune system could be turned on its own proteins or cells, in fact, when they became damaged, such as in the case of cancer. She helped groundwork for a new understanding of the immune system, one in which the powerful wrath of the immune system could be targeted inward to its own self antigen-like molecular patterns, a "damage-associated molecular pattern" or DAMP. At the time, everyone knew the immune system could sometimes go haywire and mistakenly attack its own cells, cases of auto-immune disorders. But Matzinger threw a monkey wrench into the field of immunology by suggesting a mechanism by which the immune system could turn on its own forces that was not only accidental, but sometimes ominous and purposeful. If this was valid, it meant doctors might leverage the body's own immunity to fight diseases. It turns out that cancer cells present DAMPs which trigger first-responder dendritic cells to mature, which stimulates CD8+ "killer" T-cells to send out a suite of cytokines such as interferon gamma, and granulocytes, to fight the body's pathogenic cancer cells. In the years since, it has been discovered that sickly human cells shed MHC type I molecules, the badges that all cells must carry to freely circulate in the human body, leading them to be destroyed by roving natural killer cells.

414 When I was a student in genetics at UConn, James Cole, my teacher in structural biology, told us how there had initially been great controversy over the structure of the hammerhead ribozyme, but in 2006 a complete "crystallized" structure of the molecule was obtained. I was happy to hear everything had been solved and there was nothing more to worry about. Then, the first question on the final exam: draw the hammerhead ribozyme freehand with a pencil. So, just how does it

cut itself? Electron bonds hold elements together, and they can be exchanged or broken as they jump to engage with other passerby protons. This accounts for a nucleophilic attack, a reorganization or break in electron bonds.

415 Qi LS, Larson MH, Gilbert LA *et al.* Repurposing Crispr as an RNA-guided platform for sequence-specific control of gene expression. *Cell*.2013; 152:1173–1183. doi: 10.1016/j.cell.2013.02.022.

416 Zhao Y, Dai Z, Liang Y *et al.* Sequence-specific inhibition of microRNA via Crispr/Crispri system. *Sci. Rep.* 2014; 4:3943. doi: 10.1038/srep03943.

417 Gilbert LA, Larson MH, Morsut L *et al.* Crispr-mediated modular RNA-guided regulation of transcription in eukaryotes. *Cell.* 2013; 154:442–451. doi: 10.1016/j.cell.2013.06.044.

418 Bikard D, Jiang W, Samai P *et al.* Programmable repression and activation of bacterial gene expression using an engineered Crispr-Cas system. *Nucleic Acids Res.* 2013; 41:7429–7437. doi: 10.1093/nar/gkt520.

419 The new frontier of genome engineering with Crispr-Cas9 Science. 2014 Nov 28;346(6213):1258096. Doi: 10.1126/science. 1258096d

420 Pollack. A biotech evangelist.

421 Kozubek J. FDA decision will lead to first ever genetically-modified animal for consumption. *TPM Idea Lab.* October 10, 2011.

422 Pollack A. New weapon to fight Zika: The mosquito. *The New York Times.* January 30, 2016.

423 Pollack. A biotech evangelist.

CHAPTER 10

424 Begley S. Meet one of the world's most groundbreaking scientists. He's 34. *STAT.* November 6, 2015.

425 Begley. Meet one of the world's most groundbreaking scientists.

426 Specter. The gene hackers.

427 Although it's hard to believe, there is no light inside your head. As the philosopher Daniel Dennett once quipped, "It's pitch black inside your skull and besides, you haven't any eyes in there to see colors with."

428 Begley. Meet one of the world's most groundbreaking scientists.

429 Begley. Meet one of the world's most groundbreaking scientists.

430 Baker M. Gene-editing nucleases. *Nat. Meth.*2012; 9:23–26.

431 Specter. The gene hackers.

432 "Trained as a chemist, I liked the idea of changing the restriction enzymes' ability to recognize new sequences, especially long sequences

in order to cut at specific genes within cells. Most scientists were focusing on the best-known Type II class of enzymes, which recognize and cleave DNA at the same site. Our lab decided to look into another type of enzyme, the Type IIS class, in which the recognition and cleavage sites are separated by a few base pairs. In my new lab, I flipped through the New England Biolabs catalog and found only two, GsuI and FokI. I chose to work on FokI because it was a better characterized enzyme." He used a digestive enzyme called trypsin to break the FokI restriction enzyme into two parts. Srinivasan Chandrasegaran, personal correspondence.

433 In 1981, two Japanese scientists, Sugisaki Hiroyuki and Kanazawa Susumu, first isolated FokI from the microbe.

434 Baker. Gene-editing nucleases.

435 Baker. Gene-editing nucleases.

436 Smithies O, Gregg RG, Boggs SS, Koralewski MA, Kucherlapati RS. Insertion of DNA sequences into the human chromosomal beta-globin locus by homologous recombination. *Nature*. September 19, 1985; 317 (6034):230–234.

437 Jasin M, de Villiers J, Weber F, Schaffner W. High frequency of homologous recombination in mammalian cells. *Cell*. December 1985; 43:695–703.

438 Jasin M, Berg P. Homologous integration in mammalian cells without target gene selection. *Genes Dev*. November 1988; 2(11):1353–1363.

439 Rouet P, Smih F, Jasin M. Introduction of double-strand breaks into the genome of mouse cells by expression of a rare-cutting endonuclease. *Mol. Cell Biol*. December 1994; 14(12):8096–8106.

440 In the words of journalist Helen Pearson: "The problem is that to cover all the possible combinations of key amino acids in a three-finger protein you would have to make 8×10^{24} different proteins. By the end of his postdoc his (Joung's) library-building and selection method worked – but only for finding a single finger, not a set." Pearson H. Protein engineering: The fate of fingers. *Nature*. September 10, 2008; 455:160–164. doi: 10.1038/455160a.

441 Pearson. Protein engineering.

442 Pearson. Protein engineering.

443 Chandrasegaran S, Smith J. Chimeric restriction enzymes: what is next? *Biol. Chem*. 1999; 380:841–848.

444 Baker. Gene-editing nucleases.

445 Pearson. Protein engineering.

446 Chandrasegaran and Smith. Chimeric restriction enzymes.

447 Chandrasegaran and Smith. Chimeric restriction enzymes.

448 Again, I summon the words of Helen Pearson: "He made use of a battery of small libraries, or 'pools', that each contain 100 proteins selected to bind a target sequence. One pool, for example, is full of protein domains that bind well to the sequence GAA, but only when they are the first finger in a three-finger protein. Another pool contains domains that bind to GAA when they are the second finger, and so on. To create a three-finger protein that binds at a specific sequence, three pools are combined and subjected to a second round of selection, from which the best-binding proteins are pulled out." Pearson. Protein engineering.

449 Pearson. Protein engineering.

450 Frank White and postdoc Bing Yang at Kansas State University showed the injected proteins, or TAL effectors, bound to DNA. In 2007, Ulla Bonas and Thomas Lahaye at Martin Luther University deduced the promoter regions of plant genes where TAL effectors were binding.

451 Baker. Gene-editing nucleases.

452 With Sebastian Schomack and Ulla Bonas at Martin Luther University, Bogdanove and Boch published papers showing how TALEs recognize specific regions of DNA in an issue of *Science* in 2009.

453 Eugene V. Koonin at the National Center for Biotechnology Information along with Feng Zhang of MIT in the spring of 2016 reported there are forms of Crispr which can also target RNA, suggesting the mechanisms in the microbial world have a lot of variation. Abudayyeh OO, Gootenberg JS, Konermann S *et al*. C2c2 is a single-component programmable RNA-guided RNA-targeting CRISPR effector. *Science*. June 2, 2016. doi: 10.1126/science.aaf5573.

454 Northwestern University in September 2008 (Erik Sontheimer and Luciano Marraffini, 61/099,317)

455 Specter. The gene hackers.

456 Specter. The gene hackers.

457 Specter. The gene hackers.

458 Schwank G, Koo BK, Sasselli V *et al*. Functional repair of CFTR by Crispr/Cas9 in intestinal stem cell organoids of cystic fibrosis patients. *Cell Stem Cell*. 2013; 13:653–658. doi: 10.1016/j.stem.2013.11.002.

459 The authors also identify transcription factors that likely bind to that enhancer, suggesting that "the transcriptional deregulation of SNCA is associated with sequence-dependent binding of the brain-specific transcription factors EMX2 and NKX6-1." Soldner F, Stelzer Y, Shivalila CS *et al*. Parkinson-associated risk variant in distal enhancer of α-synuclein

modulates target gene expression. *Nature.* May 5, 2016; 533 (7601):95–99. doi: 10.1038/nature17939.

460 Specter. The gene hackers.

461 UC Berkeley in May 2012 (Jennifer Doudna and others, 61/652,086).

462 Vilnius University in March 2012 (Virginijus Siksnys and others, 61/613,373).

463 Sherkow. The Crispr patent interference showdown is on.

464 USPTO granted Patent No. 8,697,359 to Broad Institute, MIT and Dr. Feng Zhang.

465 "The applications filed in 2012 by the Vilnius (Siksnys') team and the Berkeley (Doudna's) team each showed only that purified Cas9 protein and a certain purified RNA could cut a short piece of DNA in a solution in a test tube. In both cases, the applications in 2012 contained no cells, no genomes, and no editing," according to Broad Institute communication officer Lee McGuire. Crispr itself cannot be patented, he noted. Any patents issued to the Broad, refer to "engineered components and compositions specifically altered from their naturally-occurring form to be useful in methods for editing the genomes of living mammalian cells."

466 Sherkow. The Crispr patent interference showdown is on.

467 Crispr tracer guide molecules are 20 nucleotides in length and can usually tolerate one or two mismatches, and still bind to a target, or an unintended target that is similar in sequence. Technically, the reason for a reduction in off-target effects when the molecule was trimmed down to 17 bases, is that the interaction energy is lowered due to the shorter sequence, and the strength of binding of Crispr to the DNA is weaker; if the target wasn't exact (as is the case at off-target sites), it would be less likely to bind.

468 GUIDE-Seq is one of several assays developed for testing off-target effects of Crispr systems. Feng Zhang developed a tool called BLESS, and there are others: Digenome-Seq, IDLV Capture, HTGTS. What commonly happens, and what had not yet been done, is that someone in science will write a methods paper that benchmarks several comparable tools against each other, revealing which is the preferred technology, and drawing on comparative analysis to reduce false positives, providing a more accurate picture of the effects that are really happening in the biology. As with all research agendas in science, thinking outpaced the time and energy, and resources, to accomplish all that needs to be done.

469 Sp for the *Streptococcus pyogenes* bacteria, which is the source of this widely used Cas9, and HF for high-fidelity.

470 Kleinstiver BP, Pattanayak V, Prew MS *et al.* High-fidelity Crispr–Cas9 nucleases with no detectable genome-wide off-target effects. *Nature.* 2016; 529(7587):490–495. doi: 10.1038/nature16526.

471 Zetsche B, Gootenberg J, Abudayyeh O *et al.* Cpf1 is a single RNA-guided endonuclease of a Class 2 CRISPR-Cas system. *Cell.* September 25, 2015; 163(3):759–771. doi: 10.1016/j.cell.2015.09.038.

472 Yamano T, Nishimasu H, Zetsche B *et al.* Crystal structure of Cpf1 in complex with guide RNA and target DNA. *Cell.* 2016; 165(4):949–962. doi: 10.1016/j.cell.2016.04.003.

473 Mandal PK, Ferreira LM, Collins R *et al.* Efficient ablation of genes in human hematopoietic stem and effector cells using CRISPR/Cas9. *Cell Stem Cell.* November 6, 2014; 15(5):643–652. doi: 10.1016/j.stem.2014.10.004.

474 Maxmen. The Genesis Engine.

475 Sherkow. The Crispr patent interference showdown is on.

476 One count of interference was contended on, "A method, in a eukaryotic cell, of cleaving or editing a target DNA molecule or modulating transcription of at least one gene encoded thereon, the method comprising: contacting, in a eukaryotic cell, a target DNA molecule having a target sequence with an engineered and/or non-naturally-occurring Type II Clustered Regularly Interspaced Short Palindromic Repeats (Crispr)-Crispr associated (Cas) (Crispr-Cas) system comprising: a) a DNA-targeting RNA comprising i) a targeter-RNA or guide sequence that hybridizes with the target sequence, and ii) an activator-RNA or tracr sequence that hybridizes with the targeter-RNA to form a double-stranded RNA duplex of a protein-binding segment, and b) a Cas9 protein, wherein the DNA-targeting RNA forms a complex with the Cas9 protein, thereby targeting the Cas9 protein to the target DNA molecule, whereby said target DNA molecule is cleaved or edited or transcription of at least one gene encoded by the target DNA molecule is modulated."

477 Sherkow. The Crispr patent interference showdown is on.

CHAPTER 11

478 Skerrett. Experts debate.

479 The mammoth is more closely related to the Asian elephant, than the Asian is to the African elephant. The Asian elephant could therefore act as a probable surrogate.

480 Askew C. *Tmc* gene therapy restores auditory function in deaf mice. *Sci. Transl. Med.* July 8, 2015; 7(295): 295ra108. doi: 10.1126/scitranslmed.aab1996.

481 Skerrett. Experts debate

482 Chuong E, Elde N, Feschotte C. Regulatory evolution of innate immunity through co-option of endogenous retroviruses. *Science* March 4, 2016; 351(6277):1083–1087. doi: 10.1126/science.aad5497.

483 Those retrovirus in pigs are called PERV. And as Church notes, any applause should be direct to Luhan Yang. Church wrote me this chastening email: "Despite the generally nice relationships I have with journalists, it is very rare for them to include even one from the following list (that I routinely bring to them): Martin Jinek (postdoc then) was first author with Jennifer (Doudna) on her 2012 and 2013 papers and on a key patent application. Ann Ran (MCB student) and Le Cong (a BBS student in my lab and Feng's) were co-first authors on one of the 3-Jan-2013 papers. Prashant Mali (postdoc) and Luhan Yang (BBS student) were co-first authors on the other 3-Jan-2013 paper and co-inventors on our unchallenged patent # 9,023,649 on 'RNA-guided human genome engineering'. This is also true for the PERV story, for which Luhan was a very deserving first author."

484 Zimmer C. Editing of pig DNA may lead to more organs for people. *The New York Times*. October 15, 2015.

485 Martel Y. We ate the children last. *The Guardian*. July 16, 2004.

486 Scranton R. We're doomed. Now what? The Stone. *The New York Times*. December 21, 2015.

487 Greely. On science, Crispr-Cas9, and Asilomar.

488 Ainsworth C. Agriculture: A new breed of edits. *Nature*. December 3, 2015; 528:S15–S16. doi: 10.1038/528S15a.

489 Smidler AL, Terenzi O, Soichot J, Levashina EA, Marois E. Targeted mutagenesis in the malaria mosquito using TALE nucleases. *PLoS ONE*. 2013; 8:e74511.

490 Kistler KE, Vosshall LB, Matthews BJ. Genome engineering with CRISPR-Cas9 in the mosquito *Aedes aegypti. Cell Rep.* 2015; 11:51–60.

491 Windbichler N, Menichelli M, Papathanos PA *et al.* A synthetic homing endonuclease-based gene drive system in the human malaria mosquito. *Nature.* 2011; 473:212–215.

492 Gantz VM, Bier E. Genome editing. The mutagenic chain reaction: a method for converting heterozygous to homozygous mutations. *Science*. 2015; 348:442–444.

493 Ainsworth. Agriculture.

494 Esvelt K, Church G, Lunshof J. "Gene drives" and Crispr could revolutionize ecosystem management. *Scientific American*. July 17, 2014.

495 Balazs AB, Chen J, Hong CM *et al.* Antibody-based protection against HIV infection by vectored immunoprophylaxis. *Nature.* November 30, 2011; 481(7379):81–84. doi: 10.1038/nature10660.

496 Greely. On science, Crispr-Cas9, and Asilomar.

497 Ainsworth. Agriculture.

498 Montenegro M. Crispr is coming to agriculture – with big implications for food, farmers, consumers and nature. *Ensia.* January 28, 2016.

499 Doudna. Genome-editing revolution.

500 Xie K, Yang Y. RNA-guided genome editing in plants using a Crispr-Cas system. *Mol. Plant.* 2013; 6:1975–1983. doi: 10.1093/mp/sst119.

501 Jiang W, Zhou H, Bi H *et al.* Demonstration of Crispr/Cas9/sgRNA-mediated targeted gene modification in *Arabidopsis*, tobacco, sorghum and rice. *Nucleic Acids Res.* 2013; 41:e188. doi: 10.1093/nar/gkt780.

502 Upadhyay SK, Kumar J, Alok A, Tuli R. RNA-guided genome editing for target gene mutations in wheat. *G3.* 2013; 3:2233–2238. doi: 10.1534/g3.113.008847.

503 Sugano SS, Shirakawa M, Takagi J *et al.* Crispr/Cas9-mediated targeted mutagenesis in the liverwort *Marchantia polymorpha* L. *Plant Cell Physiol.* 2014; 55:475–481. doi: 10.1093/pcp/pcu014.

504 Jia H, Wang N. Targeted genome editing of sweet orange using Cas9/sgRNA. *PLoS ONE.* 2014; 9:e93806. doi: 10.1371/journal.pone.0093806.

505 Flowers GP, Timberlake AT, McLean KC, Monaghan JR, Crews CM. Highly efficient targeted mutagenesis in axolotl using Cas9 RNA-guided nuclease. *Development.* 2014; 141:2165–2171. doi: 10.1242/dev.105072.

506 Blitz IL, Biesinger J, Xie X, Cho KWY. Biallelic genome modification in F0 *Xenopus tropicalis* embryos using the Crispr/Cas system. *Genesis.* 2013; 51:827–834. doi: 10.1002/dvg.22719.

507 Nakayama T, Fish MB, Fisher M *et al.* Simple and efficient Crispr/Cas9-mediated targeted mutagenesis in *Xenopus tropicalis. Genesis.* 2013; 51:835–843. doi: 10.1002/dvg.22720.

508 Montenegro. Crispr is coming to agriculture.

509 Ainsworth. Agriculture.

510 Montenegro. Crispr is coming to agriculture.

511 Kolata G. A proposal to modify plants gives G.M.O. debate new life. *The New York Times.* May 28, 2015.

512 Montenegro. Crispr is coming to agriculture.

513 Montenegro. Crispr is coming to agriculture.

514 Ye X, Al-Babili S, Klöti A *et al.* Engineering the provitamin A (beta-carotene) biosynthetic pathway into (carotenoid-free) rice endosperm. *Science.* 2000; 287(5451): 303–305. doi: 10.1126/science.287.5451.303.

515 Paine JA, Shipton CA, Chaggar S *et al*. Improving the nutritional value of Golden Rice through increased pro-vitamin A content. *Nat. Biotech.* 2000; 23(4):482–487. doi: 10.1038/nbt1082.

516 Cyranoski D. CRISPR tweak may help gene-edited crops bypass biosafety regulation. Technique deletes plant genes without adding foreign DNA. *Nature News*. October 19, 2015. doi: 10.1038/nature.2015.18590

517 Harmon A. Open season is seen in gene editing of animals. *The New York Times*. November 26, 2015.

518 Harmon. Open season is seen.

519 Ainsworth. Agriculture.

520 Harmon. Open season is seen.

521 Kazmin A. Monsanto's India spat inflames corporate fears. *Financial Times*. March 13, 2016.

522 http://w2.vatican.va/content/francesco/en/encyclicals/documents/papa-francesco_20150524_enciclica-laudato-si.html.

523 Doudna. Genome-editing revolution.

524 Regaldo. Engineering the perfect baby.

525 Specter. The gene hackers.

CHAPTER 12

526 Skerrett. Experts debate.

527 Hellmann M. Researchers hope "super bananas" will combat vitamin A deficiency. *Time*. June 16, 2014.

528 No one guarantees us positive rights. US Senator from New Jersey Cory Booker made the subtle distinction between "acceptance" and "tolerance." Acceptance is a full embrace and support of our neighbors in our immediate community. Tolerance is the mere fact that we don't infringe upon the rights of our neighbors, but if they get killed in a car accident, we don't particularly care. In most cases, tolerance is the most that the law can provide, or insist upon, so-called negative rights, we don't take anything away from anyone, but the law can never insist we embrace each other.

529 Kac created a series of evocative works, among my favorite, the creation of a transgenic rabbit that glows a bright fluorescent green in the dark, GFP Bunny (2000)

530 Normative ethics is most often traced to the "operational" philosophy of Thomas Hobbes or Ludwig Wittgenstein, but is also evident in the oft repeated rap lyrics, "No justice, just us," which is basically to say that

engagement in the moral sphere requires negotiated agreement, or at least, protection of liberties by proxy, or grace. But, as always, when I have a question of how to approach a problem, I turn to doyen of twenty-first-century biology, Stephen Jay Gould, who, in his magnanimous tome *The Structure of Evolutionary Theory*, set us right. "I have always preferred, as guides to human action, messy hypothetical imperatives like the Golden Rule, based on negotiation, compromise and general respect, to the Kantian categorical imperatives of absolute righteousness, in whose name we so often murder and maim until we decide that we had followed the wrong instantiation of the right generality."

531 Regalado. Engineering the perfect baby.

532 Regalado. Engineering the perfect baby.

533 Taylor-Weiner H, Zivin JG. Medicine's Wild West: Unlicensed stem-cell clinics in the United States. *N. Engl. J. Med.* 2015; 373:985–987. doi: 10.1056/NEJMp1504560.

534 One thinks of the ending to the 1999 film *Man on the Moon*, which featured the comedian Andy Kaufman's desperate pursuit of a snake oil salesman in a failed attempt to cure his fatal disease.

535 Greely. On science, Crispr-Cas9, and Asilomar.

536 Greely. On science, Crispr-Cas9, and Asilomar.

537 Frodeman R, Briggle A. When philosophy lost its way. The Stone. *The New York Times.* January 11, 2016.

538 FFDCA §§ 201(g), (h), 21 USC 321(g), (h)

539 FDA Draft Guidance (June 2011).

540 *See* definitions at 21 CFR §§ 312.3(b), 812.3(p)

541 Kaiser J. CRISPR helps heal mice with muscular dystrophy. *Science.* December 31, 2015. doi: 10.1126/science.aae0169.

542 Greely. On science, Crispr-Cas9, and Asilomar.

543 Cools J. Using the hemoglobin switch for the treatment of sickle cell disease. *Haematologica.* February 2012; 97(2):156. doi: 10.3324/haematol.2012.062190.

544 Cools. Using the hemoglobin switch.

545 Wu Y, Liang D, Wang Y *et al.* Correction of a genetic disease in mouse via use of Crispr-Cas9. *Cell Stem Cell.* 2013; 13:659–662. doi: 10.1016/j.stem.2013.10.016.

546 Wu Y, Zhou H. Correction of a genetic disease by Crispr-Cas9-mediated gene editing in mouse spermatogonial stem cells. *Cell Res.* January 2015; 25(1):67–79. doi: 10.1038/cr.2014.160.

547 Regalado. Engineering the perfect baby.

548 Maron DF. "Improving" humans with customized genes sparks debate among scientists: Medicine or meddling? Researchers at a gene-editing summit grapple with the future of genetic enhancement. *Scientific American*. December 3, 2015.

549 Vanneste E, Voet T, Le Caignec C *et al*. Chromosome instability is common in human cleavage-stage embryos. *Nat Med*. May 2009; 15(5):577–583. doi: 10.1038/nm.1924.

550 Greco E, Minasi MG, Fiorentino F. Healthy babies after intrauterine transfer of mosaic aneuploid blastocysts. *N. Engl. J. Med*. November 19, 2015; 373(21):2089–2090. doi: 10.1056/NEJMc1500421.

551 A blastocyst specializes into cellular layers called an inner cell mass (which undergoes further specialization into an epiblast and endoderm, and at this stage embryonic stem cells can be plucked off from this inner cell layer) and an outer layer called a trophoblast, and undergoes further specialization into three major cell lines epiblast (epiderm), endoderm and mesoderm. In mice, many of these "commitment decisions" occur prior to the formation of the blastocyst, but not so for the human model, where cells may still reverse course. A group of genes called fibroblast growth factor, or FGF, signaling generates a MAP kinase pathway to drive the specialization; further segregation into a trophoblast and inner cell mas are regulated by Cdx2, a transcription factor which represses the transcription factors Oct4 and Nanog in the trophectoderm, allowing for the specification of the epiblast and primitive endoderm lineages. In humans, Cdx2 does not begin expression until the blastocyst stage and Oct4 is not restricted to ICM till very late blastocyst. In mice, Hippo signaling keeps Cdx2 expression to a compartment on the outside of a cell, and Cdx2 is committed to the trophectoderm by the 32-cell stage. Lineage commitment is complete by the blastocyst stage in mice, but not in humans. In mice, an inhibitor of FGF/Erk causes cells to be epiderm, while simulation with FGF/Erk causes cells to be endoderm. Treatment of human blastocysts with FGF promotes isolation of human ES cells, but FGF/Erk inhibitors do not affect primitive endoderm formation.

552 Wang H, Yang H, Shivalila CS *et al*. One-step generation of mice carrying mutations in multiple genes by Crispr/Cas-mediated genome engineering. *Cell*. May 9, 2013;153(4):910–918. doi: 10.1016/j.cell.2013.04.025.

553 Yang H, Wang H, Shivalila CS *et al*. One-step generation of mice carrying reporter and conditional alleles by Crispr/Cas-mediated genome engineering. *Cell*. August 27, 2013; 154(6):1370–1379. doi: 10.1016/j.cell.2013.08.022.

554 Regalado. Engineering the perfect baby.

555 NEMO stands for the "NF-kappa B Essential Modulator," and it is a gene that builds a protein required for the activation of the NF-kappa B family of transcription factors, an important master switch which regulates development of organ systems, especially the immune system, and mobilizes its swift response to infection. It is so critical that we humans cannot live without it. In the NEMO syndrome, the protein is only partially active, and many organ systems fail to develop normally, including the immune system, while B-cells, T-cells, neutrophils, macrophages and dendritic cells all respond poorly to infection.

556 The "Napa meeting" included a small group of scientists including Daley, Baltimore and Doudna, who set the agenda for this meeting in Washington.

557 Niu Y, Wang H, Shivalila CS *et al.* Generation of gene-modified cynomolgus monkey via Cas9/RNA-mediated gene targeting in one-cell embryos. *Cell.* February 13, 2014; 156(4):836–843. doi: 10.1016/j. cell.2014.01.027.

558 Yang H, Liu Z, Ma Y *et al.* Generation of haploid embryonic stem cells from *Macaca fascicularis* monkey parthenotes. *Cell Res.* 2013; 23:1187–1200. doi: 10.1038/cr.2013.93.

559 Vogel G. Infant monkey carries jellyfish gene. *Science.* January 12, 2001: 226.

560 Liu Z, Li X, Zhang JT *et al.* Autism-like behaviours and germline transmission in transgenic monkeys overexpressing MeCP2. *Nature.* January 25, 2016; 530(7588):98–102. doi: 10.1038/nature16533.

561 Belluck P. Monkeys built to mimic autism-like behaviors may help humans. *The New York Times.* January 25, 2016.

562 American scientists have created monkeys with the mutation for Huntington's disease, and in China, other researchers are creating monkeys with genes linked to neuromotor and psychiatric disorders.

563 Regalado. Engineering the perfect baby.

564 Harrison. Juvenescence.

565 Berger L. Being there: Heidegger on why our presence matters. The Stone. *The New York Times.* March 30, 2015.

566 Berger. Being there.

Bibliography

Abraham A. (2014) Is there an inverted-U relationship between creativity and psychopathology? *Front. Psychol.* 5:750.

Abudayyeh OO, Gootenberg JS, Konermann S *et al.* (2016) C2c2 is a single-component programmable RNA-guided RNA-targeting CRISPR effector. *Science.* doi: 10.1126/science.aaf5573.

Ainsworth C. (2015) Agriculture: A new breed of edits. *Nature.* 528: S15–S16. doi: 10.1038/528S15a.

Anticevic A, Van Snellenberg JX, Barch DM. (2012) Neurobiology of emotional dysfunction in schizophrenia: new directions revealed through metaanalyses. *BP.* 71:e23–e24. Author reply e25.

Apple S. (2016) An old idea revived: Starve cancer to death. *The New York Times.*

Arber W. (1965) Host-controlled modification of bacteriophage. *Annu. Rev. Microbiol.* 19:365–378.

Ashton CH. Anything for a quiet life? www.benzo.org.uk/afaql2.htm (accessed June 2016).

Askew C. (2015) *Tmc* gene therapy restores auditory function in deaf mice. *Sci. Transl. Med.* 7(295): 295ra108. doi: 10.1126/scitranslmed.aab1996.

Au A, Griffiths LR, Cheng KK *et al.* (2015) The influence of OLR1 and PCSK9 gene polymorphisms on ischemic stroke: Evidence from a meta-analysis. *Sci Rep.* 15(5):18224.

Baltimore D, Berg P, Botchan M *et al.* (2015) Biotechnology: A prudent path forward for genomic engineering and germline gene modification. *Science.* 348(6230):36–38. doi: 10.1126/science.aab1028.

Baker M. (2012) Gene-editing nucleases. *Nat. Meth.* 9:23–26.

Baker M. (2015) Over half of psychology studies fail reproducibility test. *Nature.* doi: 10.1038/nature.2015.18248.

Balazs AB, Chen J, Hong CM *et al.* (2011) Antibody-based protection against HIV infection by vectored immunoprophylaxis. *Nature.* 481(7379):81–84. doi: 10.1038/nature10660.

Bardwell AJ, Bardwell L, Iyer N *et al.* (1994) Yeast nucleotide excision repair proteins Rad2 and Rad4 interact with RNA polymerase II basal transcription factor b. *Mol. Cell. Biol.* 14:3569–3576.

Bardwell L, Bardwell AJ, Feaver WJ *et al.* (1994) Yeast Rad3 protein binds directly to both Ssl2 and Ssl1 proteins: implications for the structure and function of transcription/repair factor b. *Proc. Natl. Acad. Sci. USA.* 91:3926–3930.

Bardwell AJ, Bardwell L, Wang Z *et al.* Recent insights on DNA repair: the mechanism of damaged nucleotide excision in eukaryotes and its relationship to other cellular processes. *Ann. N.Y. Acad. Sci.* 726:281–291.

Barrangou R, Fremaux C, Deveau H *et al.* (2007) Crispr provides acquired resistance against viruses in prokaryotes. *Science.* 315:1709–1712.

Beck T. (2015) A vaccine for depression? *Nautilus.*

Begley CG, Ellis LM. (2012) Drug development: Raise standards for pre-clinical cancer research. *Nature.* 28;483(7391):531–533. doi: 10.1038/483531a.

Begley S. (2015) Meet one of the world's most groundbreaking scientists. He's 34. *STAT.*

Begley S. (2016) Controversial Crispr history sets off an online firestorm. *STAT News.*

Belluck P. (2016) Monkeys built to mimic autism-like behaviors may help humans. *The New York Times.*

Benyamin B, Pourcain BSt, Davis OS *et al.* (2014) Childhood intelligence is heritable, highly polygenic and associated with FNBP1L. *Mol Psychiatry.* 19(2):253–258. doi: 10.1038/mp.2012.184.

Berg P. (2000) *A Stanford Professor's Career in Biochemistry, Science Politics, and the Biotechnology Industry* (typescript of an oral history conducted in 1997 by Sally Smith Hughes). Regional Oral History Office, University of California.

Berg P. (2003) Moments of discovery: My favorite experiments. *JBC.* 278:40417–40424. doi: 10.1074/jbc.X300004200.

Berg P. (2008) Meetings that changed the world: Asilomar 1975: DNA modification secured. *Nature.* 455(7211):290–291.

Berg P, Mertz JE. (2010) Personal reflections on the origins and emergence of recombinant DNA technology. *Genetics.* 184(1):9–17. doi: 10.1534/genetics.109.112144.

Berg P, Baltimore D, Boyer HW *et al.* (1974) Potential biohazards of recombinant DNA molecules. *Science* 185:303.

Berg DE, Jackson DA, Mertz JE. (1974) Isolation of a lambda dv plasmid carrying the bacterial gal operon. *J. Virol.* 14(5):1063–1069.

Berger L. (2015) Being there: Heidegger on why our presence matters. The Stone. *The New York Times.*

Bessen J. (2016) What does it mean for researchers, journalists and the public when secrecy surrounds science? theconversation.com.

Bianconi E. (2013) An estimation of the number of cells in the human body. *Ann. Hum. Biol.* 40(6):463–471.

Bikard D, Jiang W, Samai P *et al.* (2013) Programmable repression and activation of bacterial gene expression using an engineered Crispr-Cas system. *Nucleic Acids Res.* 41:7429–7437. doi: 10.1093/nar/gkt520.

Blitz IL, Biesinger J, Xie X, Cho KWY. (2013) Biallelic genome modification in F0 *Xenopus tropicalis* embryos using the Crispr/Cas system. *Genesis.* 51:827–834. doi: 10.1002/dvg.22719.

Bloom P. (2013) The baby in the well: The case against empathy. A Critic at Large, *The New Yorker.*

Boeke JD, Church G, Hessel A *et al.* (2016) The Genome Project – Write. *Science.* doi:10.1126/science.aaf6850.

Bolotin A, Quinquis B, Sorokin A, Ehrlich SD. (2005) Clustered regularly interspaced short palindrome repeats (Crisprs) have spacers of extrachromosomal origin. *Microbiology.* 151:2551–2561.

Borenstein S. (2006) NASA chief's gamble – or calculated decision – that paid off, big time. *Associated Press.*

Botchan M, Stringer J, Mitchison T, Sambrook J. (1980) Integration and excision of SV40 DNA from the chromosome of a transformed cell. *Cell.* 20:143–152.

Boyer HW. (1994) *Recombinant DNA Research at UCSF and Commercial Application at Genentech. Interviews Conducted by Sally Smith Hughes.* The UCSF Oral History Program and the Program in the History of the Biological Sciences and Biotechnology. http://content.cdlib.org/ark:/13030/kt5d5nb0zs/.

Braskie MN, Jahanshad N, Stein JL *et al.* (2012) Relationship of a variant in the NTRK1 gene to white matter microstructure in young adults. *J. Neurosci.* 32:5964–5972.

Breivikmay J. (2016) Obama's pointless cancer "moonshot." *The New York Times.*

Brouns SJJ, Jore MM, Lundgren M *et al.* (2008) Small Crispr RNAs guide antiviral defense in prokaryotes. *Science.* 321:960–964.

Campbell AM. (1963) Episomes. *Adv. Genet.* 11:101–145.

Carey B. (2016) Scientists move closer to understanding schizophrenia's cause. *The New York Times.*

Chandrasegaran S, Smith J. (1999) Chimeric restriction enzymes: what is next? *Biol. Chem.* 380:841–848.

Chang ACY, Cohen SN. (1974) Genome construction between bacterial species *in vitro*: Replication and expression of *Staphylococcus* plasmid genes in *Escherichia coli. Proc. Natl. Acad. Sci. USA.* 71(4):1030–1034.

Chen C. (2015) These superhumans are real and their DNA could be worth billions. *Bloomberg.*

Chen J, Lipska BK, Halim N *et al.* (2004) Functional analysis of genetic variation in catechol-O-methyltransferase (COMT): effects on mRNA, protein, and enzyme activity in postmortem human brain. *Am. J. Hum. Genet.* 75:807–821.

Cheng MY, Lee IP, Jin M *et al.* (2011) An insult-inducible vector system activated by hypoxia and oxidative stress for neuronal gene therapy. *Transl Stroke Res.* 2(1):92–100.

Cheng MY, Sun G, Jin M *et al.* (2009) Blocking glucocorticoid and enhancing estrogenic genomic signaling protects against cerebral ischemia. *J. Cereb. Blood Flow Metab.* 29(1):130–136.

Chiang MC, Barysheva M, Shattuck DW *et al.* (2009) Genetics of brain fiber architecture and intellectual performance. *J. Neurosci.* 29:2212–2224.

Chiang MC, Barysheva M, Toga AW *et al.* (2011) *BDNF* gene effects on brain circuitry replicated in 455 twins. *Neuroimage.* 55:448–454.

Cho SW, Kim S, Kim JM, Kim J-S. (2013) Targeted genome engineering in human cells with the Cas9 RNA-guided endonuclease. *Nat. Biotechnol.* 31:230–232.

Chuong E, Elde N, Feschotte C. (2016) Regulatory evolution of innate immunity through co-option of endogenous retroviruses. *Science* 351 (6277):1083–1087. doi: 10.1126/science.aad5497.

Cohen SN. (2013) DNA cloning: A personal view after 40 years. *Proc. Natl. Acad. Sci. USA.* 110(39):15521–15529. doi: 10.1073/pnas.1313397110.

Cohen S, Chang A, Boyer H, Helling R. (1973) Construction of biologically functional bacterial plasmids *in vitro. Proc. Natl. Acad. Sci. USA.* 70 (11):3240–3244. doi: 10.1073/pnas.70.11.3240.

Cohen SN, Chang AC, Hsu L. (1972) Nonchromosomal antibiotic resistance in bacteria: Genetic transformation of *Escherichia coli* by R-factor DNA. *Proc. Natl. Acad. Sci. USA.* 69(8):2110–2114. doi: 10.1073/pnas.69.8.2110.

Comfort N. (2016) A Whig History of Crispr. http://genotopia.scienceblog.com/573/a-whig-history-of-Crispr/.

Comfort N. (2016) Genes are overrated. *The Atlantic.*

Cong L, Ran FA, Cox D *et al.* (2013) Multiplex genome engineering using Crispr/Cas systems. *Science.* 339:819–823.

Cools J. (2012) Using the hemoglobin switch for the treatment of sickle cell disease. *Haematologica.* 97(2):156. doi: 10.3324/haematol.2012.062190.

Crichton M. (1991) *Jurassic Park.* Century Books.

Crow JF, Dove WF (eds). (1995) *Perspectives: Anecdotal, Historical and Critical Commentaries on Genetics*. The Genetics Society of America.

Cyranoski D. (2015) CRISPR tweak may help gene-edited crops bypass biosafety regulation. Technique deletes plant genes without adding foreign DNA. *Nature News*. doi: 10.1038/nature.2015.18590.

Cyranoski D. (2015) Scientists sound alarm over DNA editing of human embryos: Experts call for halt in research to work out safety and ethics issues. *Nature News*. doi: 10.1038/nature.2015.17110.

Datta N. (1962) Transmissible drug resistance in an epidemic strain of *Salmonella typhimurium*. *J. Hygiene*. 60(3):301–310. doi: 10.1017/s0022172400020416.PMC 2134509.

Datta N, Pridie RB, Anderson ES. (2009) An outbreak of infection with *Salmonella typhimurium* in a general hospital. *J. Hygiene*. 58(02):229. doi: 10.1017/S0022172400038316.

Deltcheva E, Chylinski K, Sharma CM *et al*. (2011) Crispr RNA maturation by trans-encoded small RNA and host factor RNase III. *Nature*. 471:602–607.

Dennis EL, Jahanshad N, Rudie JD *et al*. (2011) Altered structural brain connectivity in healthy carriers of the autism risk gene, CNTNAP2. *Brain Connect*. 1:447–459.

Deveau H, Barrangou R, Garneau JE *et al*. (2008) Phage response to Crispr encoded resistance in *Streptococcus thermophilus*. *Bacteriol*. 190:1390–1400.

Dobrikova EY, Broadt T, Poiley-Nelson J *et al*. (2008) Recombinant oncolytic poliovirus eliminates glioma in vivo without genetic adaptation to a pathogenic phenotype. *Mol. Ther*. 16:1865–1872.

Doudna J. (2015) Genome-editing revolution: My whirlwind year with Crispr. *Nature*. 528(7583):469–471. doi: 10.1038/528469a.

Doudna JA, Charpentier E. (2014) Genome editing: The new frontier of genome engineering with Crispr-Cas9. *Science*. 346(6213):1258096. doi: 10.1126/science.1258096.

East EM. (1916) Studies on size inheritance in nicotiana. *Genetics*. 1:164–176.

The Economist. (2008) Cancer stem cells: The root of all evil? *The Economist*.

Edelman G. (2006) *Second Nature: Brain Science and Human Knowledge*. Yale University Press.

Egan MF, Kojima M, Callicott JH *et al*. (2003) The BDNF val66met polymorphism affects activity-dependent secretion of BDNF and human memory and hippocampal function. *Cell*. 112:257–269.

Endy D, Zoloth L. (2016) Should we synthesis a human genome? https://dspace.mit.edu/bitstream/handle/1721.1/102449/ShouldWeGenome.pdf?sequence=1. (accessed June 2016).

Esvelt K, Church G, Lunshof J. (2014) "Gene drives" and Crispr could revolutionize ecosystem management. *Scientific American.*

Farrer LA, Cupples LA, Haines JL *et al.*; APOE and Alzheimer Disease Meta Analysis Consortium. (1997) Effects of age, sex, and ethnicity on the association between apolipoprotein E genotype and Alzheimer disease: A meta-analysis. *JAMA.* 278:1349–1356.

Feaver WJ, Svejstrup JQ, Bardwell L *et al.* (1993) Dual roles of a multiprotein complex from *Saccharomyces cerevisiae* in transcription and DNA repair. *Cell.* 75:1379–1387.

Fitch WT, Hauser MD, Chomsky N. (2005) The evolution of the language faculty: clarifications and implications. *Cognition.* 97(2):179–210.

Flavahan WA, Drier Y, Liau BB *et al.* (2016) Insulator dysfunction and oncogene activation in IDH mutant gliomas. *Nature.* 529:10–114. doi: 10.1038/nature16490.

Flowers GP, Timberlake AT, McLean KC, Monaghan JR, Crews CM. (2014) Highly efficient targeted mutagenesis in axolotl using Cas9 RNA-guided nuclease. *Development.* 141:2165–2171. doi: 10.1242/dev.105072.

Fosse R, Joseph J, Richardson K. (2015) A critical assessment of the equal-environment assumption of the twin method for schizophrenia. *Front. Psychiatry.* 6:62. doi: 10.3389/fpsyt.2015.00062.

Fredrickson DS. (2001) *The Recombinant DNA Controversy: A Memoir. Science, Politics, and the Public Interest 1974–1981.* ASM Press.

Friedberg EC. (1992) Xeroderma pigmentosum, Cockayne syndrome, essential genes, helicases and DNA repair: what's the relationship? *Cell.* 71:887–889.

Friedberg EC. (2014) Master molecule, heal thyself. *J. Biol. Chem.* 289 (20):13691–13700. doi: 10.1074/jbc.X114.572115.

Friedberg EC, Goldthwait DA. (1969) Endonuclease II of *E. coli. Cold Spring Harbor Symp. Quant. Biol.* 33:271–275.

Friedberg EC, Goldthwait DA. (1969) Endonuclease II of *E. coli.* I. Isolation and purification. *Proc. Natl. Acad. Sci. USA.* 62:934–940.

Friedberg EC, Bardwell AJ, Bardwell L *et al.* (1995) Nucleotide excision repair in the yeast *Saccharomyces cerevisiae*: its relationship to specialized mitotic recombination and RNA polymerase II basal transcription. *Philos. Trans. R. Soc. Lond. B Biol. Sci.* 347:63–68.

Friedberg EC, Hadi SM, Goldthwait DA. (1969) Endonuclease II of *E. coli.* II. Enzyme properties and studies on the degradation of alkylated and native deoxyribonucleic acid. *J. Biol. Chem.* 244:5879–5889.

Frodeman R, Briggle A. (2016) When philosophy lost its way. The Stone. *The New York Times.*

Gantz VM, Bier E. (2015) Genome editing. The mutagenic chain reaction: a method for converting heterozygous to homozygous mutations. *Science.* 348:442–444.

Gasiunas G, Barrangou R, Horvath P, Siksnys V. (2012) Cas9-crRNA ribonucleoprotein complex mediates specific DNA cleavage for adaptive immunity in bacteria. *Proc. Natl. Acad. Sci. USA.* 109: E2579–E2586.

Gibson DG, Glass JI, Lartigue C *et al.* (2010) Creation of a bacterial cell controlled by a chemically synthesized genome. *Science.* 329:52–56. doi: 10.1126/science.1190719.

Gilbert LA, Larson MH, Morsut L *et al.* (2013) Crispr-mediated modular RNA-guided regulation of transcription in eukaryotes. *Cell.* 154:442–451. doi: 10.1016/j.cell.2013.06.044.

Goldberg N. (1986) *Writing Down the Bones.* Shambala.

Goldstein DB, Allen A, Keebler J, *et al.* (2013) Sequencing studies in human genetics: design and interpretation. *Nature Rev. Genet.* 14:460–470.

Gordon JW. (1999) Genetic enhancement in humans. *Science.* 283 (5410):2023–2024. doi: 10.1126/science.283.5410.2023.

Gottschall J. (2012) *The Storytelling Animal: How Stories Make Us Human.* Houghton Mifflin Harcourt.

Grady D. (2011) An immune system trained to kill cancer. *The New York Times*: D1.

Greco E, Minasi MG, Fiorentino F. (2015) Healthy babies after intrauterine transfer of mosaic aneuploid blastocysts. *N. Engl. J. Med.* 373(21):2089–2090. doi: 10.1056/NEJMc1500421.

Greely H. (2015) On Science, Crispr-Cas9, and Asilomar. Law and Biosciences Blog. *Stanford Law Rev.*

Gromeier M, Lachmann S, Rosenfeld MR, Gutin PH, Wimmer E. (2000) Intergeneric poliovirus recombinants for the treatment of malignant glioma. *Proc. Natl. Acad. Sci. USA.* 97:6803–6808.

Harada K, Kameda M, Suzuki M, Mitsuhashi S. (1964) Drug resistance of enteric bacteria. 3. Acquisition of transferability of nontransmissible R(Tc) factor in cooperation with F factor and formation of Fr(Tc). *J. Bacteriol.* 88:1257–1265.

Harmon A. (2015) Open season is seen in gene editing of animals. *The New York Times.*

Harrison RP. (2014) *Juvenescence: A Cultural History of our Age*. University of Chicago Press.

Hart J, Chabris CF. (2016) Does a "Triple Package" of traits predict success? *Personality and Individual Differences*. 94:216–222.

Hedgpeth J, Goodman HM, Boyer HW. (1972) DNA nucleotide sequence restricted by the RI endonuclease. *Proc. Natl. Acad. Sci. USA*. 69 (11):3448–3452.

Hellmann M. (2014) Researchers hope "super bananas" will combat vitamin A deficiency. *Time*.

The Hinxton Group. (2006) *An International Consortium on Stem Cells, Ethics and Law*. Consensus Statement.

Horvath P, Romero DA, Coûté-Monvoisin A-C *et al.* (2008) Diversity, activity, and evolution of Crispr loci in *Streptococcus thermophilus*. *Bacteriol*. 190:1401–1412.

Huebbe P, Nebel A, Siegert S *et al.* (2011) APOE e4 is associated with higher vitamin D levels in targeted replacement mice and humans. *FASEB J*. 25(9):3262–3270. doi: 10.1096/fj.11-180935. PMID 21659554.

Hutchison CA 3rd, Chuang RY, Noskov VN *et al.* (2016) Design and synthesis of a minimal bacterial genome. *Science*. 351:1414. doi: 10.1126/science.aad6253.

Huttlin EL, Ting L, Bruckner RJ *et al.* (2015) The BioPlex Network: A systematic exploration of the human interactome. *Cell*. 162(2):425–440. doi: 10.1016/j.cell.2015.06.043.

Hwang WY, Fu Y, Reyon D *et al.* (2013) Efficient genome editing in zebrafish using a Crispr-Cas system. *Nat. Biotechnol*. 31:227–229.

Ishino Y, Shinagawa H, Makino K, Amemura M, Nakata, AJ. (1987) Nucleotide sequence of the iap gene, responsible for alkaline phosphatase isozyme conversion in *Escherichia coli*, and identification of the gene product. *Bacteriol*. 169:5429–5433.

Jacob F, Brenner S, Cuzin F. (1963) On the regulation of DNA replication in bacteria. *Cold Spring Harb. Symp. Quant. Biol*. 28:329–348.

Jahanshad N, Kohannim O, Hibar DP *et al.* (2012) Brain structure in healthy adults is related to serum transferrin and the H63D polymorphism in the HFE gene. *Proc. Natl. Acad. Sci. USA*. 109:E851–E859.

Jahanshad N, Rajagopalan P, Thompson PM. (2013) Neuroimaging, nutrition, and iron-related genes. *Cell. Molec. Life Sci*. 70(23):4449–4461. doi: 10.1007/s00018-013-1369-2.

James W. (1956) *The Will To Believe*, Dover Publications, 21, 25.

Jansen R, Embden JDAV, Gaastra W, Schouls LM. (2002) Identification of genes that are associated with DNA repeats in prokaryotes. *Mol. Microbiol.* 43:1565–1575.

Jasin M, Berg P. (1988) Homologous integration in mammalian cells without target gene selection. *Genes Dev.* 2(11):1353–1363.

Jasin M, de Villiers J, Weber F, Schaffner W. (1985) High frequency of homologous recombination in mammalian cells. *Cell.* 43:695–703.

Jia H, Wang N. (2014) Targeted genome editing of sweet orange using Cas9/sgRNA. *PLoS ONE* 9:e93806. doi: 10.1371/journal.pone.0093806.

Jiang W, Zhou H, Bi H *et al.* (2013) Demonstration of Crispr/Cas9/sgRNA-mediated targeted gene modification in *Arabidopsis*, tobacco, sorghum and rice. *Nucleic Acids Res.* 41:e188. doi: 10.1093/nar/gkt780.

Jinek M, Chylinski K, Fonfara I *et al.* (2012) A programmable dual-RNA-guided DNA endonuclease in adaptive bacterial immunity. *Science.* 337:816–821.

Jinek M, East A, Cheng A *et al.* (2013) RNA-programmed genome editing in human cells. *eLife.* 2:e00471.

Jinek M, Jiang F, Taylor DW *et al.* (2014) Structures of Cas9 endonucleases reveal RNA-mediated conformational activation. *Science.* 343:1247997. doi: 10.1126/science.1247997; pmid: 24505130.

Kahn J. (2015) The Crispr quandry. *The New York Times Magazine.*

Kaufman JC (ed). (2014) *Creativity and Mental Illness.* Cambridge University Press.

Kaufman R. (2011) It doesn't add up. *Science.* doi: 10.1126/science.caredit. a1100139.

Kazmin A. (2016) Monsanto's India spat inflames corporate fears. *Financial Times.*

Kaiser J. (2015) CRISPR helps heal mice with muscular dystrophy. *Science.* doi: 10.1126/science.aae0169.

Kelly TJ Jr, Smith HO. (1970) A restriction enzyme from *Hemophilus influenzae. J. Mol. Biol.* 51(2):393–409.

Kim YJ, Mantel PL, June CH, Kim SH, Kwon BS. (1999) 4-1BB costimulation promotes human T cell adhesion to fibronectin. *Cell Immunol.* 192 (1):13–23.

Kistler KE, Vosshall LB, Matthews BJ. (2015) Genome engineering with CRISPR-Cas9 in the mosquito *Aedes aegypti. Cell Rep.* 11:51–60.

Kleinstiver BP, Pattanayak V, Prew MS *et al.* (2016) High-fidelity Crispr–Cas9 nucleases with no detectable genome-wide off-target effects. *Nature.* 529(7587):490–495. doi: 10.1038/nature16526.

Knight H. (2015) A metabolic master switch underlying human obesity. *MIT News.*

Knudson A. (1971) Mutation and cancer: statistical study of retinoblastoma. *Proc. Natl. Acad. Sci. USA.* 68(4):820–823.

Kochunov P, Glahn DC, Lancaster JL *et al.* (2010) Genetics of microstructure of cerebral white matter using diffusion tensor imaging. *Neuroimage.* 53:1109–1116.

Kohannim O, Jahanshad N, Braskie MN *et al.* (2012) Predicting white matter integrity from multiple common genetic variants. *Neuropsychopharmacol.* 37(9):2012–2019.

Kolata G. (2015) A proposal to modify plants gives G.M.O. debate new life. *The New York Times.*

Kolata G. (2015) Scientists discover reason brain tumors grow fast. *The New York Times.*

Kong A, Frigge ML, Masson G, *et al.* (2012) Rate of de novo mutations and the importance of father's age to disease risk. *Nature.* 488:471–475. doi: 10.1038/nature11396.

Kozubek J. (2011) FDA decision will lead to first ever genetically-modified animal for consumption. *TPM Idea Lab.*

Kozubek J. (2014) Love is not algorithmic. *The Atlantic.*

Kozubek J. (2016) An ON/OFF switch for genes. *Sci. Am.* 314:52–57. doi: 10.1038/scientificamerican0116-52.

Kozubek J. (2016) Why can't we prevent Alzheimer's? *The Atlantic.*

Kuwana Y, Asakura Y, Utsunomiya N *et al.* (1987) Expression of chimeric receptor composed of immunoglobulin-derived V regions and T-cell receptor-derived C regions. *Biochem. Biophys. Res. Commun.* 149(3): 960–968.

Lander E. (2016) The heroes of Crispr. *Cell.* 164(1–2):18–28. doi: 10.1016/j.cell.2015.12.041.

Lander ES. (2015) Brave new genome. *N. Engl. J. Med.* 373:5–8. doi: 10.1056/NEJMp1506446.

Lear J. (1978) *Recombinant DNA: The Untold Story.* Crown Publishers.

Lederberg J. (1952) Cell genetics and hereditary symbiosis. *Physiol. Rev.* 32(4): 403–430.

Lederberg J. (1996) Interview with Prof. Lederberg, Winner of the 1958 Nobel Prize in Physiology and Medicine. Conducted by Lev Pevzner.

Lederberg J, Cavalli LL, Lederberg EM. (1952) Sex compatibility in *Escherichia coli. Genetics* 37(6):720–730.

Liu B, Song M, Li J *et al.* (2010) Prefrontal-related functional connectivities within the default network are modulated by COMT val158met in healthy young adults. *J. Neurosci.* 30:64–69.

Liu X, Jiang S, Fang C *et al.* (2015) Affinity-tuned ErbB2 or EGFR chimeric antigen receptor T cells exhibit an increased therapeutic index against tumors in mice. *Cancer Res.* 75:3596. doi: 10.1158/0008-5472.CAN-15-0159.

Liu Z, Li X, Zhang JT *et al.* (2016) Autism-like behaviours and germline transmission in transgenic monkeys overexpressing MeCP2. *Nature.* 530(7588):98–102. doi: 10.1038/nature16533.

MacArthur D, Manolio TA, Dimmock DP *et al.* (2014) Guidelines for investigating causality of sequence variants in human disease. *Nature.* 508:469–476.

Mackinnon DW, Nielson G. (eds) (1962) The personality correlates of creativity: A study of American architects. *Proceedings of the XIV International Congress of Applied Psychology. Volume 2, Personality Research.* Munksgaard:11–39.

Madabhushi R, Gao F, Pfenning AR *et al.* (2015) Activity-induced DNA breaks govern the expression of neuronal early-response genes. *Cell.* 161:1592–1605.

Makari G. (2016) Notes from psychiatry's battle lines. *The New York Times.*

Makarova KS, Grishin NV, Shabalina SA, Wolf YI, Koonin EV. (2006) A putative RNA-interference-based immune system in prokaryotes: computational analysis of the predicted enzymatic machinery, functional analogies with eukaryotic RNAi, and hypothetical mechanisms of action. *Biol. Direct.* 1:7.

Mali P, Yang L, Esvelt KM *et al.* (2013) RNA-guided human genome engineering via Cas9. *Science.* 339:823–826.

Mandal PK, Ferreira LM, Collins R *et al.* (2014) Efficient ablation of genes in human hematopoietic stem and effector cells using CRISPR/Cas9. *Cell Stem Cell.* 15(5):643–652. doi: 10.1016/j.stem.2014.10.004.

Mandel M, Higa A. (1970) Calcium-dependent bacteriophage DNA infection. *J. Mol. Biol.* 53(1):159–162.

Mangold M, Siller M, Roppenser B *et al.* (2004) Synthesis of group A streptococcal virulence factors is controlled by a regulatory RNA molecule. *Mol. Microbiol.* 53:1515–1527.

Maron DF. (2015) "Improving" humans with customized genes sparks debate among scientists: Medicine or meddling? Researchers at a gene-editing summit grapple with the future of genetic enhancement. *Scientific American.*

Marraffini LA, Sontheimer EJ. (2008) Crispr interference limits horizontal gene transfer in staphylococci by targeting DNA. *Science.* 322:1843–1845.

Martel Y. (2004) We ate the children last. *The Guardian.*

Massachusetts Institute of Technology Oral History Program. (1988) *Oral History Collection on the Recombinant DNA Controversy, 1966–1978*. MC.0100.

Matfield M. (1986) New vectors for gene therapy. *New Sci.*: 32.

Matsumoto M, Weickert CS, Akil M *et al.* (2003) Catechol O-methyltransferase mRNA expression in human and rat brain: Evidence for a role in cortical neuronal function. *Neuroscience.* 116:127–137.

Maxmen A. (2015) The Genesis Engine. *Wired.*

McGregor J. (2016) Why this Wharton wunderkind wants leaders to replace their intuition with evidence. *The Washington Post.*

Merrill MK, Bernhardt G, Sampson JH *et al.* (2004) Poliovirus receptor CD155-targeted oncolysis of glioma. *Neuro-oncol.* 6:208–217.

Mertz JE, Davis RW. (1972) Cleavage of DNA by R 1 restriction endonuclease generates cohesive ends. *Proc. Natl. Acad. Sci. USA.* 69(11): 3370–3374.

Michaelson JJ. (2012) Whole-genome sequencing in autism identifies hot spots for de novo germline mutation. *Cell.* 151(7):1431–1442. doi: 10.1016/j.cell.2012.11.019.

Mitsuyasu RT. (2000) Prolonged survival and tissue trafficking following adoptive transfer of CD4zeta gene-modified autologous CD4(+) and CD8(+) T cells in human immunodeficiency virus-infected subjects. *Blood.* 96(3):785–793.

Mojica FJM, Díez-Villaseñor C, García-Martínez J, Soria EJ. (2005) Intervening sequences of regularly spaced prokaryotic repeats derive from foreign genetic elements. *Mol. Evol.* 60:174–182.

Mojica FJM, Díez-Villaseñor C, Soria E, Juez G. Biological significance of a family of regularly spaced repeats in the genomes of Archaea, bacteria and mitochondria. *Mol. Microbiol.* 2000; 36:244–246.

Mojica FJM, Ferrer C, Juez G, Rodríguez-Valera F. (1995) Long stretches of short tandem repeats are present in the largest replicons of the Archaea *Haloferax mediterranei* and *Haloferax volcanii* and could be involved in replicon partitioning. *Mol. Microbiol.* 17:85–93.

Mojica FJM, Garrett RA. *Discovery and Seminal Developments in the Crispr Field.* Springer, 1–31.

Mojica FJM, Juez G, Rodríguez-Valera F. (1993) Transcription at different salinities of *Haloferax mediterranei* sequences adjacent to partially modified PstI sites. *Mol. Microbiol.* 9:613–621.

Montenegro M. (2016) Crispr is coming to agriculture – with big implications for food, farmers, consumers and nature. *Ensia.*

Moreno J. (2011) *The Body Politic*. Bellevue Literary Press.

Morrow JF, Berg P, Kelly TJ Jr, Lewis AM Jr. (1973) Mapping of simian virus 40 early functions on the viral chromosome. *J. Virol.* 12(3):653–658.

Morrow JF, Cohen SN, Chang AC, *et al.* (1974) Replication and transcription of eukaryotic DNA in *Escherichia coli. Proc. Natl. Acad. Sci. USA.* 71(5):1743–1747.

Müller-Hill B. (1996) *The lac Operon: A Short History of a Genetic Paradigm*. Walter de Gruyter.

Mulligan RC. (2014) Development of gene transfer technology. *Hum. Gene Ther.* 25:995–1002. doi: 10.1089/hum.2014.2543.

Mulligan RC, Howard BH, Berg P. (1979) Synthesis of rabbit β-globin in cultured monkey kidney cells following infection with a SV40 β-globin recombinant genome. *Nature.* 277:108–114. doi: 10.1038/277108a0.

Nakayama T, Fish MB, Fisher M *et al.* (2013) Simple and efficient Crispr/Cas9-mediated targeted mutagenesis in *Xenopus tropicalis. Genesis.* 51:835–843. doi: 10.1002/dvg.22720.

Nature News (1974) NAS ban on plasmid engineering. *Nature.* 250:175.

Nishimasu H, Ran FA, Hsu PD *et al.* (2014) Crystal structure of Cas9 in complex with guide RNA and target DNA. *Cell.* 156:935–949. doi: 10.1016/j.cell.2014.02.001; pmid: 24529477.

Niu Y, Wang H, Shivalila CS *et al.* (2014) Generation of gene-modified cynomolgus monkey via Cas9/RNA-mediated gene targeting in one-cell embryos. *Cell.* 156(4):836–843. doi: 10.1016/j.cell.2014.01.027.

Odelberg W (ed). (1979) *Les Prix Nobel: The Nobel Prizes 1978*. Nobel Foundation.

Oettinger MA, Schwatz DG, Gorka C, Baltimore D. (1990) RAG1 and RAG2, adjacent genes that synergistically activate V(D)J recombination. *Science.* 248:1517–1523.

Open Science Collaboration. (2015) Estimating the reproducibility of psychological science. *Science.* 349(6251). doi: 10.1126/science.aac4716.

Paine JA, Shipton CA Chaggar S *et al.* (2000) Improving the nutritional value of Golden Rice through increased pro-vitamin A content. *Nat. Biotech.* 23(4):482–487. doi: 10.1038/nbt1082.

Pearson H. (2008) Protein engineering: The fate of fingers. *Nature.* 455:160–164. doi: 10.1038/455160a.

Pinker S. (2015) Steven Pinker on new advances in behavioral genetics. *The Washington Post*.

Pinker S, Jackendoff R. (2005) The faculty of language: what's special about it? *Cognition* 95(2):201–236.

Pinker S, Jackendoff R. (2005) The nature of the language faculty and its implications for evolution of language. *Cognition* 97:211–225.

Pollack A. (2016) A biotech evangelist seeks a Zika dividend. *The New York Times Magazine.*

Pollack A. (2016) New weapon to fight Zika: The mosquito. *The New York Times.*

Pollack A. (2016) Scientists talk privately about creating a synthetic human genome. *The New York Times.*

Pourcel C, Salvignol G, Vergnaud G. (2005) Crispr elements in *Yersinia pestis* acquire new repeats by preferential uptake of bacteriophage DNA, and provide additional tools for evolutionary studies. *Microbiology.* 151:653–663.

Prinz F, Schlange T, Asadullah K. (2011) Believe it or not: how much can we rely on published data on potential drug targets? *Nature Rev. Drug Discov.* 10:712. doi: 10.1038/nrd3439-c1.

Qi LS, Larson MH, Gilbert LA *et al.* (2013) Repurposing Crispr as an RNA-guided platform for sequence-specific control of gene expression. *Cell.* 152:1173–1183. doi: 10.1016/j.cell.2013.02.022.

Regalado A. (2015) Engineering the perfect baby. *Technol. Rev.*

Regalado A. (2016) A scientist's contested history of Crispr. *Technol. Rev.*

Rope AF, Wang K, Evjenth R *et al.* (2011) Using VAAST to identify an X-linked disorder resulting in lethality in male infants due to N-terminal acetyltransferase deficiency. *Am. J. Hum. Genet.* 89(1): 28–43.

Rouet P, Smih F, Jasin M. (1994) Introduction of double-strand breaks into the genome of mouse cells by expression of a rare-cutting endonuclease. *Mol. Cell Biol.* 14(12):8096–8106.

Sapolsky RM. (2015) Stress and the brain: individual variability and the inverted-U. *Nat. Neurosci.* 18(10):1344–1346. doi: 10.1038/nn.4109.

Sapranauskas R, Gasiunas G, Fremaux C *et al.* (2011) The *Streptococcus thermophilus* Crispr/Cas system provides immunity in *Escherichia coli. Nucleic Acids Res.* 39:9275–9282.

Schwank G, Koo BK, Sasselli V *et al.* (2013) Functional repair of CFTR by Crispr/Cas9 in intestinal stem cell organoids of cystic fibrosis patients. *Cell Stem Cell.* 13:653–658. doi: 10.1016/j. stem.2013.11.002.

Scranton R. (2015) We're doomed. Now what? The Stone. *The New York Times.*

Sekar A. (2016) Schizophrenia risk from complex variation of complement component 4. *Nature.* 530(7589):177–183. doi: 10.1038/nature16549.

Sgaramella V. (1972) Enzymatic oligomerization of bacteriophage P22 DNA and of linear Simian virus 40 DNA. *Proc. Natl. Acad. Sci. USA.* 69(11):3389–3393.

Shapin S. (2015) The desire to know: Scientific virtue is worth saving. *The Boston Review*: 32.

Shenk JW. (2014) The end of "genius." *The New York Times.*

Sherkow J. (2015) The Crispr patent interference showdown is on: How did we get here and what comes next? Law and Biosciences Blog. *Stanford Law Review.*

Skerrett P. (2015) Experts debate: Are we playing with fire when we edit human genes? *STAT News.*

Smidler AL, Terenzi O, Soichot J, Levashina EA, Marois E. (2013) Targeted mutagenesis in the malaria mosquito using TALE nucleases. *PLoS ONE.* 8:e74511.

Smithies O, Gregg RG, Boggs SS, Koralewski MA, Kucherlapati RS. (1985) Insertion of DNA sequences into the human chromosomal beta-globin locus by homologous recombination. *Nature.* 317(6034):230–234.

Soldner F, Stelzer Y, Shivalila CS *et al.* (2016) Parkinson-associated risk variant in distal enhancer of α-synuclein modulates target gene expression. *Nature.* 533(7601):95–99. doi: 10.1038/nature17939.

Specter M. (2015) The Gene Hackers: A powerful new technology enables us to manipulate our DNA more easily than ever before. *The New Yorker.*

Sternberg SH, Redding S, Jinek M, Greene EC, Doudna JA. (2014) DNA interrogation by the Crispr RNA-guided endonuclease Cas9. *Nature.* 507:62–67. doi: 10.1038/nature13011; pmid: 24476820.

Sugano SS, Shirakawa M, Takagi J *et al.* (2014) Crispr/Cas9-mediated targeted mutagenesis in the liverwort *Marchantia polymorpha* L. *Plant Cell Physiol.* 55:475–481. doi: 10.1093/pcp/pcu014.

Taylor-Weiner H, Zivin JG. (2015) Medicine's Wild West: Unlicensed stem-cell clinics in the United States. *N. Engl. J. Med.* 373:985–987. doi: 10.1056/NEJMp1504560.

Thompson PM, Ge T, Glahn DC, Jahanshad N, Nichols TE. (2013) Genetics of the connectome. *Neuroimage.* 80:475–488.

Tomlinson I. (2002) How many mutations in a cancer? *Am. J. Pathol.* 160(3): 755–758. doi: 10.1016/S0002-9440(10)64896-1.

Tucker A. (2006) Obituary: ES Anderson. *The Guardian.*

Tunbridge EM, Harrison PJ, Weinberger DR. (2006) Catechol-o-methyltransferase, cognition, and psychosis: Val158Met and beyond. *BP.* 60:141–151.

Upadhyay SK, Kumar J, Alok A, Tuli R. (2013) RNA-guided genome editing for target gene mutations in wheat. *G3* 3:2233–2238. doi: 10.1534/g3.113.008847.

Vanneste E, Voet T, Le Caignec C *et al.* (2009) Chromosome instability is common in human cleavage-stage embryos. *Nat. Med.* 15(5):577–583. doi: 10.1038/nm.1924.

Vence T. (2016) "Heroes of Crispr" disputed. *The Scientist.*

Vogel G. (2001) Infant monkey carries jellyfish gene. *Science.* 226.

Walker RE, Bechtel CM, Natarajan V *et al.* (2000) Long-term in vivo survival of receptor-modified syngeneic T cells in patients with human immunodeficiency virus infection. *Blood.* 96(2):467–474.

Wang H, Isaacs F, Carr P *et al.* (2009) Programming cells by multiplex genome engineering and accelerated evolution. *Nature.* 460(7257): 894–898.

Wang H, Yang H, Shivalila CS *et al.* (2013) One-step generation of mice carrying mutations in multiple genes by Crispr/Cas-mediated genome engineering. *Cell.* 153(4):910–918. doi: 10.1016/j.cell.2013.04.025.

Wang Z, Svejstrup JQ, Feaver WJ *et al.* (1994) Requirement for RNA polymerase II transcription factor b (TFIIH) during nucleotide excision repair in the yeast *Saccharomyces cerevisiae. Nature.* 368:74–76.

Watanabe T, Fukasawa T. (1961) Episome-mediated transfer of drug resistance in Enterobacteriaceae. I. Transfer of resistance factors by conjugation. *J. Bacteriol.* 81:669–678.

Watanabe T, Ogata C, Sato S. (1964) Episome-mediated transfer of drug resistance in Enterobacteriaceae. 8. Six-drug-resistance R factor. *J. Bacteriol.* 88:922–928.

Whitfield-Gabrieli S, Thermenos HW, Milanovic S *et al.* (2009) Hyperactivity and hyperconnectivity of the default network in schizophrenia and in first-degree relatives of persons with schizophrenia. *Proc. Natl. Acad. Sci. USA.* 106:1279–1284.

Wilson J. (2013) Oxidants, antioxidants and the current incurability of metastatic cancers. *Open Biol.* 3(1):120144. doi: 10.1098/rsob.120144.

Wilson JH, Berget PB, Pipas JM. (1982) Somatic cells efficiently join unrelated DNA segments end-to-end. *Mol. Cell Biol.* 2:1258–1269.

Windbichler N, Menichelli M, Papathanos PA *et al.* (2011) A synthetic homing endonuclease-based gene drive system in the human malaria mosquito. *Nature.* 473:212–215.

Winocour E, Keshet I. (1980) Indiscriminate recombination in simian virus 40-infected monkey cells. *Proc. Natl. Acad. Sci. USA.* 77:4861–4865.

Wray H. (2011) On the trail of the Orchid Child. *Sci. Am. Mind.*

Wright AV, Doudna JA. (2016) Biology and applications of Crispr systems: harnessing nature's toolbox for genome engineering. *Cell.* 164(1):29–44.

Wu Y, Zhou H. (2015) Correction of a genetic disease by Crispr-Cas9-mediated gene editing in mouse spermatogonial stem cells. *Cell Res.* 25(1):67–79. doi: 10.1038/cr.2014.160.

Wu Y, Liang D, Wang Y *et al.* (2013) Correction of a genetic disease in mouse via use of Crispr-Cas9. *Cell Stem Cell.* 13:659–662. doi: 10.1016/j.stem.2013.10.016.

Xie K, Yang Y. (2013) RNA-guided genome editing in plants using a Crispr-Cas system. *Mol. Plant.* 6:1975–1983. doi: 10.1093/mp/sst119.

Yamano T, Nishimasu H, Zetsche B *et al.* (2016) Crystal structure of Cpf1 in complex with guide RNA and target DNA. *Cell.* 165(4):949–962. doi: 10.1016/j.cell.2016.04.003.

Yang H, Liu Z, Ma Y *et al.* (2013) Generation of haploid embryonic stem cells from *Macaca fascicularis* monkey parthenotes. *Cell Res.* 23:1187–1200. doi: 10.1038/cr.2013.93.

Yang H, Wang H, Shivalila CS *et al.* (2013) One-step generation of mice carrying reporter and conditional alleles by Crispr/Cas-mediated genome engineering. *Cell.* 154(6):1370–1379. doi: 10.1016/j.cell.2013.08.022.

Yang J, Benyamin B, McEvoy BP *et al.* (2010) Common SNPs explain a large proportion of the heritability for human height. *Nat. Genet.* 42:565–569.

Ye X, Al-Babili S, Klöti A *et al.* (2000). Engineering the provitamin A (beta-carotene) biosynthetic pathway into (carotenoid-free) rice endosperm. *Science.* 287(5451): 303–305. doi: 10.1126/science.287.5451.303.

Zalocusky KA, Ramakrishnan C, Lerner TN *et al.* (2016) Nucleus accumbens D2R cells signal prior outcomes and control risky decision-making. *Nature.* 531(7596):642–646. doi: 10.1038/nature17400.

Zetsche B, Gootenberg J, Abudayyeh O *et al.* (2015) Cpf1 Is a single RNA-guided endonuclease of a Class 2 CRISPR-Cas system. *Cell.* 163(3): 759–771. doi: 10.1016/j.cell.2015.09.038.

Zhao Y, Dai Z, Liang Y *et al.* (2014) Sequence-specific inhibition of microRNA via Crispr/Crispri system. *Sci. Rep.* 4:3943. doi: 10.1038/srep03943.

Zimmer C. (2015) Editing of pig DNA may lead to more organs for people. *The New York Times.*

Zinder ND, Lederberg J. (1952) Genetic exchange in *Salmonella. J. Bacteriol.* 64(5):679–699.

Zizek S. (2003) *The Puppet and the Dwarf: The Perverse Core of Christianity.* The MIT Press.

Index